Cardiovascular Disease I

Cardiovascular Disease I

Publisher: iConcept Press Ltd.
Cover design: Pineapple Design Ltd.
Interior design: iConcept Press Ltd.
Typesetting and copy editing: iConcept Press Ltd. and Pineapple Design Ltd.

ISBN: 978-1-922227-54-6

Printed in the United States of America

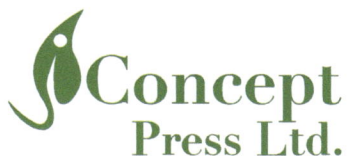

iConcept
Press Ltd.

www.iconceptpress.com

Contents

Preface

Cardiovascular disease is a class of diseases that involve the heart or blood vessels, such as arteries, capillaries and veins. Cardiovascular diseases remain the biggest cause of deaths worldwide, though over the last two decades, cardiovascular mortality rates have declined in many high-income countries. At the same time, cardiovascular deaths and disease have increased at a fast rate in low- and middle-income countries. The causes of cardiovascular disease are diverse but atherosclerosis and/or hypertension are the most common ones.

This book is targeted for researchers, scholars or other health care providers who need a ready reference for cardiovascular disease ranging from causes, signs and symptoms, and diagnosis through treatment and special considerations. There are two volumes. This book is the first volume.

There are totally 12 chapters in this book. Chapter 1 proposes that the renal artery diameter could represents a marker of non-traditional cardiovascular risk factors in selected populations. A pathophysiological explanation, including main biophysical background, and clinical implication of this new finding has been critically discussed. Bicuspid aortic valve (BAV) is the commonest congenital cardiac disease and is characterized by the aortic valve only having two leaflets rather than the usual three. Chapter 2 provides a comprehensive review of the condition, from epidemiology and etiology to diagnosis and management. In the case of coronary artery disease, cardiomyocytes' oxygen supply and thus the heart's contractility diminishes with the consequence that the oxygen demands of the whole organism are no longer fulfilled. Chapter 3 focuses on retroperfusion and it is shown that it is possible to perform a regional venous retrobypass in a long term pig model. Chapter 4 discusses the FGF23/Klotho system, which is a new biological system with a pivotal role in normal regulation of phosphorus homeostasis. In addition, this system have important implications regarding cardiovascular health and disease.

Chapter 5 assesses the effect of high-intensity and moderate intensity exercise on the exercise efficiency of ischaemic heart disease patients. Although ischemic heart disease patients were more inefficient during high-intensity exercise, this type of exercise may provide greater benefits for this population group due to eliciting a higher physiological response and energy expenditure. Chapter 6 presents the characteristics of cardiovascular manifestations, including cardiac manifestations, cerebrovascular disease, pulmonary vascular involvement, renal vascular involvement, intestinal vasculitis, and cutaneous vasculitis. All of them are analyzed and described using a retrospective review of the medical records of 1125 SLE patients examined in Juntendo University Hospital between 1955 and 2002 Chapter 7 shows that serotonin, angiotensin II, urotensin II, cardiotrophin-1 and salusin-β exert proatherogenic effects, whereas adiponectin, GLP-1, GIP, heregulin-β1 and salusin-α have antiatherogenic effects. Based on this finding, it proposes emerging roles of these novel vasoactive agents as biomarkers and therapeutic targets for atherosclerotic cardiovascular diseases. Chapter 8 highlights the role mutations of mitochondrial genome in atherosclerosis. The understanding of the role mutations of mitochondrial genome in atherogenesis is of direct clinical relevance because increased mitochondrial DNA damage represents an emerging target of therapeutic strategies against atherosclerosis.

Chapter 9 reviews the relationship between thiamine and MI. Genetic studies provide opportunities to determine which proteins link thiamine to MI pathology. Thiamine is also able to act through numerous non-genomic mechanisms, including protein expression, oxidative stress, inflammation, and cellular metabolism. These findings suggest that thiamine may play an important role in MI. Chapter 10 illustrates a variety types of peripheral vascular disease including from etiology to endovascular treatment. Especially, venous vascular disease are shown as not only endovascular treatment but pharmaceutical therapy. Chapter 11 proposes conventional and new techniques/methods for diagnosis and treatment of the cardiovascular disease. In addition, the chapter explain the comparison of conventional formulation and new nanomedicine therapy of cardiovascular disease. Chapter 12 describes all aspects of cardiogenic shock, especially as the complication of acute myocardial infarction.

Editing and publishing a book is never an easy task. Each chapter in this book has gone through a peer review, a selection and an editing process so as to guarantee its quality. Without the supports and contributions of the authors and reviewers, this book can never be able to complete. We would like to thank all of the authors in this book and all of the reviewers who participated in the reviewing process: Pasquale Abete, Abdulkareem A. Al-Othman, Ruby Alexander-Lindo, Sorour Amirhaeri, Madhu B Anand-Srivastava, Polychronis Antonitsis, Inês Araújo, Jaroslav Benedik, María J. Blanco-Prieto, Federico Cacciapuoti, Alejandro R. Chade, Yuh-Lien Chen, Yung-Chang Chen, Marco Matteo Ciccone, Kirk P. Conrad, Bibhu R. Das, Brenda Dawley, Lisa A. DeRoo, Luca Di Lullo, Sandra Donnini, AMIT NANDAN DHAR DWIVEDI, Vitor Engracia Valenti, Hardik Gandhi, Vidu Garg, Bagavad Gita, Wolfgang F. Graier, Mohammad H. Haddadzadeh, Nienke Hoeve, Peter Hofmann, Shih-Yi Huang, Keiichi Ikeda, Kenji Inoue, Takeo Isozaki, M. P. Jadhav, Pudur Jagadeeswaran, Neerod K Jha, R Kalyani, Balaji Kannan, Ali Karami, Lakshmi Sudha Prasanna Karanam, Tomohiro Katsuya, Sebastian Kelle, Kee Sik Kim, Sejoong Kim, Akira Kohsaka, Shyam S Kothari, George Kouvelos, Graciela Krikun, Hiroshi Kubota, Sikiru. Lamina, Timothy R. Larsen, Conor C. Lynch, Masha Maharaj, Giuseppe Maltese, paulo marcelino, Ju-Young Moon, Piotr Musialek, Manuel F. Navedo, Shaoping Nie, Chike Nzerue, Basil Okeahialam, Evangelia Papadimitriou, Athanasia K Papazafiropoulou, A. N. Patnaik, Ilka Pinz, Prabhakara Prabhu, Athina Pyrpasopoulou, Ruomei Qi, Prabhakar Rajiah, S. Ramakrishnan, Adam Reich, S. A. M. Said, Miklos Santha, Thorsten Schinke, Danny J. Schust, Thomas Seidel, Sang-Hoon Seol, Raffaele Serra, Nobuyuki Shimohata, Il-Suk Sohn, Z Sun, Jan L Svennevig, J. Nasehi Tehrani, Venkataswarup Tiriveedhi, Kimimasa Tobita, László Vígh, Hong-Sheng Wang, Shaoxiao Wang, Menachem M. Weiner, Weirong Xing, Kyung Lim Yoon, Luca Zanoli, Junping Zhang and Shetuan Zhang. We hope that you, the reader, will find this book interesting and useful. Any advices please feel free and are always welcome to tell us.

iConcept Press Ltd
August 2014

Renal Artery Diameter:
A "New" Parameter Beyond an Old Disease –
The Renal Artery Stenosis

Luca Zanoli, Stefania Rastelli
Department of Medical and Pediatric Sciences
University of Catania, Catania, Italy

Paolo Lentini
Department of Nephrology & Dialysis
San Bassiano Hospital, Bassano del Grappa, Italy

Carmelita Marcanoni
Department of Nephrology
Cannizzaro Hospital, Catania, Italy

Davide Capodanno
Cardiovascular Department
Ferrarotto Hospital, Catania, Italy

Enzo Saretto Dante Vicari, Aldo Eugenio Calogero
Section of Endocrinology, Andrology and Internal Medicine
Department of Medical and Pediatric Sciences
University of Catania, Catania, Italy

Antonio Granata
Department of Nephrology
Presidio Ospedaliero Agrigento, Agrigento, Italy

Francesco Rapisarda, Pasquale Fatuzzo
Section of Nephrology, Department of Medical and Pediatric Sciences
University of Catania, Catania, Italy

Pietro Castellino
Department of Medical and Pediatric Sciences
University of Catania, Catania, Italy

1   Prolog

Recently, taking advantage of the cohort of the RAS-CAD (Renal Artery Stenosis in Coronary Artery Disease) Study (NCT 01173666), a large randomized controlled trial designed to determine whether the stenting of the renal artery is of benefit in reducing the left ventricular mass, our group reported that small renal arteries, for the first time defined by a low reference diameter or minimal luminal diameter, (*a*) are associated with low GFR and resistant hypertension independently of the degree of stenosis and major confounders, (*b*) predict the development of contrast-induced nephropathy better than the unspecific baseline reduction of GFR independently of major confounders and (*c*) could impact the prognosis of patients with ischemic heart disease and non-significant renal artery stenosis (10-70%) independently of major confounders. These results are clinically relevant and suggest that the renal artery diameter could represents a marker of non-traditional cardiovascular risk factors in selected populations. In the present chapter, these results will be presented, and a pathophysiological explanation, including main biophysical background, and the clinical implication of these new findings will be critically discussed.

2   Epidemiology of Renal Artery Stenosis

Few topics generate more controversy between nephrologists and interventional cardiologists than the management of atherosclerotic renal artery stenosis. Atherosclerotic disease of the renal arteries is common in the elderly and in subjects with a high cardiovascular risk (Conlon *et al.*, 2001). Many lesions of the renal artery occur in ostial segments and represent extension of adjacent aortic atherosclerotic plaque. The prevalence of such lesions is a function of both age and atherosclerotic risk factors. Although it has been long recognized that renal artery stenosis can initiate or accelerate hypertension, the role of renal artery disease as an important contributor to renal failure is a concept emphasized mainly since the 1980s (Novick *et al.*, 1983).

Renal artery stenosis is often associated with a higher cardiovascular risk (Conlon *et al.*, 2001), as well as a high frequency of alterations in left ventricular mass and function (Wright *et al.*, 2005) with a rate of death of about 16% per year (Kalra *et al.*, 2005; Cheung *et al.*, 2002; Guo *et al.*, 2007), and is a potentially modifiable clinical condition. In addition, RAS is associated with progression and loss of renal function (Dean *et al.*, 1981; Guzman *et al.*, 1994; Crowley *et al.*, 1998). The association between renal artery stenosis and systemic atherosclerosis is well established, and there is evidence that patients affected by ischemic heart disease and peripheral vascular disease are at increased risk for renal artery stenosis (Harding *et al.*, 1992; Rihal *et al.*, 2002; Buller *et al.*, 2004; Weber-Mzell *et al.*, 2002; Olin *et al.*, 1990; Mui *et al.*, 2006; De Mast & Beutler, 2009; Marcantoni *et al.*, 2011; Shukla *et al.*, 2013). In high-risk population, such as patients undergoing screening renal artery angiography at the time of cardiac catheterization, the prevalence of significant RAS ranges from 5-14% (Marcantoni *et al.*, 2011; Buller *et al.*, 2004; Shukla *et al.*, 2013) whereas the prevalence of atherosclerotic renovascular disease, regardless on its severity, could be significantly higher (up to 39%, Buller *et al.*, 2004). Atherosclerotic RAS is a progressive disease (Conlon *et al.*, 2000). Temporal progression of the degree of stenosis occurred in up to 71% of patients, and renal artery occlusion occurred in 16% (Wollenweber *et al.*, 1968; Meaney *et al.*, 1968; Schreiber *et al.*, 1984; Tollefson *et al.*, 1991). RAS progression may account for 5% to 15% of all patients developing end-stage renal disease each year (Rimmer & Gennari, 1993). Therefore, the identification of subjects with this condition may be useful to clinician to establish a closer surveillance, and to refine the clinical decision making process.

For these reasons, in the recent past several scoring systems were suggested to select patients at higher risk for renal artery stenosis. One of the most accepted score was provided by the DRASTIC study (Krijnen *et al.*, 1998). In this study, authors emphasize the predictive value of clinical variables, including age, symptomatic vascular disease, elevated cholesterol, and the presence of an abdominal bruit, as the most powerful predictors of detecting renal artery lesions of at least 50% vessel occlusion and developed a scoring system with which one could estimate the pre-angiographic probability of finding such a lesion with accuracy at least equal to radionuclide angiography. Even if interesting, this score was developed in a selected population with a high prevalence of risk factors for renal artery stenosis (hypertensive patients who underwent renal angiography because they had drug-resistant hypertension or an increase in serum creatinine concentration during therapy with angiotensin-converting enzyme inhibitors) and was never validated in an external unselected population.

Parameters	Score for RAS>50%
Peripheral vascular disease	
Present	3
Absent	1
Glomerular filtration rate	
<67 ml/min/1.73 m^2	3
≥67 ml/min/1.73 m^2	1
Age	
>66 years	2
≤66 years	1
Dyslipidemia	
Present	3
Absent	1
Coronary artery disease	
≥2 stenotic coronary vessels	2
<2 stenotic coronary vessels	1
Pulse pressure	
>52 mmHg	2
≤52 mmHg	1

Table 1: Scoring system for the detection of renal artery stenosis > 50%. Data are expressed as odds ratios. Adapted from Marcantoni et al., 2011.

Behold to the prevalence of atherosclerotic renal artery stenosis in patients undergoing coronary angiography, most of the available data derive from American populations. Moreover, data on the prevalence of renal artery stenosis in several population studies and in different populations varies considerably, suggesting an influence of lifestyle in the onset and development of this disease. At present, few data are available in Mediterranean populations (Marcantoni *et al.*, 2011; Buller *et al.*, 2004; Shukla *et al.*, 2013). Further, data interpretation is often biased by the presence of additional selection criteria such as resistant hypertension, peripheral vascular disease or renal insufficiency. Recently, a recent study performed on a Mediterranean population in a large cohort of high cardiovascular risk patients undergoing non emergent coronary angiography was designed to look at the prevalence of renal artery stenosis in unselected population of subjects undergoing screening renal artery angiography at the time of cardiac catheterization (Marcantoni *et al.*, 2011). In this study it was reported that renal artery stenosis >50% is an infrequent complication (5.4%) and that the presence of peripheral vascular disease, reduced renal function, older age, dyslipidemia, severity of coronary artery disease and increased pulse pressure are independent predictors of renal artery stenosis >50%. Furthermore, the authors indicates that a risk score based on these few clinical variables, readily available in cardiac catheterization laboratories, has a good predictive performance, and may be useful to select patients to undergo screening renal angiography at the end of cardiac catheterization (Table 1).

It is important to remember that whether the stenting of the stenotic renal artery is more favourable than the strict medical treatment is still debated (see chapter 2.2 - Is the renal artery stenting effective for the renal and blood pressure endpoint? and chapter 2.3 - Is the renal artery stenting effective for the cardiac endpoint?) and that the selection of the subjects to treat with revascularization should be improved. For these reasons, although renal artery stenosis is a potentially evolutive lesion, its screening in asymptomatic patients during coronary angiography is still a matter for debate. Available data on treatment and outcome (Textor *et al.*, 2001; ASTRAL investigators, 2009; Kumbhani *et al.*, 2011) as well as the low prevalence of renal artery stenosis in unselected patients (Marcantoni *et al.*, 2011) do not support a routinely "drive by" screening for renal artery stenosis in all subjects undergoing non-emergent coronary angiography. In this regard, the validation of a predictive model for the onset of cardiovascular events in subjects with renal artery stenosis may provide support for a more accurate patient selection. However, a distinction should be made between identifying patients with renal artery stenosis who are at high risk of cardiovascular events and need closer surveillance, and the selection of patients for revascularization, which implicates a risk-to benefit balance. In this regard, the recent finding that the minimal diameter of the stenotic renal artery and the reduction of reference diameter in subjects with or without renal artery stenosis predict the onset of major adverse coronary events better than the percentage of stenosis (Zanoli *et al.*, 2013) and that the minimal diameter of the stenotic renal artery predicts the GFR 1 month after renal artery stenting (Yu H *et al.*, 2011) suggests the presence of a new parameter widely ignored in the literature (the minimal renal artery diameter in subjects with renal artery stenosis and the reference renal artery diameter in subjects without renal artery stenosis) to consider in the selection of patients that need a closer surveillance or a renal artery revascularization (see chapter 2.2 - Is the renal artery stenting effective for the renal and blood pressure endpoint? and chapter 5 - Renal artery diameter and cardiovascular events).

2.1   Vascular Imaging for the Study of Renal Arteries

Vascular imaging of renal artery study is a rapidly evolving field, in both clinical and experimental aspects (Granata A *et al.*, 2009). Even if nowadays radiology plays a large part in the diagnosis, with a variety of imaging techniques available, it is reasonable to predict that there will be in the near future new non-invasive techniques to study the renal artery structure and function (i.e. echotracking techniques. Laurent *et al.*, 2006). Each has relative advantages and disadvantages depending on each unique clinical setting.

Ultrasound is a non-invasive, first-line method for screening RAS. The assessment can be carried out relatively quickly and is safe. Duplex ultrasound evaluates renal morphology and the presence of significant stenosis. The flow in the normal renal artery produces an early peak systolic velocity that ranges from 60-100 cm/s. In subjects with RAS, the reduced cross-sectional area of the stenotic renal artery causes increased blood velocity in attempt to maintain appropriate flow. The increased velocity causes turbulence of blood flow immediately distal to the stenosis. A threshold of >3.5 renal artery to aorta velocities suggests RAS (Soulez *et al.*, 2000). Moreover, since it is technically difficult to directly image the site of stenosis due to obscuration by overlying bowel gas, most experts assess the intra-renal arteries. Distal to the stenotic segment the pulse is "late" and "weak" - "tardus parvus". Ultrasounds have 95% sensitivity and 90% specificity to detect significant RAS when performed in dedicated laboratories (Rabbia & Valpreda, 2003) and significantly lower (57% sensitivity) when performed by less experienced operators (Hashemi *et al.*, 2011). The limiting factors of ultrasounds are (1) the operator dependency, (2) suboptimal patient breath-holding, (3) obesity and (4) intervening bowel gas (Turi *et al.*, 2003).

Another well accepted technique to detect RAS is the nuclear medicine. The diagnosis is made using either static or dynamic renography by detecting a significant change in renal split function following ACE inhibitor administration. The sensitivity of this technique is 76% and specificity is 90% (Cosgriff, 2005).

Computed tomography angiography with administration of intravenous iodinated contrast medium. Due to the potential risk of contrast-induced nephropathy, administration of contrast media should be carefully considered based on a risk-benefit assessment in subjects with serum creatinine >150 mmol/l. Computer tomography angiography is quoted as having a 94-100% sensitivity and 79-97% specificity (Rountas *et al.*, 2007; Echevarria *et al.*, 2008; Fraioli *et al.*, 2006).

Magnetic resonance angiography post-gadolinium administration provides sensitivities ranging from 88-100% and specificities ranging from 71-100% (Dong *et al.*, 1999). Unlike computed tomography angiography, this method does not involve ionizing radiation; however, in patients with renal impairment, it does introduce the potential risk of nephrogenic systemic fibrosis (Igreja *et al.*, 2012). Therefore, an estimated glomerular filtration rate of no less than 30 ml/min is required before administering intravenous gadolinium. Unenhanced magnetic resonance angiography has reported sensitivities ranging from 53-100% and specificities ranging from 47-97% (Dong *et al.*, 1999; Xu *et al.*, 2011).

Angiography is the reference standard for the diagnosis of RAS due to its high sensitivity (Tullus, 2011). However, since a iodinated contrast medium is administered during the procedure, there is a potential risk of contrast-induced nephropathy.

Echotracking technique is the gold standard for the study of superficial arteries, such as carotid and brachial artery (Laurent *et al.*, 2006). With this technique it is possible to measure diameter, distension and intima-media thickness with a high spatial resolution (2-10 micron) at least ten times better than classical ultrasound devices (Laurent *et al.*, 2006). The current limit of this technique is that it actually works only with high-resolution probes and, consequently, only superficial arteries can be studied.

In conclusion, developments in vascular imaging, including echotracking techniques, magnetic resonance angiography, doppler ultrasound, and nontoxic contrast angiography make the identification of renal artery stenosis more readily possible. Therefore, even if today invasive tests are necessary for a detailed study of the renal arteries, it is reasonable to expect in the near future that non-invasive techniques will be preferred and that the study of the renal artery function will be available even routinely, similarly to what happens in carotid and brachial arteries (Laurent *et al.*, 2006).

2.2 Is the Renal Artery Stenting Effective for the Renal and Blood Pressure Endpoint?

Given the potential benefits of early detection of renal artery stenosis, the 2005 guidelines of the American Heart Association/American College of Cardiology recommended, in patients at increased risk for atherosclerotic renal artery stenosis, to perform a renal angiography at the time of cardiac catheterization

(Hirsch *et al.*, 2006; White *et al.*, 2006). Thanks to this strong recommendation, the number of renal angiographies performed during a non-emergent coronary angiography has therefore increased considerably in the last decade, as suggested by the increased number of citations in Pubmed of the phrase "renal artery stenting" (<5 citations/year before 1990; 5-80 citations/year during nineties; 84-234 citations/year from 2000). However whether the renal artery revascularization is effective for the improvement of glomerular filtration rate and reduction of hypertension is highly debated even after the recent publication of the Angioplasty and Stenting for Renal Artery Lesions (ASTRAL) trial, a landmark study testing the effect of renal revascularization on rate of kidney function loss in patients with renal artery stenosis (ASTRAL investigators, 2009). The ASTRAL and STAR trials showed no evidence for a worthwhile clinical benefit of revascularization in patients with atherosclerotic renovascular disease, but rather a small number of significant procedure-related complications (ASTRAL investigators, 2009; Bax *et al.*, 2009). However, it is important to underline that the authors of the ASTRAL study correctly reported that some subjects with significant renal artery stenosis beneficiates of the renal artery revascularization. This observation could suggest that other factors than the percentage of the renal artery stenosis should be involved in the selection of subjects to be treated with revascularization, such as renal translesional pressure gradient (Leesar *et al.*, 2009) or minimal renal artery diameter (Yu *et al.*, 2011), and explain why it has been suggested that the failure of ASTRAL and STAR trials to demonstrate an improvement in kidney function could be explained by the enrolment of subjects who a priori were unlikely to benefit (White, 2010; Rooke *et al*, 2011). Therefore, the question that still needs to be answered is how to select patients most likely to benefit from stenting while avoiding the procedure and its associated risks in those least likely to benefit (Mann & Sos, 2010). A recent meta-analysis of randomized controlled trials in patients with RAS reported that percutaneous renal revascularization in addition to medical therapy may result in a lower requirement for antihypertensive medications, but not with improvements in serum creatinine or clinical outcomes, as compared with medical management (Kumbhani *et al.*, 2011). The 2011 ACCF/AHA update of the guidelines for the management of patients with peripheral artery disease (Rooke *et al.*, 2011) concluded that, "although the specific recommendations for renal disease did not change, the writing group acknowledges that some new studies support a more limited role for renal revascularization and that ongoing studies such as the CORAL (Cardiovascular Outcomes in Renal Atherosclerotic Lesions) trial (Cooper *et al.*, 2006) will provide additional evidence relevant to these recommendations in the near future". The currently indications for endovascular management in significant RAS (greater than 70% stenosis) are (1) progressive or acute decline in renal function - with or without the introduction of ACE inhibitors; (2) malignant and/or recalcitrant hypertension; (3) solitary kidney; and (4) recurrent flash pulmonary oedema or other cardiac disturbance syndromes (Henry *et al.*, 2010; Rabbia & Pini, 2010).

2.3   Is the Renal Artery Stenting Effective for the Cardiac Endpoint?

It is well known that atherosclerotic renal artery stenosis is associated with premature cardiovascular events and confers a high mortality risk in patients with coronary artery disease (Conlon *et al.*, 2001). The cardiovascular burden of renal artery stenosis is reflected in the high frequency of left ventricular hypertrophy in patients with this condition (Wright *et al.*, 2005). The prevalence of left ventricular hypertrophy was 79% in a large survey of subjects with renal artery stenosis whereas only 5% of patients with renal artery stenosis had normal cardiac structure and function (Wright *et al.*, 2005), a figure close to that observed in a high-risk condition such as end-stage renal disease (Zoccali *et al.*, 2002). Moreover, left ventricular hypertrophy is considered the strongest indicator for cardiovascular risk in patients with advanced chronic kidney disease (Middleton *et al.*, 2001), and it is well shown that both progression and regression of left ventricular hypertrophy signal parallel changes in the underlying risk of death and cardiovascular complications (London *et al.*, 2001; Zoccali *et al.*, 2004; Zhang *et al.*, 2003). Recently, in the ASTRAL trial (ASTRAL investigators, 2009; Bax *et al.*, 2009) no difference in mortality and cardiovascular events (secondary end point) emerged between medical treatment and medical treatment associated with angioplasty/stenting. Therefore, information for the effect of these interventions on a solid surrogate end point elected as a primary end point is of relevance to further investigate the impact of renal revascularization on the cardiovascular system.

Whether the renal artery stenting is effective for the reversion of left ventricular hypertrophy was never clearly studied until the recent publication of the RAS-CAD Study (Marcantoni *et al.*, 2012). The possibility that angioplasty/stenting of renal artery stenosis might prevent the evolution of left ventricular hypertrophy emerged in three small uncontrolled studies (Denolle *et al.*, 1993; Symonides *et al.*, 1999; Corriere *et al.*, 2010) and a case-series (Zeller *et al.*, 2007). Recently, the RAS-CAD study, a clinical trial aimed at testing whether renal artery revascularization compared with medical therapy, affects left ventricular hypertrophy progression, left ventricular systolic dysfunction and clinical outcomes, was unable to detect a clinically significant benefit of renal revascularization on left-ventricular mass in patients with coronary artery disease and renal artery stenosis of 50-80% (Marcantoni *et al.*, 2012). In particular, the authors of the RAS-CAD study reported that there was a mild but statistically significant regression of left ventricular mass in patients on medical therapy alone and in those who underwent both renal revascularization and medical therapy. The parallel partial regression of left ventricular hypertrophy in the two study arms was associated with a small decrease in arterial pressure. Furthermore, the incidence of death and cardiovascular events during follow-up was almost identical in patients randomly assigned to revascularization and those maintained on medical therapy. Hypothetical mechanisms whereby renal revascularization may increase cardioprotection in patients with renal artery stenosis include superior control of hypertension and full correction of renin-angiotensin system overactivity, which is an alteration frequently seen in subjects with renal artery stenosis (Pradhan & Rossi, 2013). The authors explain the lack of such hypothetical cardioprotection by revascularization noted in the RAS-CAD study with fact that renal artery stenosis could have been functionally irrelevant in at least some patients. Identifying patients with (functionally) significant renal artery stenosis is a complex undertaking (Dworkin & Muphy, 2010). Other factors than the ratio between reference and minimal diameter (Figure 1) were proposed for the evaluation of the severity of renal artery stenosis with poor results. For example, measuring the pressure gradient, a criterion considered the most potent predictor of the effect of angioplasty/stenting, fails to correctly classify the response to revascularization in almost 30% of patients (Mangiacapra *et al.*, 2010). Interestingly, the authors of the RAS-CAD study suggest that the RAS-CAD study did not find greater regression of left ventricular hypertrophy in patients classified as blood pressure responders to revascularization compared with non-responders because the angiotensin-converting enzyme inhibitors and angiotensin II receptor blockers, two classes of drugs used by most patients in this trial, allow a degree of cardioprotection that overshadows any additional effect on the renin-angiotensin system by renal artery stenosis correction.

3   Renal Artery Diameter, GFR and Resistant Hypertension

In a recent paper (Zanoli *et al.*, 2012), it was reported that small renal arteries, defined by a low reference diameter in subjects with or without renal artery stenosis or minimal diameter in subjects with renal artery

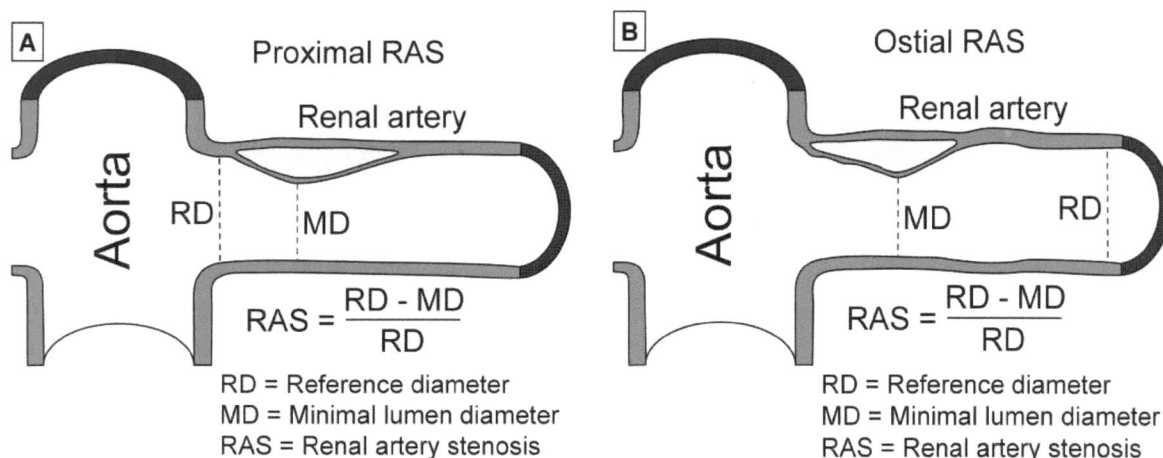

Figure 1: Renal artery diameters measurements in subjects with proximal/distal RAS (Panel A) or ostial RAS (Panel B) In case of ostial RAS, reference diameter was measured at least 2 cm after the stenosis and always after the post-stenotic dilatation. Adapted from Zanoli *et al.*, 2012.

stenosis (Figure 1), are more likely to be associated with low glomerular filtration rate than larger renal arteries (even in the absence of luminal narrowing). Moreover, in the presence of low-to-moderate renal artery stenosis (10-70%), small reference diameter and minimal diameter were more predictive of chronic kidney disease than the percentage of renal artery stenosis (Figure 2 Panel A-C). Finally, in subjects with renal artery stenosis, small renal arteries (defined as low reference diameter or low minimal diameter) are more likely to be associated with resistant hypertension than larger renal arteries in the presence of low-to-moderate renal artery stenosis (Figure 4). These findings were in accordance with the results of the RESIST trial (Yu *et al.* 2011), a multi-center study of patients undergoing renal artery stenting that evaluated the utility of embolic protection and or abciximab (a platelet glycoprotein inhibitor), showing that minimal renal artery diameter is a better determinant of renal function at baseline and 1 month after renal artery stenting than the percentage of RAS in patients with RAS 50-100%.

Renal artery stenosis, a common condition with high rate of cardiovascular mortality (Kalra *et al.*, 2005; Cheung *et al.*, 2002; Guo *et al.*, 2007), is usually associated with chronic kidney disease and hypertension, although the causal relationship is discussed (Cheung CM *et al.*, 2005). Reduction of minimal diameter of the renal artery may alter renal function hemodynamically, causing global renal ischemia, by lowering glomerular pressure and filtration especially when renal artery stenosis is above 70%. At this regard, Gobe *et al.* (Gobe *et al.*, 1990) described that a combination of necrosis and apoptosis are important in the loss of renal function during and after an ischemic insult. Moreover, reduction of minimal diameter of the renal artery may alter renal function biochemically, through activation of inflammation, the renin-angiotensin system and oxidative stress, or structurally by inducing cell death and fibrosis of the kidney (Meyer *et al.*, 1998; Chonchol & Linas, 2006; Lerman *et al.*, 2009). Before occurrence of hemodynamic significant stenosis, the burden of atherosclerosis at the site of renal arteries contributes to renal failure because of recurrent migration of plaque content and/or thrombosis to the kidney. At early stages, the atherosclerotic plaque develops outward (Glagov *et al.*, 1987).

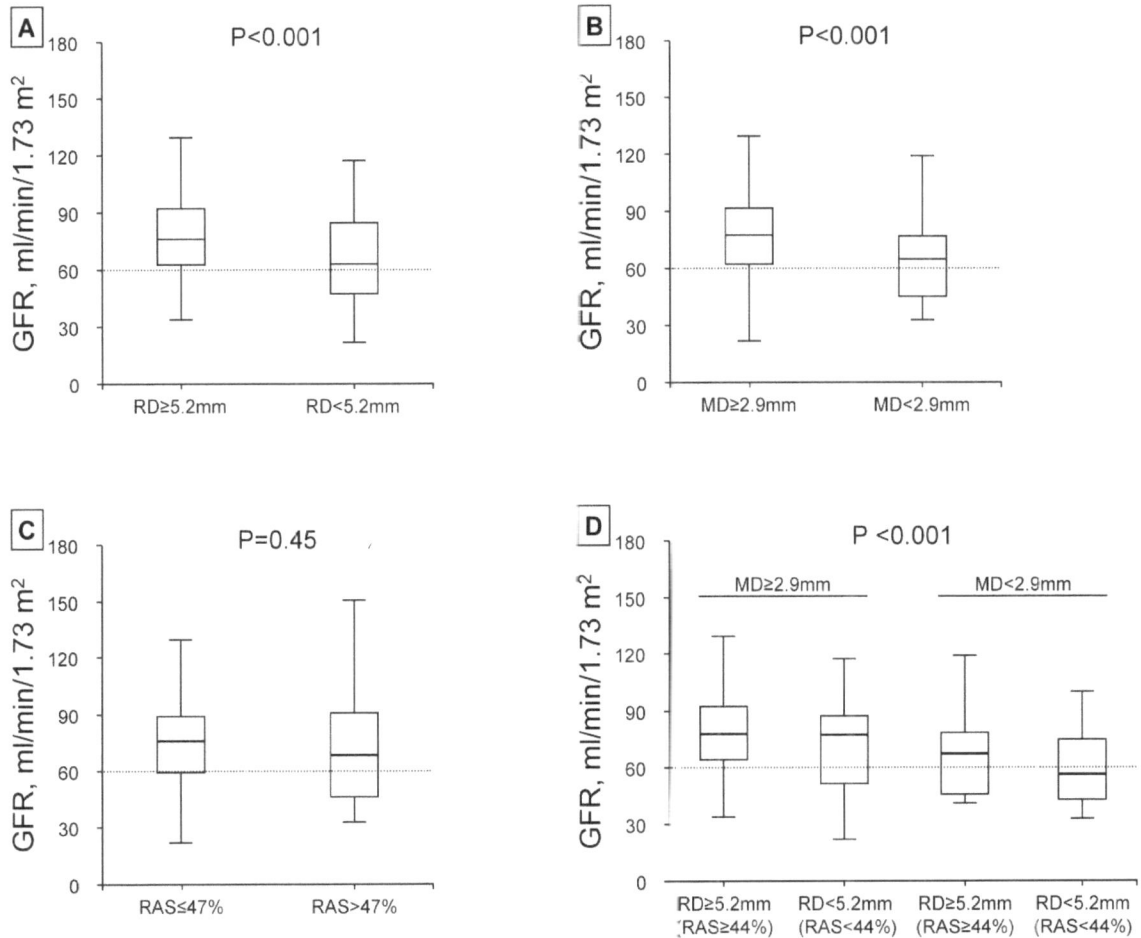

Figure 2: Patients with luminal narrowing, box plot of glomerular filtration rate. GFR, glomerular filtration rate; RD, mean reference vessel diameter; MD, minimal diameter; RAS, renal artery stenosis referred to changes in vascular diameter. Panel A. Patients in the lower quartile of reference vessel diameter (RD<5.2mm) have lower GFR. Panel B. Patients in the lower quartile of minimal diameter (MD<2.9mm) have lower GFR. Panel C. The GFR of patients in the higher quartile of renal artery stenosis (RAS>47%) did not differs significantly than GFR of patients in the 1-3 quartiles of renal artery stenosis (RAS≤47%). Panel D. Reference and minimal diameter, together, are strongly associated with a lower GFR. RAS=44% corresponds at the ratio between MD=2.9mm and RD=5.2mm. Boxes represent interquartile range (IQR, i.e. 50% of the distribution); the horizontal bar is the median; upper whisker represents the 75th percentile + 1.5 IQR; lower whisker 25th percentile – 1.5 IQR; Circles outside the whiskers are mild outliers. P values are given for the global ANOVA. Adapted from Zanoli *et al.*, 2012

Reference diameter could be influenced by reduction in blood flow through flow-induced decrease in shear stress and inward arterial remodeling (Langille & O'Donnell, 1986). Reference diameter reduction can be associated with resistant hypertension by an increase in the renal nerve activation, chronic kidney damage, or a nitric oxide deficiency (Khawaja *et al.*, 2011).

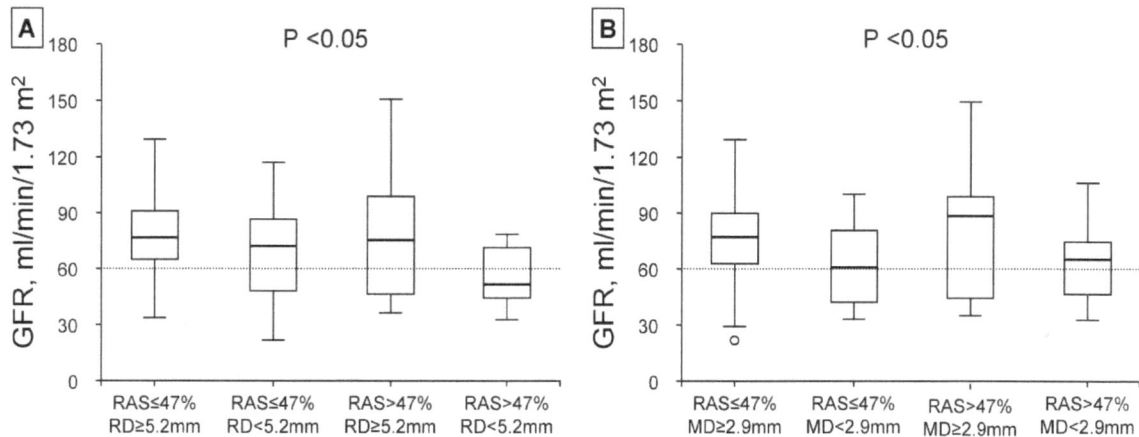

Figure 3: Panel A. A lower reference renal artery diameter is strongly associated with a lower glomerular filtration rate in each renal artery stenosis category and is able to stratify for renal function above and beyond the renal artery stenosis. Panel B. A lower minimal renal artery diameter is strongly associated with a lower glomerular filtration rate in each luminal narrowing category and is able to stratify for renal function above and beyond the renal artery stenosis. Boxes represent interquartile range (IQR, i.e. 50% of the distribution); the horizontal bar is the median; upper whisker represents the 75th percentile + 1.5 IQR; lower whisker 25th percentile − 1.5 IQR; Circles outside the whiskers are mild outliers. P values are given for the global ANOVA. RAS, renal artery stenosis; MD, minimal renal artery diameter; RD, reference renal artery diameter. Adapted from Zanoli et al,. 2012.

3.1   Renal Artery Diameter and GFR

Zanoli and colleagues (Zanoli *et al.*, 2012) divided the patients according to the presence of renal artery stenosis >10% or not. Patients with renal artery stenosis were divided into quartile for the maximal degree of renal artery stenosis and compared the upper quartile (i.e. stenosis >47%) against the other 3 quartiles. Accordingly, patients were classified according to the minimal diameter (MD) ≥2.9 or <2.9 mm, where 2.9 mm represents the lower quartile of minimal diameter, and according to the reference diameter (RD) ≥5.2 or <5.2 mm, where 5.2 mm represents the lower quartile of reference diameter. An important finding of this study was that kidneys with small renal arteries (RD<5.2 mm) were more likely associated with low glomerular filtration rate than larger renal arteries (even in the absence of renal artery stenosis). Both reference diameter and minimal diameter could be related to glomerular filtration rate by several mechanisms. In case of severe stenosis, minimal diameter could represent the limiting factor for renal blood flow. In case of no stenosis or low-to-moderate stenosis, reference diameter could be determined by blood flow through flow-mediated dilation.

Moreover, the reference diameter reduction may be the consequence of a decreased renal blood flow. Arterial diameter is dependent upon several dynamic factors, among the level of vascular tone on the short-term and vascular remodelling on the long-term. It is well known that long-term changes in local hemodynamic forces induce arterial remodelling that is critical to vascular adaptation and to the progression of cardiovascular disease (Langille, 1993). Sustained reductions in blood flow lead to flow-induced decreases in shear stress and inward arterial remodelling with a narrowing of lumen diameter

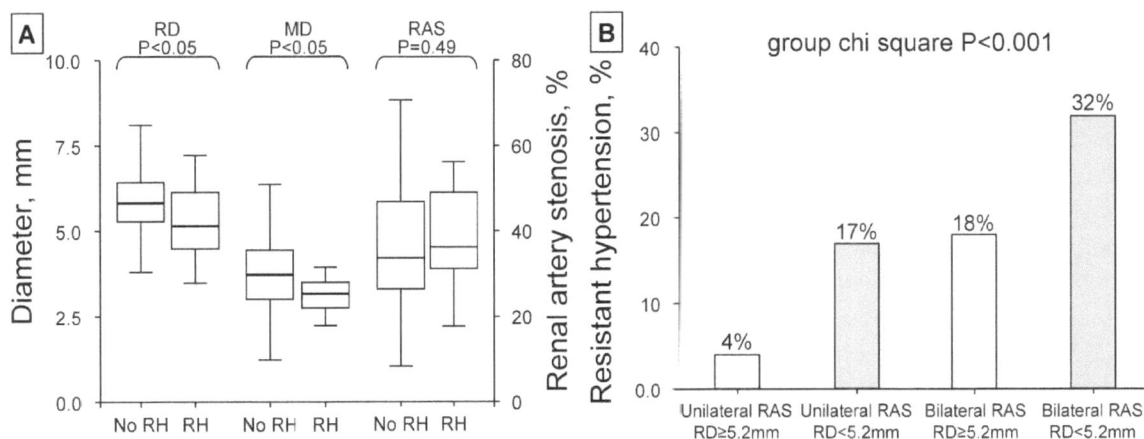

Figure 4: Patients with luminal narrowing. Panel A: Box plot of reference vessel diameter, minimal luminal diameter and luminal narrowing. Patients with resistant hypertension have a lower reference vessel diameter and a lower minimal luminal diameter; the luminal narrowing was not significantly different between patients with and without resistant hypertension. Boxes represent interquartile range (IQR, i.e. 50% of the distribution); the horizontal bar is the median; upper whisker represents the 75th percentile + 1.5 IQR; lower whisker 25th percentile − 1.5 IQR; Circles outside the whiskers are mild outliers. P values are given for the global ANOVA. Panel B: Prevalence of resistant hypertension combining unilateral/bilateral luminal narrowing with reference diameter. RAS, renal artery stenosis; MD, minimal renal artery diameter; No RH, patients without resistant hypertension; RD, reference renal artery diameter; RH, patients with resistant hypertension. Adapted from Zanoli *et al,*. 2012.

(Langille & O'Donnell, 1986). Clinically significant arterial occlusive disease depressurizes the arterial tree downstream from the occlusion site and reduces the wall shear stress. Arterial remodelling limits change in wall shear stress (Langille & O'Donnell, 1986). Animal models suggested that the minimal diameter and renal artery stenosis were related to pressure and flow (Morel *et al.*, 1990) and that the relation between renal artery stenosis and renal blood flow could be not linear (Rognant *et al.*, 2010).

Several investigators reported the absence of association between percentage of renal artery stenosis and glomerular filtration rate (Suresh *et al.*, 2000; Cheung *et al.*, 2002; Wright *et al.*, 2002) or that minimal renal artery diameter is a better predictor of GFR than the percentage of stenosis (Yu *et al.* 2011). Our group has recently furnished a possible explanation at this lack of association (Zanoli *et al.*, 2012). We reported that, in the presence of low-to-moderate renal artery stenosis, small reference diameter and small minimal diameter are both more predictive of chronic kidney disease than the percentage of renal artery stenosis (Figure 2 Panel A-C). Moreover, since data of the work recently published by Zanoli *et al.* (Zanoli *et al.*, 2012) are referred to high risk patients with ischemic heart disease and several cardiovascular risk factors, including an high prevalence of hypertension (88% in all study cohort; 95% in subjects with renal artery stenosis) and since it is well known that subjects with hypertension, and in particular those with several concomitant cardiovascular risk factors, had increased arterial stiffness (The Task Force for the management of arterial hypertension of the European Society of Hypertension and of the European Society of Cardiology, 2013), these findings are also in accordance with the Poiseuille's law in rigid vessels, demonstrating that a small reduction in radius produces a great increase in resistance. Consequently, the smaller the reference diameter and the minimal diameter the more significant the hemodynamic effect of stenosis should be. By definition, the percentage of renal artery stenosis is mathematically correlated with reference diameter (positively) and minimal diameter (negatively) (Figure 1). Indeed, since the percentage of renal artery stenosis results from the ratio of minimal diameter and reference diameter, since both are negatively associated with glomerular filtration rate (Figure 2 Panel A-B), it is evident that little or no association there should be between the percentage of renal artery stenosis and glomerular filtration rate decline, as previously reported (Suresh *et al.*, 2000; Cheung *et al.*, 2002), and that minimal renal artery diameter could be a better predictor of GFR than the percentage of stenosis (Yu *et al.* 2011). In support of this hypothesis, our group demonstrated that the use of the percentage of stenosis to predict the GFR could be questionable (Figure 2 Panel D), reporting that in subjects with similar minimal diameter (i.e. MD<2.9mm) there was a lower glomerular filtration rate in presence of low reference diameter (RD<5.2mm) and, therefore, low percentage of renal artery stenosis (RAS<44%) rather than in presence of high reference diameter (RD≥5.2mm) and, therefore, higher percentage of renal artery stenosis (RAS≥44%). At the light of the results of the paper of Zanoli (Zanoli *et al.*, 2012), it might be not surprising that association between altered renal function and diameter exists for diameters far off the definition of stenosis. This association could be also partly explained by the evidence that, when an overt atherosclerotic plaque is present (with consequent narrowing of the lumen of any degree) in the renal artery most likely the smaller vessels distal to the stenosis are also compromised (function and structure) (Lerman LO *et al.*, 2009; Eirin A & Lerman, 2013). Furthermore, even in the absence of plaques, significant renal functional and structural damage may develop. Finally, this study, in conjunction with several other factors reported in chapter 3, may potentially help to explain why the use of the percentage of stenosis for the selection of the patients produced inconclusive results on renal artery revascularization (see chapter 2.2 - Is the renal artery stenting effective for the renal and blood pressure endpoint?). Other study is needed to solve this question.

3.2   RAS and GFR

Recently (Zanoli *et al.*, 2012), an increased association between reference diameter and glomerular filtration rate according to the severity of the percentage of renal artery stenosis has been reported (Figure 3). Even if patients with severe renal artery stenosis (>70%) were excluded from this report, the relationships between reference diameter and renal function became steeper in patients with low-moderate renal artery stenosis and, among these patients, in the higher quartile of renal artery stenosis (47-70%). These finding suggest that the burden of atherosclerosis at the site of renal arteries could play a role on the association of small renal arteries and reduced renal function even in low-moderate renal artery stenosis. Whether low-to-moderate renal artery stenosis is associated with a reduction in glomerular filtration rate is not clear. In another work, it has been demonstrated that increments of systolic pressure gradient (difference between blood pressure before and after renal artery stenosis) develop in an exponential manner even at not severe renal artery stenosis, with a renal artery stenosis of 50% indicating a significant (22 mm Hg) systolic pressure gradient (Gross *et al.*, 2001). In agreement with Cheung (Cheung *et al.*, 2002) Zanoli reported that, after univariate analysis, a moderate RAS (47-70%) was not significantly associated with chronic kidney disease. Interestingly, in fully adjusted model renal artery stenosis 47-70% and minimal diameter <2.9 mm appeared non independently associated with glomerular filtration rate whereas reference diameter was significantly and independently associated with glomerular filtration rate. These findings demonstrate that, in subjects with renal artery stenosis, reference diameter is useful to select patients with chronic kidney disease.

3.3   Renal Artery Diameter and Resistant Hypertension

Another important clinical finding of the study by Zanoli (Zanoli *et al.*, 2012) is that patients with resistant hypertension have smaller renal arteries, especially in the presence of low-to-moderate renal artery stenosis (Figure 4). This is the first time that reference diameter was tested as determinant of resistant hypertension and compared with minimal diameter and percentage of renal artery stenosis. In a recent paper, performed in a small cohort of patients, angiographic minimal diameter, and not the percentage of renal artery stenosis, was associated with hypertension improvement after stenting of renal artery stenosis at 12 months follow-up (Leesar *et al.*, 2009).

Reference diameter reduction can be associated with resistant hypertension by an increase in the renal nerve activation, with consequent renal vasoconstriction, chronic reductions in renal blood flow and flow-induced decreases in shear stress (Langille & O'Donnell, 1986) or, alternatively, by chronic kidney damage, with consequent decreased renal blood flow, increased renin activity, blunted pressure natriuresis and increased extracellular fluid volume (Khawaja *et al.*, 2011). Moreover, both RD reduction and resistant hypertension could be due to a nitric oxide deficiency, with consequent reduced NO-dependent vasodilatation (Langille & O'Donnell, 1986; Khawaja *et al.*, 2011; Langille, 1993). Taking together, these studies support the role of kidney in the pathophysiology of resistant hypertension (Calhoun DA *et al.*, 2008) and suggest that the renal vascular bed could be a marker of kidney damage even in not-severe renal artery stenosis (see chapter 3 - Renal artery diameter, GFR and resistant hypertension). Future studies are needed to clarify the role of reference diameter in the treatment of resistant hypertension.

3.4   Take-home message

In a population with a high prevalence of mild-moderate renal artery stenosis, small renal arteries are more associated with low glomerular filtration rate than larger renal arteries, even in the absence of stenosis. In the presence of low-to-moderate renal artery stenosis, small reference and minimal diameter are more associated with chronic kidney disease than the percentage of renal artery stenosis. Small renal arteries are more likely associated with resistant hypertension than larger renal arteries in the presence of low-to moderate renal artery stenosis.

4   Renal Artery Diameter and Contrast Induced Nephropathy

Contrast-induced nephropathy is a common and serious complication of contrast used in imaging studies, and is the third leading cause of acute kidney injury in hospitalized patients (Nash *et al.*, 2002). The incidence of contrast-induced nephropathy is low in patients without cardiovascular risk factors (Rihal *et al.*, 2002) and increases in patients with high cardiovascular risk (Senoo *et al.*, 2010). Patients who develop contrast-induced nephropathy after percutaneous coronary intervention sustain an increase in both short- and long-term mortality (Senoo *et al.*, 2010; McCullough *et al.*, 1997). Therefore, it is important to identify high-risk patients to reduce the incidence of contrast-induced nephropathy.

Many individual risk factors for the development of contrast-induced nephropathy have been detected and chronic kidney disease is one of the most important. However, Zanoli (Zanoli *et al.*, 2011) recently reported that patients with low-moderate renal artery stenosis have an increased risk of contrast-induced nephropathy and that reference diameter, a factor highly associated with glomerular filtration rate (see Chapter 3.1 - Renal artery diameter and glomerular filtration rate), was a stronger predictor of contrast-induced nephropathy than the presence of chronic kidney disease, suggesting that, at least in subjects with ischemic cardiac disease, the state of the renal vascular bed was most important than the unspecific chronic reduction in glomerular filtration rate.

5   Renal Artery Diameter and Cardiovascular Events

Numerous studies performed in the past decade have identified severe renal artery stenosis as a novel cardiovascular disease risk marker (Kalra et al., 2005; Cheung et al., 2002; Guo et al., 2007). Reduction of the renal artery diameter can induce global renal ischemia, especially when the RAS is above 70%. This is also a proxy for severity and extension of atherosclerosis. Renal injury distal to an atherosclerotic renovascular obstruction reflects multiple intrinsic factors producing parenchymal tissue injury. Atherosclerotic disease pathways superimposed on renal arterial obstruction may aggravate damage to the kidney and other target organs, and some of the factors activated by renal artery stenosis may in turn accelerate the progression of atherosclerosis. This cross-talk is mediated through amplified activation of renin-angiotensin system, oxidative stress, inflammation, and fibrosis-pathways notoriously involved in renal disease progression (Lerman et al, 2009). To date, even if there are no evidences that a moderate renal artery stenosis is associated with increased risk for cardiovascular events, it is well known that arterial diameters, either reference diameter or minimal diameter are dependent on several dynamic factors (Langille & O'Donnell, 1986; Khawaja et al., 2011; Langille, 1993), among the level of vascular tone on the short-term and vascular remodeling on the long term, and are associated with many cardiovascular risk factors (Zanoli et al., 2011; Zanoli et al., 2012; Dinenno et al., 2000; Zoccali et al., 2002). In addition, it is well known that long-term changes in local hemodynamic forces induce arterial remodeling that is critical to vascular adaptation in relation to the progression of cardiovascular disease (Langille, 1993). Minimal diameter reduction could be a marker of subclinical atherosclerosis, which significantly correlates with the development of coronary or cerebro-vascular disease, as well as suggested for another measure of structural abnormalities in carotid district, the carotid intima-media thickness.

Recently it has been demonstrated that low minimal renal artery diameter is significantly associated with an increased risk of cardiovascular events independently to standard cardiovascular risk factors including chronic kidney disease and hypertension (Zanoli et al., 2013) (Figure 5). Moreover, when minimal renal artery diameter was added to a model that includes a standard set of cardiovascular risk factor, integrated discrimination improves of 2.2%. Finally, it has been previously reported that subjects with renal artery stenosis demonstrated a significantly greater prevalence of clinical and subclinical manifestation of cardiovascular disease such as angina, previous myocardial infarction, ≥25% diameter-reducing internal carotid artery stenosis, increased carotid intima-media thickness and major electrocardiographic abnormalities (Edwards MS et al., 2004). Taking together, these findings indicate that the link between renal vascular bed and cardiovascular events could be partly independent to the reduction of the renal function and the onset of hypertension, and suggest that the renal vascular bed could be a marker of non-traditional cardiovascular risk factors (including subclinical atherosclerosis).

5.1   Take Home Message

In patients with ischemic heart disease and non-significant renal artery stenosis (RAS 10-70%), low minimal renal artery diameter is associated with an increased risk for a first cardiovascular event and improves risk prediction when added to standard risk factors. In these high risk subjects a comprehensive

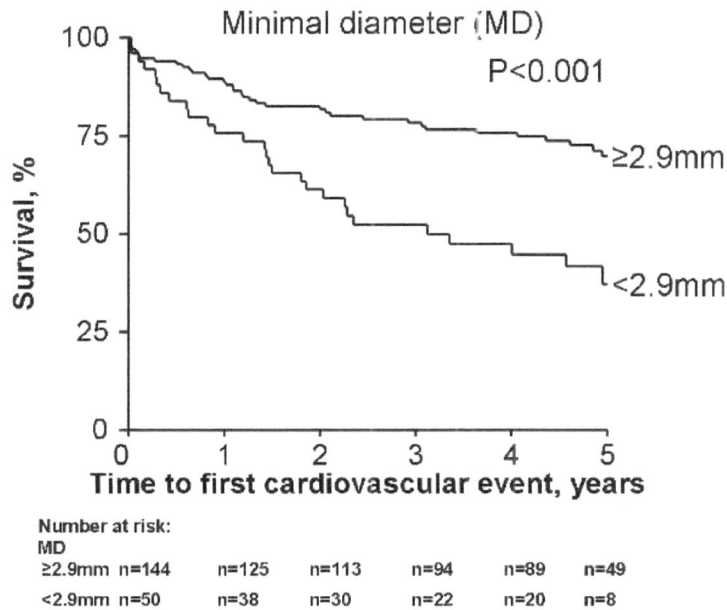

Figure 5: Kaplan–Meier plot of cumulative probability of a first major CVD event when participants were grouped according to minimal renal artery diameter. Adapted from Zanoli *et al.*, 2013.

evaluation of the cardiovascular risk, including asymptomatic organ damage, should be performed and focused on the detection and treatment of modifiable cardiovascular risk factors. Moreover, a recent study suggested that low minimal renal artery diameter may represent a valuable biomarker of cardiovascular disease risk (Zanoli *et al.*, 2012). Other studies are needed to confirm this data.

6   Conclusions

The reduction of renal artery diameter, either minimal or reference diameter, is associated with low glomerular filtration rate and resistant hypertension, predicts the onset of contrast induced nephropathy better than the unspecific chronic reduction of glomerular filtration rate and could represents a marker of non-traditional cardiovascular risk factors in subjects with ischemic heart disease.

References

ASTRAL Investigators, Wheatley K, Ives N, Gray R, Kalra PA, Moss JG, Baigent C, Carr S, Chalmers N, Eadington D, Hamilton G, Lipkin G, Nicholson A, Scoble J. Revascularization versus medical therapy for renal-artery stenosis. N Engl J Med 2009;361:1953–1962.

Bax L, Woittiez AJ, Kouwenberg HJ, Mali WP, Buskens E, Beek FJ, Braam B, Huysmans FT, Schultze Kool LJ, Rutten MJ, Doorenbos CJ, Aarts JC, Rabelink TJ, Plouin PF, Raynaud A, van Montfrans GA, Reekers JA, van den Meiracker AH, Pattynama PM, van de Ven PJ, Vroegindeweij D, Kroon AA, de Haan MW, Postma CT, Beutler JJ. Stent placement in patients with atherosclerotic renal artery stenosis and impaired renal function. A randomized trial. Ann Intern Med 2009;150:840-848.

Buller CE, Nogareda JG, Ramanathan K, Ricci DR, Djurdjev O, Tinckam KJ, Penn IM, Fox RS, Stevens LA, Duncan JA, Levin A. The profile of cardiac patients with renal artery stenosis. J Am Coll Cardiol 2004;43:1606-1613.

Calhoun DA, Jones D, Textor S, Goff DC, Murphy TP, Toto RD, White A, Cushman WC, White W, Sica D, Ferdinand K, Giles TD, Falkner B, Carey RM; American Heart Association Professional Education Committee. Resistant hypertension: diagnosis, evaluation, and treatment: a scientific statement from the American Heart Association Professional Education Committee of the Council for High Blood Pressure Research. Circulation. 2008;117(25):e510-26.

Cheung CM, Wright JR, Shurrab AE, Mamtora H, Foley RN, O'Donoghue DJ, Waldek S, Kalra PA. Epidemiology of renal dysfunction and patient outcome in atherosclerotic renal artery occlusion. J Am Soc Nephrol 2002;13:149-157.

Cheung CM, Hegarty J, Kalra PA. Dilemmas in the management of renal artery stenosis. Br Med Bull 2005;73-74:35-55.

Chonchol M, Linas S. Diagnosis and management of ischemic nephropathy. Clin J Am Soc Nephrol 2006;1:172–181.

Conlon PJ, O'Riordan E, Kalra PA. New insights into the epidemiologic and clinical manifestations of atherosclerotic renovascular disease. Am J Kidney Dis 2000;35:573-587.

Conlon PJ, Little MA, Pieper K, Mark DB. Severity of renal vascular disease predicts mortality in patients undergoing coronary angiography. Kidney Int 2001;60:1490-1497.

Cooper CJ, Murphy TP, Matsumoto A, Steffes M, Cohen DJ, Jaff M, Kuntz R, Jamerson K, Reid D, Rosenfield K, Rundback J, D'Agostino R, Henrich W, Dworkin L. Stent revascularization for the prevention of cardiovascular and renal events among patients with renal artery stenosis and systolic hypertension: rationale and design of the CORAL trial. Am Heart J. 2006;152:59–66.

Corriere MA, Hoyle JR, Craven TE, D'Agostino RB Jr, Edwards MS, Moore PS, Hansen KJ. Changes in left ventricular structure and function following renal artery revascularization. Ann Vasc Surg. 2010;24(1):80-84.

Cosgriff PS. The urinary tract. In: Practical nuclear medicine. 3rd ed. London: Springer; 2005. p. 222e3.

Crowley JJ, Santos RM, Peter RH, Puma JA, Schwab SJ, Phillips HR, Stack RS, Conlon PJ. Progression of renal artery stenosis in patients undergoing cardiac catheterization. Am Heart J 1998;136:913-8.

Dean RH, Kieffer RW, Smith BM, Oatet JA, Nadeau JH, Hollifield JW, DuPont WD. Renovascular hypertension: anatomic and renal function changes during drug therapy. Arch Surg 1981;116:1408-15.

De Mast Q, Beutler JJ. The prevalence of atherosclerotic renal artery stenosis in risk groups: a systematic literature review. J Hypertens 2009;27:1333-1340.

Denolle T, Chatellier G, Julien J, Battaglia C, Luo P, Plouin PF. Left ventricular mass and geometry before and after etiologic treatment in renovascular hypertension, aldosterone producing adenoma, and pheochromocytoma. Am J Hypertens. 1993;6:907-913.

Dinenno FA, Jones PP, Seals DR, Tanaka H. Age-associated arterial wall thickening is related to elevations in sympathetic activity in healthy humans. Am J Physiol Heart Circ Physiol. 2000;278(4):H1205-10.

Dong Q, Schoenberg SO, Carlos RC, Neimatallah M, Cho KJ, Williams DM, Kazanjian SN, Prince MR. Diagnosis of renal vascular disease with MR angiography. RadioGraphics 1999;19:1535-54.

Dworkin LD, Muphy T. Is there any reason to stent atherosclerotic renal artery stenosis. Am J Kidney Dis. 2010;56:259-263.

Echevarria JJ, Miguelez JL, Lopez-Romero S, Pastor E, Ontoria JM, Alustiza JM, Fernandez-Ruanova B. Arteriographic correlation in 30 patients with renal vascular disease diagnosed with multislice CT. Radiologia 2008;50:393-400.

Edwards MS, Hansen KJ, Craven TE, Bleyer AJ, Burke GL, Levy PJ, Dean RH. Associations between renovascular disease and prevalent cardiovascular disease in the elderly: a population-based study. Vasc Endovascular Surg. 2004;38(1):25-35.

Eirin A, Lerman LO. Darkness at the end of the tunnel: poststenotic kidney injury. Physiology (Bethesda). 2013;28(4):245-53.

Fraioli F, Catalano C, Bertoletti L, Danti M, Fanelli F, Napoli A, Cavacece M, Passariello R. Multidetector-row CT angiography of renal artery stenosis in 50 consecutive patients: prospective interobserver comparison with DSA. Radiol Med 2006;111:459-68.

Kalra PA, Guo H, Kausz AT, Gilbertson DT, Liu J, Chen SC, Ishani A, Collins AJ, Foley RN. Atherosclerotic renovascular disease in United States patients aged 67 years or older: risk factors, revascularization, and prognosis. Kidney Int 2005; 68:293–301.

Khawaja Z, Wilcox CS. Role of the kidneys in resistant hypertension. Int J Hypertens 2011; 2011:143471.

Krijnen P, van Jaarsveld BC, Steyerberg EW, Man in't Veld AJ, Schalekamp MADH, Habbema JKF: A clinical prediction rule for renal artery stenosis. Ann Intern Med 1998;129: 705-711.

Kumbhani DJ, Bavry AA, Harvey JE, de Souza R, Scarpioni R, Bhatt DL, Kapadia SR. Clinical outcomes after percutaneous revascularization versus medical management in patients with significant renal artery stenosis: a meta-analysis of randomized controlled trials. Am Heart J. 2011;161(3):622-630.e1.

Gobe G, Axelsen R, Searle JW. Cellular events in experimental unilateral ischemic renal atrophy and in regeneration after contralateral nephrectomy. Lab Invest 1990;63:770-779.

Glagov S, Weisenberg E, Zarins CK, Stankunavicius R, Kolettis GJ. Compensatory enlargement of human atherosclerotic coronary arteries. N Engl J Med 1987; 316:1371–1375.

Granata A, Fiorini F, Andrulli S, Logias F, Gallieni M, Romano G, Sicurezza E, Fiore CE. Doppler ultrasound and renal artery stenosis: An overview. J Ultrasound 2009;12(4):133-43.

Gross CM, Kramer J, Weingartner O, Uhlich F, Luft FC, Waigand J, Dietz R. Determination of renal arterial stenosis severity: comparison of pressure gradient and vessel diameter. Radiology 2001;220:751-756.

Guo H, Kalra PA, Gilbertson DT, Liu J, Chen SC, Collins AJ, Foley RN. Atherosclerotic renovascular disease in older US patients starting dialysis, 1996 to 2001. Circulation 2007; 115:50–58.

Guzman RP, Zierler RE, Isaacson JA, Bergelin RO, Strandness DE Jr. Renal atrophy and arterial stenosis. A prospective study with duplex ultrasound. Hypertension 1994;23:346-50.

Harding MB, Smith LR, Himmelstein SI, Harrison K, Phillips HR, Schwab SJ, Hermiller JB, Davidson CJ, Bashore TM. Renal artery stenosis: prevalence and associated risk factors in patients undergoing routine cardiac catheterization. J Am Soc Nephrol 1992; 2:1608-1616.

Hashemi Jazi M, Arasteh M, Shamsolketabi H, Tavassoli A, Nilforoush P, Gharipour M. Comparing diagnostic techniques of magnetic resonance angiography (MRA) and Doppler ultrasonography in determining severity of renal artery stenosis. ARYA Atheroscler 2011;7:58-62.

Henry M, Benejelloun A, Henry I, Polydorou A, Hugel M. Renal angioplasty and stenting: is it still indicated after ASTRAL and STAR studies. J Cardiovasc Surg 2010;51:701e20.

Hirsch AT, Haskal ZJ, Hertzer NR, Bakal CW, Creager MA, Halperin JL, Hiratzka LF, Murphy WR, Olin JW, Puschett JB, Rosenfield KA, Sacks D, Stanley JC, Taylor LM Jr, White CJ, White J, White RA, Antman EM, Smith SC Jr, Adams CD, Anderson JL, Faxon DP, Fuster V, Gibbons RJ, Hunt SA, Jacobs AK, Nishimura R, Ornato JP, Page RL, Riegel B; American Association for Vascular Surgery; Society for Vascular Surgery; Society for Cardiovascular Angiography and Interventions; Society for Vascular Medicine and Biology; Society of Interventional Radiology; ACC/AHA Task Force on Practice Guidelines Writing Committee to Develop Guidelines for the Management of Patients With Peripheral Arterial Disease; American Association of Cardiovascular and Pulmonary Rehabilitation; National Heart, Lung, and Blood Institute; Society for Vascular Nursing; TransAtlantic Inter-Society Consensus; Vascular Disease Foundation. ACC/AHA 2005 Practice Guidelines for the management of patients with peripheral arterial disease (lower extremity, renal, mesenteric, and abdominal aortic): a collaborative report from the American Association for Vascular Surgery/Society for Vascular Surgery, Society for Cardiovascular Angiography and Interventions, Society for Vascular Medicine and Biology, Society of Interventional Radiology, and the ACC/AHA Task Force on Practice Guidelines (Writing Committee to Develop Guidelines for the Management of Patients With Peripheral Arterial Disease): endorsed by the American Association of Cardiovascular and Pulmonary Rehabilitation;

National Heart, Lung, and Blood Institute; Society for Vascular Nursing; TransAtlantic Inter-Society Consensus; and Vascular Disease Foundation. Circulation 2006;113:e463–e654.

Igreja AC, Mesquita Kde C, Cowper SE, Costa IM. Nephrogenic systemic fibrosis: concepts and perspectives. An Bras Dermatol 2012;87:597-607.

Langille BL, O'Donnell F. Reductions in arterial diameter produced by chronic decreases in blood flow are endothelium dependent. Science 1986; 231:405–407.

Langille BL. Remodelling of developing and mature arteries: endothelium, smooth muscle and matrix. J Cardiovasc Pharmacol 1993;21:S11-S17.

Laurent S, Cockcroft J, Van Bortel L, Boutouyrie P, Giannattasio C, Hayoz D, Pannier B, Vlachopoulos C, Wilkinson I, Struijker-Boudier H; European Network for Non-invasive Investigation of Large Arteries. Expert consensus document on arterial stiffness: methodological issues and clinical applications. Eur Heart J. 2006;27(21):2588-605.

Leesar MA, Varma J, Shapira A, Fahsah I, Raza ST, Elghoul Z, Leonard AC, Meganathan K, Ikram S. Prediction of hypertension improvement after stenting of renal artery stenosis: comparative accuracy of translesional pressure gradients, intravascular ultrasound, and angiography. J Am Coll Cardiol 2009;53:2363-2371.

Lerman LO, Textor SC, Grande JP. Mechanisms of tissue injury in renal artery stenosis: ischemia and beyond. Prog Cardiovasc Dis 2009; 52:196–203.

London GM, Pannier B, Guerin AP, Blacher J, Marchais SJ, Darne B, Metivier F, Adda H, Safar ME. Alterations of left ventricular hypertrophy in and survival of patients receiving hemodialysis: follow-up of an interventional study. J Am Soc Nephrol. 2001;12(12):2759-2767.

Mangiacapra F, Trana C, Sarno G, Davidavicius G, Protasiewicz M, Muller O, Ntalianis A, Misonis N, Van Vlem B, Heyndrickx GR, De Bruyne B. Translesional pressure gradients to predict blood pressure response after renal artery stenting in patients with renovascular hypertension. Circ Cardiovasc Interv. 2010;3(6):537-542.

Mann SJ, Sos TA. Misleading results of randomized trials: the example of renal artery stenting. J Clin Hypertens (Greenwich). 2010;12(1):1-2.

Marcantoni C, Zanoli L, Rastelli S, Tripepi G, Matalone M, Mangiafico S, Capodanno D, Scandura S, Di Landro D, Tamburino C, Zoccali C, Castellino P. Effect of renal artery stenting on left ventricular mass: a randomized clinical trial. Am J Kidney Dis. 2012;60(1):39-46.

Marcantoni C, Rastelli S, Zanoli L, Tripepi G, Di Salvo M, Monaco S, Sgroi C, Capodanno D, Tamburino C, Castellino P. Erratum to: Prevalence of renal artery stenosis in patients undergoing cardiac catheterization. Intern Emerg Med. 2011 Jun 26 [Epub ahead of print].

McCullough PA, Wolyn R, Rocher LL, Levin RN, O'Neill WW. Acute renal failure after coronary intervention: incidence, risk factors, and relationship to mortality. Am J Med 1997;103:368-75.

Meaney TF, Dustan HP, McCormack LJ. Natural history of renal arterial disease. Radiology 1968;91:881-7.

Meyrier A, Hill GS, Simon P. Ischemic renal diseases: new insights into old entities. Kidney Int 1998;54: 2–13.

Middleton RJ, Parfrey PS, Foley RN. Left ventricular hypertrophy in the renal patient. J Am Soc Nephrol. 2001;12:1079-1084.

Morel P, Alexander-Williams J, Rohner A. Relation between flowpressure- diameter studies in experimental stenosis of rabbit and human small bowel. Gut 1990;31:875-878.

Mui KW, Sleeswijk M, van den Hout H, van Baal J, Navis G, Woittiez AJ. Incidental renal artery stenosis is an independent predictor of mortality in patients with peripheral vascular disease. J Am Soc Nephrol 2006;17:2069-2074.

Nash K, Hafeez A, Hou S. Hospital-acquired renal insufficiency. Am J Kidney Dis. 2002;39:930-936.

Novick AC, Pohl MA, Schrieber M, Gifford RW Jr, Vidt DG. Revascularization for preservation of renal function in patients with atherosclerotic renovascular disease. J Urol 1983;129: 907-912.

Olin JW, Melia M, Young JR, Graor RA, Risius B. *Prevalence of atherosclerotic renal artery stenosis in patients with atherosclerosis elsewhere. Am J Med 1990;88:46N-51N.*

Pradhan N, Rossi NF. *Interactions between the sympathetic nervous system and Angiotensin system in renovascular hypertension. Curr Hypertens Rev. 2013 May;9(2):121-9.*

Rabbia C, Valpreda S. *Duplex scan sonography of renal artery stenosis. Int Angiol 2003;22:101-15.*

Rabbia C, Pini R. *Evidence-based medicine in renal artery stenting. J Cardiovasc Surg 2010;51:755-63.*

Rihal CS, Textor SC, Breen JF, McKusick MA, Grill DE, Hallett JW, Holmes DR Jr. *Incidental renal artery stenosis among a prospective cohort of hypertensive patients undergoing coronary angiography. Mayo Clin Proc 2002;77:309-318.*

Rihal CS, Textor SC, Grill DE, Berger PB, Ting HH, Best PJ, Singh M, Bell MR, Barsness GW, Mathew V, Garratt KN, Holmes DR Jr. *Incidence and prognostic importance of acute renal failure after percutaneous coronary intervention. Circulation 2002;105:2259-64.*

Rimmer JM, Gennari FJ. *Atherosclerotic renovascular disease and progressive renal failure. Ann Intern Med. 1993;118(9):712-9.*

Rognant N, Rouvie`re O, Janier M, Le^ QH, Barthez P, Laville M, Juillard L. *Hemodynamic responses to acute and gradual renal artery stenosis in pigs. Am J Hypertens 2010;23:1216-1219.*

Rooke TW, Hirsch AT, Misra S, Sidawy AN, Beckman JA, Findeiss LK, Golzarian J, Gornik HL, Halperin JL, Jaff MR, Moneta GL, Olin JW, Stanley JC, White CJ, White JV, Zierler RE; Society for Cardiovascular Angiography and Interventions; Society of Interventional Radiology; Society for Vascular Medicine; Society for Vascular Surgery. *2011 ACCF/AHA Focused Update of the Guideline for the Management of Patients With Peripheral Artery Disease (updating the 2005 guideline): a report of the American College of Cardiology Foundation/American Heart Association Task Force on Practice Guidelines. J Am Coll Cardiol. 2011;58(19):2020-45.*

Rountas C, Vlychou M, Vassiou K, Liakopoulos V, Kapsalaki E, Koukoulis G, Fezoulidis IV, Stefanidis I. *Imaging modalities for renal artery stenosis in suspected renovascular hypertension: prospective intraindividual comparison of color Doppler US, CT, angiography, GD-enhanced MR angiography and digital subtraction angiography. Ren Fail 2007;29:295-302.*

Schreiber MJ, Pohl MA, Novick AC. *The natural history of atherosclerotic and fibrous renal artery disease. Urol Clin North Am 1984;11:383-92.*

Senoo T, Motohiro M, Kamihata H, Yamamoto S, Isono T, Manabe K, Sakuma T, Yoshida S, Sutani Y, Iwasaka T. *Contrast-induced nephropathy in patients undergoing emergency percutaneous coronary intervention for acute coronary syndrome. Am J Cardiol. 2010;105(5):624-628.*

Soulez G, Oliva VL, Turpin S, Lambert R, Nicolet V, Therasse E. *Imaging of renovascular hypertension: respective values of renal scintigraphy, renal doppler US and MR angiography. RadioGraphics 2000;20:1355-68.*

Suresh M, Laboi P, Mamtora H, Kalra PA. *Relationship of renal dysfunction to proximal arterial disease severity in atherosclerotic renovascular disease. Nephrol Dial Transplant 2000; 15:631–636.*

Symonides B. *Effects of the correction of renal artery stenosis on blood pressure, renal function and left ventricular morphology. Blood Press. 1999;8:141-150.*

Textor SC, Wilcox CS: *Renal artery stenosis: A common, treatable cause of renal failure? Annu Rev Med 2001;52: 421-442.*

Tollefson DF, Ernst CB. *Natural history of atherosclerotic renal artery stenosis associated with aortic disease. J Vasc Surg 1991;14:327-31.*

Tullus K. *Renal artery stenosis: is angiography still the gold standard in 2011? Paediatr Nephrol 2011;26:833-7.*

Turi ZG, Jaff RM. *Renal artery stenosis: searching for the algorithms for diagnosis and treatment. J Am Coll Cardiol 2003;41:1312e5.*

Weber-Mzell D, Kotanko P, Schumacher M, Klein W, Skrabal F. Coronary anatomy predicts presence or absence of renal artery stenosis. A prospective study in patients undergoing cardiac catheterization for suspected coronary artery disease. Eur Heart J 2002;23:1684-1691.

White CJ. Kiss my astral: one seriously flawed study of renal stenting after another. Catheter Cardiovasc Interv 2010;75:305–307.

White CJ, Jaff MR, Haskal ZJ, Jones DJ, Olin JW, Rocha-Singh KJ, Rosenfield KA, Rundback JH, Linas SL; American Heart Association Committee on Diagnostic and Interventional Cardiac Catheterization, Council on Clinical Cardiology; American Heart Association Council on Cardiovascular Radiology and Intervention; American Heart Association Council on Kidney in Cardiovascular Disease. Indications for Renal Arteriography at the Time of Coronary Arteriography A Science Advisory From the American Heart Association Committee on Diagnostic and Interventional Cardiac Catheterization, Council on Clinical Cardiology, and the Councils on Cardiovascular Radiology and Intervention and on Kidney in Cardiovascular Disease. Circulation 2006;114:1892–1895.

Wollenweber J, Sheps SG, Davis GD. Clinical course of atherosclerotic renovascular disease. Am J Cardiol 1968;21:60-71.

Wright JR, Shurrab AE, Cheung C, Waldek S, O'Donoghue DJ, Foley RN, Mamtora H, Kalra PA. A prospective study of the determinants of renal functional outcome and mortality in atherosclerotic renovascular disease. Am J Kidney Dis 2002; 39: 1153–1161.

Wright JR, Shurrab AE, Cooper A, Kalra PR, Foley RN, Kalra PA. Left ventricular morphology and function in patients with atherosclerotic renovascular disease. J Am Soc Nephrol 2005;16:2746-2753.

Xu JL, Shi DP, Li YL, Zhang JL, Zhu SC, Shen F. Non-enhanced MR angiography of renal artery using inflow-sensitive inversion recovery pulse sequence: a prospective comparison with enhanced CT angiography. Eur J Radiol 2011;80:57-63.

Yu H, Zhang D, Haller S, Kanjwal K, Colyer W, Brewster P, Steffes M, Shapiro JI, Cooper CJ. Determinants of renal function in patients with renal artery stenosis. Vasc Med. 2011;16(5):331-8.

Zhang R, Crump J, Reisin E. Regression of left ventricular hypertrophy is a key goal of hypertension management. Curr Hypertens Rep. 2003;5:301-308.

Zanoli L, Rastelli S, Marcantoni C, Tamburino C, Laurent S, Boutouyrie P, Castellino P. Renal artery diameter, renal function and resistant hypertension in patients with low-to-moderate renal artery stenosis. J Hypertens. 2012;30(3):600-7.

Zanoli L, Rastelli S, Marcantoni C, Tamburino C, Castellino P. Reference renal artery diameter is a stronger predictor of contrast-induced nephropathy than chronic kidney disease in patients with high cardiovascular risk. Nephron Extra 2011;1:38-44.

Zanoli L, Rastelli S, Marcantoni C, Blanco J, Tamburino C, Castellino P. Minimal renal artery diameter and cardiovascular events in subjects with ischemic heart disease and nonsignificant renal artery stenosis. 23rd European meeting on hypertension & cardiovascular protection Abstract book 2013. Abstract.

Zoccali C, Mallamaci F, Finocchiaro P. Atherosclerotic renal artery stenosis: epidemiology, cardiovascular outcomes, and clinical prediction rules. J Am Soc Nephrol. 2002;13(suppl 3):S179-S183.

Zoccali C, Benedetto FA, Mallamaci F, Tripepi G, Giacone G, Stancanelli B, Cataliotti A, Malatino LS. Left ventricular mass monitoring in the follow-up of dialysis patients: prognostic value of left ventricular hypertrophy progression. Kidney Int. 2004;65(4):1492-1498.

Zoccali C, Mallamaci F, Parlongo S, Cutrupi S, Benedetto FA, Tripepi G, Bonanno G, Rapisarda F, Fatuzzo P, Seminara G, Cataliotti A, Stancanelli B, Malatino LS. Plasma norepinephrine predicts survival and incident cardiovascular events in patients with end-stage renal disease. Circulation. 2002;105(11):1354-9.

Zeller T, Rastan A, Schwarzwälder U, Muller C, Frank U, Burgelin K, Sixt S, Schwarz T, Noory E, Neumann FJ. Regression of left ventricular hypertrophy following stenting of renal artery stenosis. J Endovasc Ther. 2007;14:189-197.

Bicuspid Aortic Valve Disease

Ify Mordi
Institute of Cardiovascular and Medical Sciences
University of Glasgow, United Kingdom

Nikolaos Tzemos
Institute of Cardiovascular and Medical Sciences
University of Glasgow, United Kingdom

1   Introduction

Bicuspid aortic valve (BAV) is the commonest congenital cardiac anomaly, with a prevalence thought to be between 1-2% in the general population (Mordi & Tzemos, 2012; Ward, 2000). It is 3 times more common in males, although gender is not a prognostic indicator in the natural history of BAV (Tutar, Ekici, Atalay, & Nacar, 2005). It is commonly an isolated finding; however it is also associated with other congenital cardiac disease. BAV is not just a valvular anomaly, but is also associated with aortic disease, commonly described as aortopathy, typically characterised by dilatation of the ascending aorta. While many people with BAV have aortic valves that function normally throughout life, complications are frequent in the BAV population. It is estimated that complications related to the aortic valve or ascending aorta requiring surgery occur in around a third of all patients with BA (Vallely, Semsarian, & Bannon, 2008). Because these complications are common in the BAV population, there is a large burden of morbidity and mortality in comparison to many other congenital diseases as a percentage of the general population. The main causes of adverse outcome in BAV patients are either related to the valve itself (stenosis, regurgitation or endocarditis) or to the aortopathy (leading to aneurysm and dissection). Given the high incidence of adverse events, routine screening is recommended for BAV patients to allow for timely intervention.

2   Embryology and Anatomy

The definitive fetal cardiac structure is developed by 8 weeks. The normal aortic valve consists of three valve cusps, sinuses, the aorto-ventricular junction and the sinotubular junction (Angelini *et al.*, 1989). The semi-lunar valves form from the division of the truncus arteriosus into two separate channels which form the aortic and pulmonary trunks. The channels are created by the fusion of two truncal ridges across the lumen. Small swellings appear on the inferior margins of each of the truncal ridges forming the basis of the adult valve leaflets. In each channel a third swelling occurs opposite the first two which forms the 3rd leaflet. In the normal aortic valve the left and right leaflets of the adult valve are formed from the respective swellings while the posterior leaflet is formed from a swelling in the aortic trunk (Anderson, Webb, Brown, Lamers, & Moorman, 2003; Restivo, Piacentini, Placidi, Saffirio, & Marino, 2006). Simultaneously, the coronary arteries are formed from buds which arise from the coronary sinuses of the aorta. Usually however, only two buds establish a connection with the epicardial tree to form future coronary arteries. This associated timing explains the frequent association between the aortic valve and coronary artery abnormalities.

Despite our knowledge of the formation of normal aortic valves, the exact pathogenesis that leads to the formation BAV is not yet fully understood. It does however appear to be more complex than just a simple fusion of two valve cusps. The bicuspid valve is composed of two leaflets, of which one is usually larger, although the fused valve leaflet in BAV is actually smaller in area than the total area of two separate leaflets would be if the valve were tricuspid. (Roberts, 1970, 1992). Commonly the larger of the two cusps (the conjoined leaflet) has a ridge or "raphe" which is the site of the valve fusion. This can make the valve appear tricuspid on echocardiography, requiring optimal imaging to be certain of the diagnosis. A number of systems have been proposed to classify BAVs according to their orientation (Schaefer *et al.*, 2008; Sievers & Schmidtke, 2007). The commonest method used is to classify the valvular anatomy into type 1, 2 and 3 (or A-C) according to the site of leaflet fusion (Schaefer *et al.*, 2008) (figure 1). Type 1,

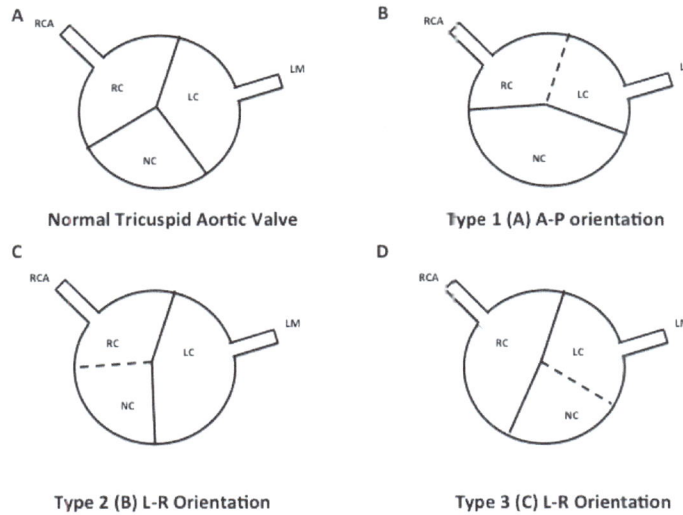

Normal Tricuspid Aortic Valve

Type 1 (A) A-P orientation

Type 2 (B) L-R Orientation

Type 3 (C) L-R Orientation

Figure 1: The anatomy of the bicuspid aortic valve (BAV). A – The normal tricuspid aortic valve; B – Type 1 (A) BAV with fusion of the right and left coronary cusps; C – Type 2 (B) BAV with fusion of the right and non-coronary cusps; D – Type 3 (C) BAV with fusion of the left and non-coronary cusps. The dotted line represents the fused cusps and signifies the potential presence of a raphe at the site of fusion. LC – left coronary cusp; LM – left main coronary artery; NC – non-coronary cusp; RC – right coronary cusp; RCA – right coronary artery.

Type 1 BAV	Type 2 BAV
More likely to become stenotic in adulthood	Valvular complications at a younger age
More common in males	Equal sex distribution
More likely to have aortic dilation at the sinus of Valsalva	More likely to have aortic dilatation at ascending aorta and aortic arch

Table 1: Bicuspid aortic valve types and their associations

the commonest configuration of the bicuspid is fusion of the left and right coronary cusps. Type 2 BAVs are caused by fusion of the right and non-coronary cusps. Type 3 BAV, the most rare, occurring in less than 1% of patients is due to fusion of the left and non-coronary cusps. The relevance of classification of BAV has been demonstrated in studies looking at the natural history of the valve. A study by Calloway et al, examining 1,128 patients, suggested that, with the suggestion that type 1 BAVs are more likely to become stenotic as adults while patients with type 2 valves tended to have valve complications as children or adolescents (Calloway *et al.*, 2011). Schaefer et al studied the link between the valve morphology and aortic disease in 191 patients (Schaefer *et al.*, 2008). In this study, the authors found that type 1 BAVs were more common in males and aortic dilatation at the sinus of Valsalva, while type 2 BAVs were associated with ascending aortic dilatation, aortic arch disease and myxomatous mitral valve disease. This pattern was also seen in study by Khoo et al (Khoo, Cheung, & Jue, 2013). This certainly may have implications for monitoring of BAV aortopathy. Finally, a study by Fernandes et al suggested that type 1 BAV was associated with coarctation of the aorta, in contrast to type 2 valves which were associated with more significant valvular disease than type 1 (Fernandes *et al.*, 2004).

Aortopathy is the commonest abnormality associated with BAV. While the altered aortic blood flow explains some of the dilatation of the aorta, there is evidence that there are other contributory mechanisms. Several studies have suggested that the pathogenesis of aortopathy is somewhat similar to that seen in Marfan syndrome, with the presence of cellular structural abnormalities including decreased fibrillin, causing smooth muscle cell detachment and cell death (de Sa, Moshkovitz, Butany, & David, 1999; Fedak *et al.*, 2002; Parai, Masters, Walley, Stinson, & Veinot, 1999). What is clear is that the development of aortopathy in BAV is fairly heterogeneous throughout the population – many patients may not develop any aortic disease throughout their life, whereas a small subset of patients develop aortic complications at a very young age, suggesting that there is a genetic component to the development of BAV aortopathy (Nistri *et al.*, 1999). Recently, Kang *et al* have also shown that the development and progression of BAV aortopathy differs in patients dependent on the orientation of the valves (i.e. which valves are fused) (Kang *et al.*, 2013). The development of BAV aortopathy and the influence of genetic and hemodynamic factors in its progression are further discussed in section 5.3.

Another major abnormality associated with BAV disease is coarctation of the aorta. This occurs in at least 20% of cases and perhaps up to 85% (Bonderman *et al.*, 1999; Presbitero *et al.*, 1987; Stewart, Ahmed, Travill, & Newman, 1993). BAV is also associated with other congenital cardiac disease such as hypoplastic left heart syndrome, and BAV is also found in other developmental diseases, for example Turner and Williams' syndrome (Siu & Silversides, 2010).

The final major association regards abnormalities of the coronary arterial circulation. Most patients with BAV disease have a left dominant coronary circulation (Roberts, 1970). The left main can also be up to 50% shorter than in normal in up to 90% of cases (Fedak *et al.*, 2002). This is an important consideration for any aortic valve surgery to ensure that steps are taken to avoid coronary artery damage during any valvular operation.

3 Genetics

It is now generally accepted that there is a heritable component to BAV disease. Initially, it was postulated that abnormal blood flow across the embryonic aortic valve may lead to BAV, however there is no convincing evidence to support this hypothesis. Meanwhile, the connection of BAV and the association of BAV with other congenital abnormalities such as coarctation of the aorta and ventricular septal defect again suggests that there may be a developmental, and therefore genetic, link (Duran *et al.*, 1995).

There have been several studies that appear to show episodes of familial clustering of BAV, again supporting the genetic theory (Glick & Roberts, 1994; Huntington, Hunter, & Chan, 1997). Huntington et al screened 190 first-degree relatives of patients with congenital BAV and reported BAV prevalence in this group of 9.1% (Huntington *et al.*, 1997). The high prevalence in this study suggests that BAV might be an autosomal dominant disorder with variable penetrance. It seems more likely however that BAV has polygenic inheritance, though few of these pathways have as yet been completely identified. A more recent study by Robledo-Carmona et al reported lower rates of BAV in people with affected first-degree relatives (Robledo-Carmona *et al.*, 2013). The authors studied 553 patients from 100 families and only found a BAV rate of 4.6% in patients with affected first-degree relatives. This is certainly lower than reported in the Huntington study. The study by Robledo-Carmona et al was conducted within a Mediterranean population however, perhaps suggesting a variable world-wide distribution – this might add further support to a heritable component to BAV.

Despite the increasing observational evidence suggesting that there is a genetic link to the development of BAV, discovery of the majority of genetic pathways leading to BAV has been elusive. Mutations in a gene called *NOTCH1*, a trans-membrane receptor that has a role in determining cell outcome in organogenesis, were noted in two families with BAV (Garg *et al.*, 2005). This seems to be the strongest genetic link discovered yet with further discoveries of missense *NOTCH1* mutations causing impaired Notch signalling (Foffa *et al.*, 2013; McKellar *et al.*, 2007; Mohamed *et al.*, 2006). Several other genetic loci have been postulated including chromosomes 18q, 5q and 13q, though no specific causative genes have been found. Not only are mutations in *NOTCH1* associated with abnormal valve morphology, but also they are also associated with accelerated calcium deposition within the valve, perhaps providing a mechanism for the advanced early calcific disease seen in the condition (Acharya *et al.*, 2011; Garg *et al.*, 2005). Work is being done to find other genes that might be associated with BAV. Recent data has linked the Gata5 gene with BAV and the development of aortopathy (Laforest, Andelfinger, & Nemer, 2011; Padang, Bagnall, Richmond, Bannon, & Semsarian, 2012).

Recent guidance from the American College of Cardiology/American Heart Association takes account of the evidence supporting a genetic component and recommend that all patients with a 1st degree relative with BAV should be evaluated for BAV and aortopathy using echocardiography (Hiratzka *et al.*, 2010). No studies have been done as yet however to prove an economic benefit to screening, however recent guidance suggests that first-degree relatives of BAV patients should be screened (Hiratzka *et al.*, 2010).

4   Diagnosis

Non-invasive testing plays an important role in the diagnosis and management of BAV patients.

Clinical findings are usually limited to auscultation with most patients having an ejection systolic murmur heard loudest at the apex (Mills, Leech, Davies, & Leathan, 1978). There may also be clinical signs of aortic stenosis (or incompetence) and coarctation of the aorta if associated. The electrocardiogram is usually normal however there may be signs of left ventricular hypertrophy.

The mainstay of diagnosis is echocardiography (transthoracic or transesophageal) which can provide a definitive diagnosis in the majority of patients. Echocardiography is the current gold-standard for diagnosis (Warnes, Williams, Bashore, Child, Connolly, Dearani, del Nido, Fasules, Graham, Hijazi, Hunt, King, Landzberg, Miner, Radford, Walsh, & Webb, 2008). Figures of 92% sensitivity and 96% specificity have been reported when images are adequate, although due to the natural history of BAV to lead to heavily calcified stenotic valves, the accuracy of transthoracic echocardiography can be reduced (Chan, Stinson, & Veinot, 1999; Tanaka *et al.*, 2010). Because of this, transesophageal echocardiography may be required. 3-dimensional transesophageal echocardiography is a newer technique which may add further detailed information, although this technique is not usually required (Koh, 2013).

Using transthoracic echocardiography, the parasternal short axis view allows for direct visualization of the valve cusps and allows diagnostic confirmation. In this view the normal triangular opening shape is lost, becoming more "fish mouth"-like in appearance, more akin to the mitral valve (figure 2). This is especially pronounced in systole, as in diastole the raphe can appear similar to a commissure of the third cusp. Other views (parasternal long axis and apical views) can show turbulent flow and eccentric lines of valve closure. If necessary, transesophageal echocardiography can be carried out to confirm the diagnosis. Because of the eccentricity of the valve jet in patients with aortic stenosis, it is recommended

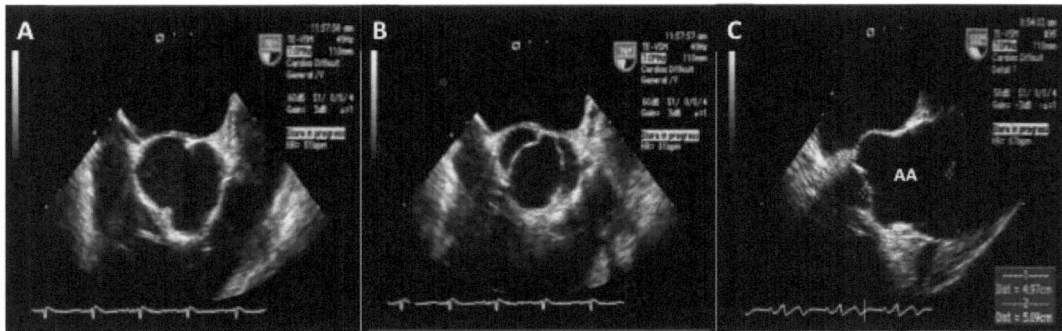

Figure 2: Type 2 bicuspid aortic valve evaluated with transthoracic echocardiography in diastole (A) and systole (B). There is concomitant ascending aortopathy with the ascending aorta (AA) measuring 51mm (C).

that aortic valve area is calculated using the continuity equation rather than by direct planimetry (Donal *et al.*, 2005). Regurgitation can be measured using routine parameters such as pressure half time, regurgitant fraction and width of the vena contracta. 3-D echocardiography may also provide even more accurate diagnosis and characterization of the valve (figure 3) (Sadron Blaye-Felice *et al.*, 2012). The severity of aortic valve disease as measured by echocardiography has been shown to be predictive of future valve repair in BAV patients (Ahmed *et al.*, 2007).

It is also important to assess the aorta in BAV patients, given the prevalence of aortopathy. The proximal ascending aorta can usually be assessed satisfactorily using echocardiography, however, as described earlier, aortopathy can often affect the ascending aorta above the level of the root, and so complimentary imaging modalities are often needed for complete vascular assessment, especially if the suprasternal windows using transthoracic echocardiography are not satisfactory. This is most commonly conducted by computed tomography (CT) or cardiovascular magnetic resonance (CMR).

CT is widely available, fast and non-invasive. It offers excellent spatial resolution and allows 3-D evaluation of the whole aorta (figure 4). Retrospective ECG-gated CT study acquisition allows visualization of the valve is both systole and diastole, allowing clear diagnosis of the valve. CT has been shown to have diagnostic accuracy for differentiation of BAV and tricuspid aortic valves with both sensitivity and specificity ranging from 94-100% in recent studies (Alkadhi *et al.*, 2010; Lee *et al.*, 2012; Tanaka *et al.*, 2010). CT can offer coronary artery evaluation, which could aid surgical planning in the case of anomalous coronary arteries, which as described earlier are common in BAV patients. Also, in older patients evaluation of the coronary arteries is mandatory prior to cardiac surgery. Finally, the use of retrospective gating also enables calculation of left ventricular volumes and ejection fraction. The main drawback of CT is its use of ionizing radiation, which means that it may not be practical to use it for serial assessment of the aorta, although scanners continue to improve and radiation doses continue to decline.

CMR is increasingly used in the assessment of BAV and enables views of the valve to be obtained without interference from calcification. It also allows for excellent assessment of the aorta. A recent study of 123 patients with confirmed BAV found that 10% of the patients were misidentified as having a tricuspid valve using transthoracic echo and 28% had a non-diagnostic study, in comparison to 4% being misidentified as having a tricuspid valve by magnetic resonance imaging and 2% having a non-diagnostic study (Malaisrie *et al.*, 2012). Using cine imaging and phase-contrast imaging, the severity of any valvular disease can also be assessed with reasonable accuracy, although echocardiography remains

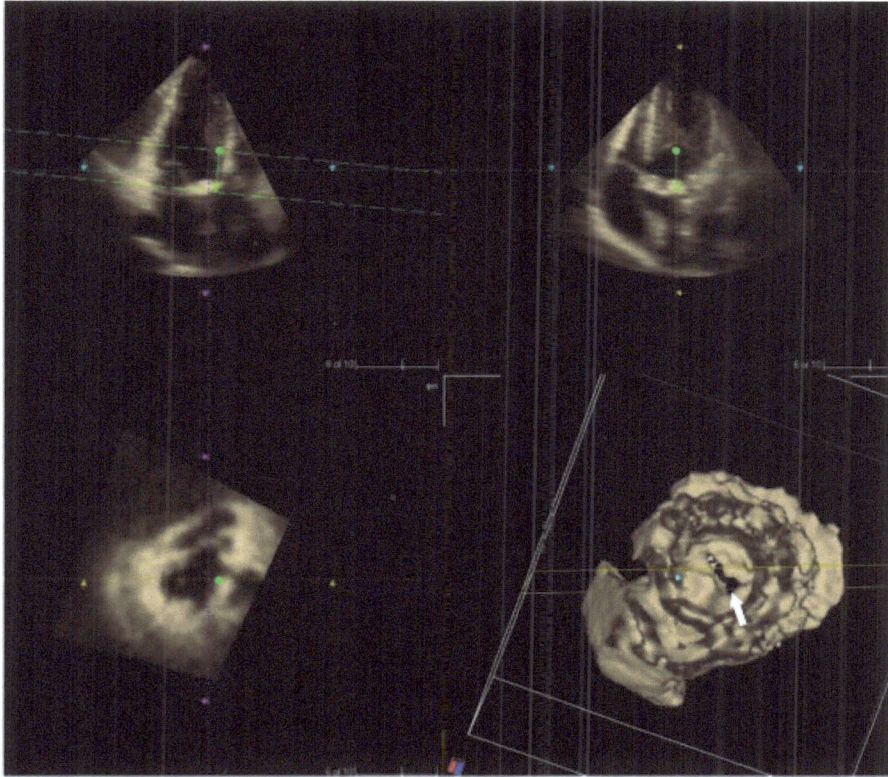

Figure 3: Bicuspid aortic valve seen using 3-dimensional echocardiography. The aortic valve is severely stenosed with area measured by direct planimetry of 0.9cm^2 (arrow).

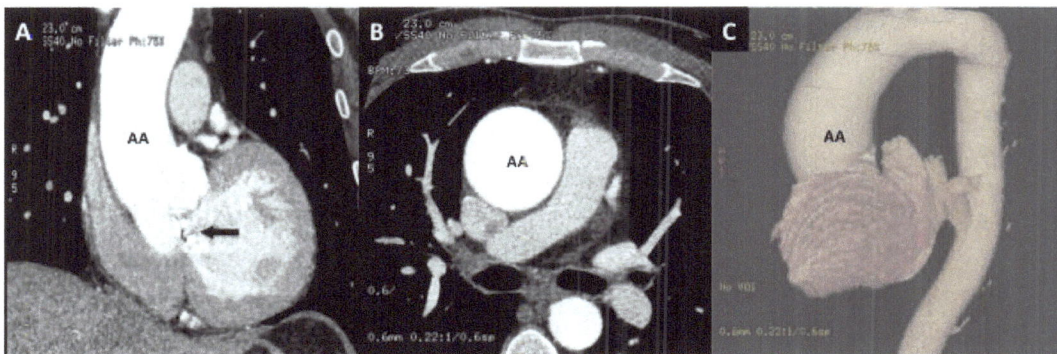

Figure 4: Computed tomography in the assessment of bicuspid aortic valve. A heavily calcified aortic valve is seen (A, arrow), as well as ascending aortopathy (AA, panels A and B). CT allows complete 3-dimensional reconstruction of the whole aorta allowing evaluation of the extent of aortopathy and assessment of any coarctation (C).

the mainstay for diagnosis. There are limitations however – not least its limited availability and higher technical requirements (both for the technician and the reporting cardiologist/radiologist). The limited temporal resolution of CMR also means that measurements of peak velocity can be inaccurate, although there is reasonable correlation with echocardiographic values (Caruthers *et al.*, 2003; Cawley, Maki, & Otto, 2009).

The main advantage of CMR lie in its accurate assessment of ventricular volumes and function, for which it is the non-invasive gold-standard, and, perhaps more importantly, its ability to completely characterise the extent and nature of any aortopathy (Tsai, Trivedi, & Daniels, 2012) (figure 5). Furthermore, its lack of ionizing radiation confers an advantage over CT, particularly for surveillance, although certainly CT can also accurately image both the valve and the aorta (Joo *et al.*, 2012).

In summary, all 3 non-invasive techniques have advantages and disadvantages. A recent study evaluated 262 patients undergoing aortic valve surgery and found all 3 non-invasive techniques to have high diagnostic accuracy (>95%) for assessment of valve morphology (Lee *et al.*, 2012). Echocardiography remains the mainstay for diagnosis and surveillance, however both CT and CMR can provide clearer images and are also able to provide complete aortic evaluation.

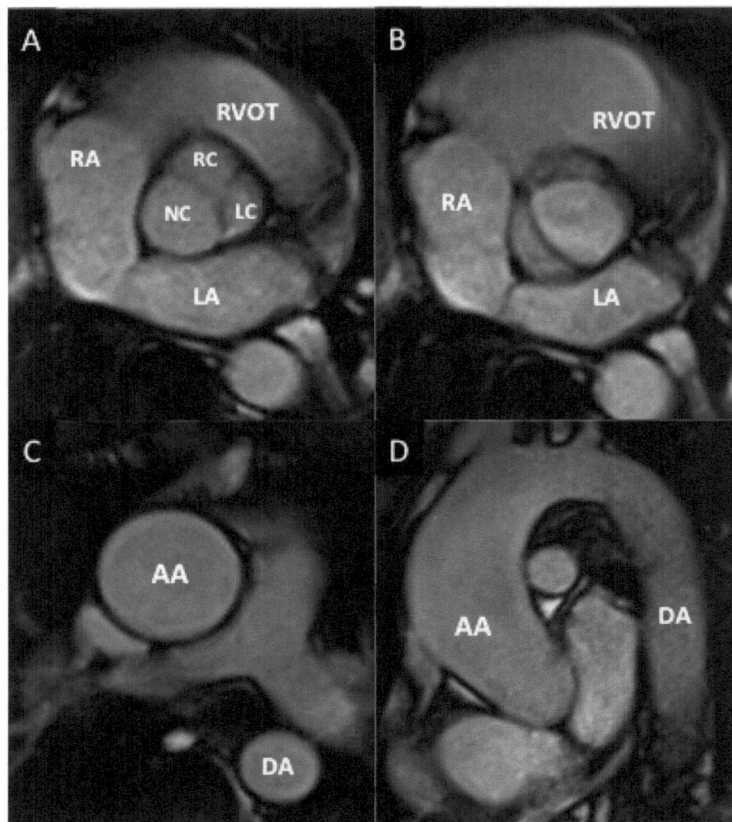

Figure 5: Type 1 bicuspid aortic valve seen in diastole (A) and systole (B) using cardiovascular magnetic resonance imaging allowing excellent visualization of proximal aortopathy (C and D). AA – ascending aorta; DA – descending aorta; LA – left atrium; LC – left coronary cusp; NC – non-coronary cusp; RA – right atrium; RC – right coronary cusp; RVOT – right ventricular outflow tract.

5   Clinical Progression

The natural history of BAV has been evaluated a several cohort studies. It is known to be variable and of course somewhat dependent on associated abnormalities. In some patients there is the appearance of severe aortic stenosis in childhood, however many patients (forming the majority) are asymptomatic until adulthood. Indeed, there have been reports of incidental findings of a minimally calcified BAV in patients in their 70s (Fenoglio, McAllister, DeCastro, Davia, & Cheitlin, 1977). More commonly however (in around 75% of patients) there is progressive fibro-calcific stenosis of the valve eventually requiring surgery. This usually leads to presentation in middle age – only around 2% of children have clinically significant BAV disease (Bonow *et al.*, 2006).

Until recently, there had been few recent studies investigating the natural clinical course of the BAV. The first large cohort study was by Michelena *et al* (Michelena *et al.*, 2008). In this study, the authors examined a cohort of 212 asymptomatic patients with BAV (age 32+/-20 years) and followed them up for a mean of 15 years. The authors found that the BAV group had the same 20 year survival rate as the normal population (around 90%) but also an increased frequency of cardiac events including aortic valve surgery, ascending aorta surgery and any other cardiovascular surgery. Predictive factors for cardiovascular events were found to be age ≥50 years and valve degeneration at diagnosis while an ascending aorta ≥40 mm at baseline independently predicted surgery for aorta dilatation.

The largest study in BAV patients was conducted by Tzemos et al (Tzemos *et al.*, 2008). The authors examined outcomes in 642 patients with both symptomatic and asymptomatic BAV (mean age 35+/-16 years) and followed them up for a mean of 9 years, again with a 10-year survival rate similar to the normal population (96%). One or more primary cardiac events occurred in 25% including cardiac death in 3%, intervention on the aortic valve or ascending aorta in 22%, aortic dissection or aneurysm in 2% and congestive heart failure requiring hospital admission in 2%. Independent predictors of primary cardiac events were age older than 30 years, moderate or severe aortic stenosis and moderate or severe aortic regurgitation (figure 6).

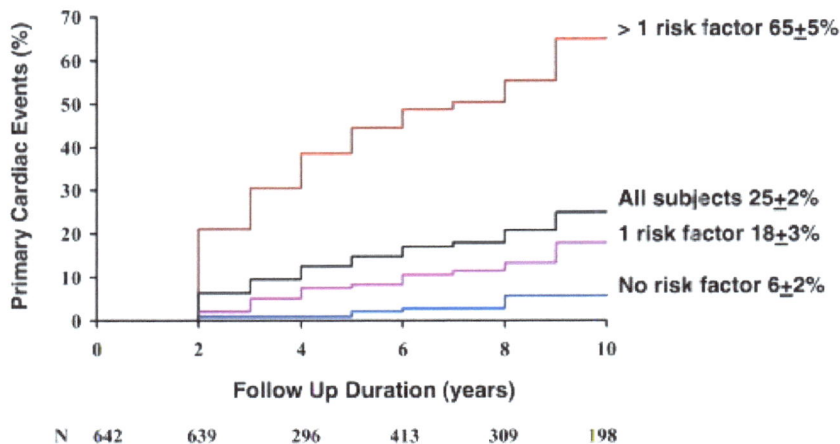

Figure 6: Outcomes in Bicuspid Aortic Valve Patients (from Tzemos *et al.*)

A more recent study has looked at the incidence of aortic complications in 416 BAV patients (mean age 35 years) (Michelena *et al.*, 2011). Incidence of aortic dissection was found to be 1.5% in all patients regardless of the progression of BAV; however this increased markedly in patients aged 50 or older at baseline to 17.4% and even more in those found to have aneurysm formation at baseline (44.9%). 25 year rate for aortic surgery was 25% and there was a significant burden of progression of disease to cause aortic dissection with 49 of the 384 patients without baseline aneurysms developing them during follow-up, giving an age-adjusted relative risk of 86.2 and an incidence of 84.9 cases per 10000 patient-years.

The common denominator in all three of these large outcome studies is the independent prognostic significance of age, suggesting that over time, many patients will require some sort of intervention. This has lead to the increased drive towards surveillance of BAV patients.

All in all, life expectancy in patients with BAV is not significantly different from the general population – Tzemos *et al* reported a 10-year survival of 96% in patients with a spectrum of valve dysfunction (Tzemos *et al.*, 2008). Despite this, there are several complications which have been identified in BAV patients. These can be divided into two groups: valvular complications (aortic stenosis, aortic incompetence and endocarditis) and vascular complications i.e. aortopathy.

5.1   Aortic Stenosis

The symptoms of the BAV tend to worsen with increasing stenosis severity and measurements of the valve orifice. The main symptoms are (exertional) dyspnea, syncope and chest pain. These patients should be evaluated and managed similarly to patients with tricuspid aortic valve stenosis, but of course the patients will generally present much earlier as described previously.

The fetus can generally survive with severe aortic stenosis due to blood flow through the right side of the heart, however in infancy there is usually a sudden decline in cardiovascular status. One study indicated that children with a valve gradient greater or equal to 50mmHg had a risk of adverse cardiovascular events of 1.2% per year (J. F. Keane *et al.*, 1993). In infants, due to the lack of valvular calcification, balloon valvuloplasty is the chosen treatment rather than valve replacement (Tworetzky *et al.*, 2004). Re-operation is common however, with one study reporting further intervention in 26% of patients within 10 years (Janatuinen, Vanttinen, Saraste, & Ingberg, 1989).

In adults with BAV, stenosis occurs by similar methods to the process in patients with tricuspid aortic valves i.e. leaflet calcification (Subramanian, Olson, & Edwards, 1984). Similarly to tricuspid aortic valve stenosis, it is felt to be an active process with inflammation and endothelial dysfunction (Wallby, Janerot-Sjoberg, Steffensen, & Broqvist, 2002).Indeed, it has been suggested that up to 50% of adults with aortic stenosis have a congenitally BAV and that it is the commonest cause of aortic stenosis in patients under 70 (Pomerance, 1972; Ward, 2000). Echocardiographic data has suggested that sclerosis of the valve begins to occur at the age of 20, with calcification prominent at age 40. The valve gradient is estimated to increase by an average of 18mmHg per decade (Beppu *et al.*, 1993). Some studies have also suggested that leaflet orientation may be a predictive factor in the rate of valve stenosis, although this was not replicated in the larger studies by Tzemos and Michelena (Beppu *et al.*, 1993; Fernandes, Khairy, Sanders, & Colan, 2007). A further recent study in 167 patients using CT and echocardiography found that patients with type 1 BAV were more likely to have stenotic valves than those with type 2 (Kang *et al.*, 2013). The variability of stenotic valves with BAV orientation was also found in another study by Huang et al (Huang & Le Tan, 2013).

5.2   Aortic Incompetence

This is relatively common in BAV and is often independent of aortic stenosis (M. G. Keane *et al.*, 2000; Sadee, Becker, Verheul, Bouma, & Hoedemaker, 1992). One cohort of 118 BAV patients found that of 70 patients without aortic stenosis, 28 (40%) had moderate to severe aortic regurgitation. The mechanisms of aortic incompetence in children are usually due to prolapsing cusps, post-valve surgery or endocarditis, while as the patients age dilatation of the ascending aorta can lead to a functionally regurgitant valve. Tzemos *et al* (Tzemos *et al.*, 2008) however suggested that rates of intervention in BAV patients with solitary aortic incompetence tended to be low. Another important cause of aortic incompetence is myxoid degeneration of the valve. This is where the connective tissue of the valve is replaced by acid mucopolysaccharides disrupting the structural integrity of the valve. One case series included 27 patients with BAV who had pure aortic incompetence – 16 of these had severe myxoid degeneration and required earlier intervention than the other 11 (average 40 years v 52) (Yotsumoto *et al.*, 1998).

The prevalence of aortic regurgitation in adults with BAV has varied – one study reported rates of 13% (Sabet, Edwards, Tazelaar, & Daly, 1999) whereas the large study by Michelena et al reported almost half of their cohort to have some aortic regurgitation. Intervention rates for pure aortic incompetence were low in both this study and that conducted by Tzemos et al. Patients who undergo intervention for this indication tend to be younger however, perhaps due to the association of aortic incompetence with infective endocarditis and aortic coarctation (Ward, 2000).

5.3   Aortopathy/Aortic Dissection

BAV is often associated with dilatation of the aortic root and the ascending aorta (Nistri *et al.*, 1999). This is otherwise known as aortopathy. This can lead to aneurysm and dissection. In BAV patients, the risk of aortic dissection is 8-fold. Furthermore, the risk of aortic aneurysm is 26% over 25 years and around a quarter of patients will require aortic surgery over this same time frame (Michelena *et al.*, 2011). The dilatation has been reported during childhood, and it has also been suggested that increased aortic size at baseline is predictive for earlier dilatation and worse outcomes (Dore, Brochu, Baril, Guertin, & Mercier, 2003; Holmes *et al.*, 2007). The aorta is generally larger in patients with BAV compared to those with tricuspid aortic valves (Morgan-Hughes, Roobottom, Owens, & Marshall, 2004). The most likely risk factor for progression of aortopathy is felt to be age. Aortic root size itself is related to valve morphology and the presence of significant disease (Schaefer, Lewin, Stout, Byers, & Otto, 2007; Thanassoulis *et al.*, 2008) however, a recent study did suggest that while most patients with BAV and ascending aortic aneurysm had severe valve dysfunction, there was a small proportion of patients (5%) who did have aneurysm formation without any aortic valve dysfunction (Aydin *et al.*, 2013).

Many theories have been postulated for the mechanism of BAV aortopathy. For a long time it has been thought to be predominantly genetic in origin, however there is increasing evidence for the contribution of a hemodynamic mechanism (Padang *et al.*, 2013). Recent work using CMR has shown abnormal flow in the proximal ascending aorta in BAV patients which may lead to shear stress and promotion of aortic dilatation, with variable patterns of aortic dilation seen with different valve orientations (Hope *et al.*, 2011). It is felt that it is due to defects in the aortic media, such as elastin fragmentation, loss of smooth muscle cells, and an increase in collagen (Bonderman *et al.*, 1999; Fedak *et al.*, 2003; Michelena *et al.*, 2011; Niwa *et al.*, 2001). Systemic features have also been noted in BAV patients that may predispose to aneurysm formation including systemic endothelial dysfunction and higher plasma levels of matrix metalloproteinases (Tzemos *et al.*, 2010). Also noted has been an increased amount of wall stress in the ascending aorta (Nathan *et al.*, 2011).

Aortic dissection is a devastating concern in these patients however reported incidence of this in the literature has been variable, from no events and 0.1% in the larger studies, up to 4% in pooled earlier studies (Guntheroth, 2008; Michelena *et al.*, 2008; Tzemos *et al.*, 2008). Risk stratification for BAV and development of aortopathy still has a long way to go as there has so far appeared to be little correlation between echocardiographic and histologic findings and development of aortic disease (Leone *et al.*, 2012). Recent advances in echocardiography may help to identify at-risk patients in future (Santarpia *et al.*, 2012). The incidence of aortic dissection is actually much higher in patients with Marfan syndrome, however due to the increased prevalence of BAV in comparison it is by far the commoner etiology (Larson & Edwards, 1984).

There is still a lot of evidence pointing towards a genetic origin. 4 "important lines of evidence" have been identified for the genetic theory (Bonow, 2008): 1. Greater aortic size in patients with BAVs and aortic stenosis compared with those with tricuspid valves and aortic stenosis who are matched for hemodynamic severity (Novaro *et al.*, 2003); 2. Enlarged aortas are found in patients (including children) with BAVs but without any aortic stenosis or aortic regurgitation, compared with age-matched normal controls (Cecconi *et al.*, 2005; Pachulski, Weinberg, & Chan, 1991); 3. Studies have demonstrated progressive enlargement of the aorta after aortic valve replacement (AVR) in patients with BAVs (Borger *et al.*, 2004; Russo *et al.*, 2002) and 4. Studies have demonstrated degeneration of the extracellular matrix of the aorta in patients with BAVs, including elastic fiber fragmentation, increased metalloproteinase expression, decreased expression of tissue inhibitors of metalloproteinases, and smooth muscle cell apoptosis as mentioned previously.

5.4   Infective Endocarditis

Endocarditis is more common in BAV. The estimated incidence is 0.16% per year in unoperated children and adolescents (Gersony *et al.*, 1993). In adults the two large case series by Tzemos and Michelena give an incidence of 0.3% and 2% per year respectively.

Outcomes in BAV patients with infective endocarditis tend to be worse than in those with normal valves. A recent observational study of 310 patients with infective endocarditis found that the 50 patients with BAV were younger at presentation and had a higher incidence of aortic perivalvular abscess (Bonow *et al.*, 2008). Early surgery was also performed in most of the BAV patients (72%) with similar perioperative mortality to those with tricuspid aortic valves. In-hospital mortality and 5 year survival was also comparable to patients with normal valves. Infective endocarditis associated with BAV is more common in children, and indeed in one cohort was the cause of death in over half the patients under 30, whereas it was the cause of death in only 13% of over 70s (Ward, 2000).

6   Management

The only treatments to offer any sort of curative option are surgical. Medical therapies are to try and alleviate symptoms and slow progression.

6.1   Screening and Surveillance

Given the possible genetic link we described earlier, and the clearer evidence of increased familial clustering, there has been increased interest in screening for the condition (Kerstjens-Frederikse *et al.*, 2011). As an asymptomatic disease with a relatively easy non-invasive method of diagnosis and defined treatments it is a disease that certainly meets WHO criteria for adoption of screening. Recent guidance from the ACC/AHA have recommended screening first degree family members of patients with BAV, however this has not been adopted in European guidelines as yet (Warnes, Williams, Bashore, Child, Connolly, Dearani, del Nido, Fasules, Graham, Hijazi, Hunt, King, Landzberg, Miner, Radford, Walsh, Webb, *et al.*, 2008).

Once diagnosed, patients with BAV should undergo yearly transthoracic echocardiograms if aortic root diameter is >40mm or there is significant valve disease, or every 2 years if less than 40mm (Warnes, Williams, Bashore, Child, Connolly, Dearani, del Nido, Fasules, Graham, Hijazi, Hunt, King, Landzberg, Miner, Radford, Walsh, & Webb, 2008).

6.2   Medical

It is generally felt that blood pressure should be aggressively controlled to try and slow the progression of aortopathy. Small studies in patients with Marfan syndrome and ascending aortic dilatation have shown some benefit in reduction of cardiac events in the use of beta-blockers (Ladouceur *et al.*, 2007; Shores, Berger, Murphy, & Pyeritz, 1994). Nevertheless, the role of beta-blockers in BAV aortopathy is as yet unproven. The joint ACC/AHA guidelines have however suggested use of beta-blockers as first-line therapy in BAV patients with dilated aortic roots (>4.0cm) who are not candidates for surgery and have no more than mild aortic regurgitation (Bonow *et al.*, 2008).

Extrapolating from patients with aortopathy in Marfan syndrome there is also a suggestion that ACE inhibitors and angiotensin receptor blockers may have a role to play, however the evidence in BAV is still lacking (Ahimastos *et al.*, 2007; Brooke *et al.*, 2008; Yetman, Bornemeier, & McCrindle, 2005). There is interest in the use of angiotensin receptor blockers in patients with aortopathy based on positive results in mouse models of aortopathy (Habashi *et al.*, 2006) – there are two trials presently being conducted in patients with Marfan syndrome which may provide insight into the mechanisms behind BAV aortopathy also (Detaint *et al.*, 2010; Radonic *et al.*, 2010).

Of course, concomitant conditions and risk factors should be treated as in the normal population.

6.3   Surgical

Indications for valve surgery in patients with BAV are similar to those with tricuspid aortic valves and are summarized in table 2. Due to the variation in patient characteristics and pathology an individual approach must be taken to all surgical decisions. In children it is usually not practical to do AVR as they outgrow the prosthetic valve. Due to the lack of valve calcification in children balloon valvuloplasty is possible and is the management strategy of choice. Studies have shown good follow-up in both the immediate and medium-terms, with 50% of patients in one series (the majority of whom had BAV) requiring no intervention at 38 months (Rosenfeld *et al.*, 1994).

The Ross procedure can be used in BAV patients with very good outcome. In this operation first described in 1962, the patient's aortic valve is replaced with their own pulmonary valve ("autograft"), while the pulmonary graft valve is replaced by a cadaveric pulmonary valve ("allograft") (Ross, 1962). This is the operation of choice in children. The main advantages of this procedure are thought to be an

	Indication for Surgery
Aortic Stenosis (AS)	Surgery is indicated in symptomatic patients with severe AS, patients with severe AS undergoing CABG, other valvular or aortic surgery, asymptomatic patients with LV ejection fraction ≤50% not due to any other cause and asymptomatic patients with severe AS and exercise related symptoms (on exercise testing)*. Echocardiographic criteria: <ul><li>Valve area <1cm^2</li><li>Mean gradient >40cm^2</li><li>Maximum jet velocity >4m/s</li></ul>
Aortic Incompetence (AI)	Surgery is indicated in symptomatic patients with severe AI, asymptomatic patients with resting LV ejection fraction ≤50% or patients undergoing CABG, other valvular surgery or aortic surgery. Echocardiographic criteria: <ul><li>Effective Regurgitant Orifice Area ≥30mm^2</li><li>Regurgitant Volume ≥60ml</li><li>Pressure half time <200ms</li><li>Vena Contracta width >6mm</li></ul>
Aortopathy	Aortic root repair or replacement if >5cm or rate of increase in diameter ≥0.5cm/year. Aortic root repair or replacement if >4.5cm and undergoing AVR for severe AS or AI. Yearly screening (by echocardiography, CT or CMR) if aortic root diameter >4cm.

* Class 2b in ACC/AHA guidelines, Class I in ESC guidelines.

Table 2: Class I indications for surgery in patients with BAV (adapted from ACC/AHA 2008 guidelines (Bonow *et al.*, 2008) and the ESC guidelines (Vahanian *et al.*, 2012) for valvular heart disease).

improvement in hemodynamics, the growth of the valve with the patient (allowing the use of the procedure in children) and the use of tissue for the valve. The major disadvantage is that the patient has to undergo double valve operation despite the fact that only one valve is diseased. Despite this, the operation is associated with low mortality and morbidity (David, Woo, Armstrong, & Maganti, 2010; El-Hamamsy *et al.*, 2010). There are some concerns regarding long-term outcome however (David *et al.*, 2000; Mokhles *et al.*, 2012).

In adults, the favoured operations are AVR and aortic valve repair. Although AVR is associated with excellent outcomes, because BAV patients tend to be younger, valve sparing repair surgery tends to be favoured so as to avoid complications of prosthetic valves. Patients with 180° orientated valves with minimal calcification/stenosis are ideal candidates for aortic valve repair. Aortic root surgery can also be carried with excellent results (Boodhwani *et al.*, 2009; Schafers, Kunihara, Fries, Brittner, & Aicher, 2010). Prior to any surgery in adults coronary angiography (either invasive or by CT) is mandatory.

The 2008 AHA/ACC guidelines recommend aortic root repair or replacement if the root is greater than 50mm or the rate of increase in diameter is 5mm or more per year. The guidelines also suggest that patients with BAV undergoing aortic valve surgery should also have concomitant replacement of the ascending aorta if it is greater than 45mm in diameter(Bonow *et al.*, 2008). This has been supported by evidence looking at outcomes in over 200 patients with varying aortic diameters (Borger *et al.*, 2004). Estimated 15 year freedom from complications was 86% in patients with an aortic diameter less than 40mm, dropping down to 81% in those with diameter 40-44 and 43% in patients with a diameter 45mm or greater. Once the ascending aorta reaches 50mm or greater, it is also appropriate to carry out aortic root replacement with a tube graft.

New techniques of repair such as transcatheter aortic valve implantation (TAVI) have also been reported in BAV with promising results (Kochman, Huczek, Koltowski, & Michalak, 2012). Recently, Hayashida et al evaluated a cohort of 229 patients undergoing TAVI, of which 21 had BAV and found that there was no appreciable difference in outcome between the BAV group and those with tricuspid valves with similar device success, rate of annulus rupture, mean post-operative gradient and 30-day mortality in both groups (Hayashida *et al.*, 2013).

7 Conclusion

BAV is the commonest congenital cardiac abnormality, and presents a significant burden on cardiac services. Recent cohort studies have given us knowledge of the clinical progression of the disease and when to operate, however there is still a need for further evidence for screening and for medical therapies to be evaluated. Surgical techniques will also continue to be refined, with the advent of transcatheter aortic valve implantation holding significant promise in this group of patients. The roles of CT and CMR as imaging tools will continue to enlarge. Much remains to be discovered about the genetics behind BAV, and as we discover more about this area we may be able to identify which patients are more likely to require early intervention and perhaps pick them up earlier. As our understanding of the pathogenesis of valve degeneration and aortopathy improves, this will allow us to identify new targets for treatment such as angiotensin receptor blockers which hold some promise in slowing the progression of aortopathy.

References

Acharya, A., Hans, C. P., Koenig, S. N., Nichols, H. A., Galindo, C. L. Garner, H. R., . . . Garg, V. (2011). *Inhibitory role of Notch1 in calcific aortic valve disease. [Research Support, N.I.H., Extramural Research Support, Non-U.S. Gov't]. PLoS One, 6(11), e27743. doi: 10.1371/journal.pone.0027743.*

Ahimastos, A. A., Aggarwal, A. D'Orsa, K. M., Formosa, M. F., White A. J., Savarirayan, R., . . . Kingwell, B. A. (2007). *Effect of perindopril on large artery stiffness and aortic root diameter in patients with Marfan syndrome: a randomized controlled trial. [Randomized Controlled Trial Research Support, Non-U.S. Gov't]. JAMA, 298(13), 1539-1547. doi: 10.1001/jama.298.13.1539.*

Ahmed, S., Honos, G. N., Walling, A. D., Michel, C. M., Sebag, I. A., Rudski, L. G., & Therrien, J. (2007). *Clinical outcome and echocardiographic predictors of aortic valve replacement in patients with bicuspid aortic valve. [Controlled Clinical Trial]. J Am Soc Echocardiogr, 20(8), 998-1003. doi: 10.1016/j.echo.2007.01.003.*

Alkadhi, H., Leschka, S., Trindade, P. T., Feuchtner, G., Stolzmann, P., Plass, A., & Baumueller, S. (2010). *Cardiac CT for the differentiation of bicuspid and tricuspid aortic valves: comparison with echocardiography and surgery. [Comparative Study]. AJR Am J Roentgenol, 195(4), 900-908. doi: 10.2214/AJR.09.3813.*

Anderson, R. H., Webb, S., Brown, N. A., Lamers, W., & Moorman, A. (2003). *Development of the heart: (3) formation of the ventricular outflow tracts, arterial valves, and intrapericardial arterial trunks. [Research Support, Non-U.S. Gov't Review]. Heart, 89(9), 1110-1118.*

Angelini, A., Ho, S. Y., Anderson, R. H., Devine, W. A., Zuberbuhler, J. R., Becker, A. E., & Davies, M. J. (1989). *The morphology of the normal aortic valve as compared with the aortic valve having two leaflets. [Comparative Study Research Support, Non-U.S. Gov't]. J Thorac Cardiovasc Surg, 98(3), 362-367.*

Aydin, A., Desai, N., Bernhardt, A. M., Treede, H., Detter, C., Sheikhzadeh, S., . . . von Kodolitsch, Y. (2013). Ascending aortic aneurysm and aortic valve dysfunction in bicuspid aortic valve disease. Int J Cardiol, 164(3), 301-305. doi: 10.1016/j.ijcard.2011.07.018.

Beppu, S., Suzuki, S., Matsuda, H., Ohmori, F., Nagata, S., & Miyatake, K. (1993). Rapidity of progression of aortic stenosis in patients with congenital bicuspid aortic valves. [Research Support, Non-U.S. Gov't]. Am J Cardiol, 71(4), 322-327.

Bonderman, D., Gharehbaghi-Schnell, E., Wollenek, G., Maurer, G., Baumgartner, H., & Lang, I. M. (1999). Mechanisms underlying aortic dilatation in congenital aortic valve malformation. Circulation, 99(16), 2138-2143.

Bonow, R. O. (2008). Bicuspid aortic valves and dilated aortas: a critical review of the ACC/AHA practice guidelines recommendations. [Editorial Review]. Am J Cardiol, 102(1), 111-114. doi: 10.1016/j.amjcard.2008.01.058.

Bonow, R. O., Carabello, B. A., Chatterjee, K., de Leon, A. C., Jr., Faxon, D. P., Freed, M. D., . . . Shanewise, J. S. (2008). 2008 Focused update incorporated into the ACC/AHA 2006 guidelines for the management of patients with valvular heart disease: a report of the American College of Cardiology/American Heart Association Task Force on Practice Guidelines (Writing Committee to Revise the 1998 Guidelines for the Management of Patients With Valvular Heart Disease): endorsed by the Society of Cardiovascular Anesthesiologists, Society for Cardiovascular Angiography and Interventions, and Society of Thoracic Surgeons. [Practice Guideline]. Circulation, 118(15), e523-661. doi: 10.1161/CIRCULATIONAHA.108.190748.

Bonow, R. O., Carabello, B. A., Kanu, C., de Leon, A. C., Jr., Faxon, D. P., Freed, M. D., . . . Riegel, B. (2006). ACC/AHA 2006 guidelines for the management of patients with valvular heart disease: a report of the American College of Cardiology/American Heart Association Task Force on Practice Guidelines (writing committee to revise the 1998 Guidelines for the Management of Patients With Valvular Heart Disease): developed in collaboration with the Society of Cardiovascular Anesthesiologists: endorsed by the Society for Cardiovascular Angiography and Interventions and the Society of Thoracic Surgeons. [Practice Guideline Review]. Circulation, 114(5), e84-231. doi: 10.1161/CIRCULATIONAHA.106.176857.

Boodhwani, M., de Kerchove, L., Glineur, D., Poncelet, A., Rubay, J., Astarci, P., . . . El Khoury, G. (2009). Repair-oriented classification of aortic insufficiency: impact on surgical techniques and clinical outcomes. J Thorac Cardiovasc Surg, 137(2), 286-294. doi: 10.1016/j.jtcvs.2008.08.054.

Borger, M. A., Preston, M., Ivanov, J., Fedak, P. W., Davierwala, P., Armstrong, S., & David, T. E. (2004). Should the ascending aorta be replaced more frequently in patients with bicuspid aortic valve disease? J Thorac Cardiovasc Surg, 128(5), 677-683. doi: 10.1016/j.jtcvs.2004.07.009.

Brooke, B. S., Habashi, J. P., Judge, D. P., Patel, N., Loeys, B., & Dietz, H. C., 3rd. (2008). Angiotensin II blockade and aortic-root dilation in Marfan's syndrome. [Clinical Trial Research Support, N.I.H., Extramural Research Support, Non-U.S. Gov't]. N Engl J Med, 358(26), 2787-2795. doi: 10.1056/NEJMoa0706585.

Calloway, T. J., Martin, L. J., Zhang, X., Tandon, A., Benson, D. W., & Hinton, R. B. (2011). Risk factors for aortic valve disease in bicuspid aortic valve: a family-based study. [Research Support, N.I.H., Extramural]. Am J Med Genet A, 155A(5), 1015-1020. doi: 10.1002/ajmg.a.33974.

Caruthers, S. D., Lin, S. J., Brown, P., Watkins, M. P., Williams, T. A., Lehr, K. A., & Wickline, S. A. (2003). Practical value of cardiac magnetic resonance imaging for clinical quantification of aortic valve stenosis: comparison with echocardiography. [Clinical Trial Comparative Study Controlled Clinical Trial Research Support, Non-U.S. Gov't Research Support, U.S. Gov't, P.H.S.]. Circulation, 108(18), 2236-2243. doi: 10.1161/01.CIR.0000095268.47282.A1.

Cawley, P. J., Maki, J. H., & Otto, C. M. (2009). Cardiovascular magnetic resonance imaging for valvular heart disease: technique and validation. [Research Support, Non-U.S. Gov't Review Validation Studies]. Circulation, 119(3), 468-478. doi: 10.1161/CIRCULATIONAHA.107.742486.

Cecconi, M., Manfrin, M., Moraca, A., Zanoli, R., Colonna, P. L., Bettuzzi, M. G., . . . Perna, G. P. (2005). Aortic dimensions in patients with bicuspid aortic valve without significant valve dysfunction. Am J Cardiol, 95(2), 292-294. doi: 10.1016/j.amjcard.2004.08.098.

Chan, K. L., Stinson, W. A., & Veinot, J. P. (1999). Reliability of transthoracic echocardiography in the assessment of aortic valve morphology: pathological correlation in 178 patients. Can J Cardiol, 15(1), 48-52.

David, T. E., Omran, A., Ivanov, J., Armstrong, S., de Sa, M. P., Sonnenberg, B., & Webb, G. (2000). Dilation of the pulmonary autograft after the Ross procedure. [Comparative Study]. J Thorac Cardiovasc Surg, 119(2), 210-220.

David, T. E., Woo, A., Armstrong, S., & Maganti, M. (2010). When is the Ross operation a good option to treat aortic valve disease? J Thorac Cardiovasc Surg, 139(1), 68-73; discussion 73-65. doi: 10.1016/j.jtcvs.2009.09.053.

de Sa, M., Moshkovitz, Y., Butany, J., & David, T. E. (1999). Histologic abnormalities of the ascending aorta and pulmonary trunk in patients with bicuspid aortic valve disease: clinical relevance to the ross procedure. [Research Support, Non-U.S. Gov't]. J Thorac Cardiovasc Surg, 118(4), 588-594.

Detaint, D., Aegerter, P., Tubach, F., Hoffman, I., Plauchu, H., Dulac, Y., . . . Jondeau, G. (2010). Rationale and design of a randomized clinical trial (Marfan Sartan) of angiotensin II receptor blocker therapy versus placebo in individuals with Marfan syndrome. [Multicenter Study Randomized Controlled Trial Research Support, Non-U.S. Gov't]. Arch Cardiovasc Dis, 103(5), 317-325. doi: 10.1016/j.acvd.2010.04.008.

Donal, E., Novaro, G. M., Deserrano, D., Popovic, Z. B., Greenberg, N. L., Richards, K. E., . . . Garcia, M. J. (2005). Planimetric assessment of anatomic valve area overestimates effective orifice area in bicuspid aortic stenosis. [Randomized Controlled Trial Research Support, Non-U.S. Gov't]. J Am Soc Echocardiogr, 18(12), 1392-1398. doi: 10.1016/j.echo.2005.04.005.

Dore, A., Brochu, M. C., Baril, J. F., Guertin, M. C., & Mercier, L. A. (2003). Progressive dilation of the diameter of the aortic root in adults with a bicuspid aortic valve. Cardiol Young 13(6), 526-531.

Duran, A. C., Frescura, C., Sans-Coma, V., Angelini, A., Basso, C., & Thiene, G. (1995). Bicuspid aortic valves in hearts with other congenital heart disease. [Research Support, Non-U.S Gov't]. J Heart Valve Dis, 4(6), 581-590.

El-Hamamsy, I., Eryigit, Z., Stevens, L. M., Sarang, Z., George, R., Clark, L., . . . Yacoub, M. H. (2010). Long-term outcomes after autograft versus homograft aortic root replacement in adults with aortic valve disease: a randomised controlled trial. [Comparative Study Randomized Controlled Trial Research Support, Non-U.S. Gov't]. Lancet, 376(9740), 524-531. doi: 10.1016/S0140-6736(10)60828-8.

Fedak, P. W., de Sa, M. P., Verma, S., Nili, N., Kazemian P., Butany, J., . . . David, T. E. (2003). Vascular matrix remodeling in patients with bicuspid aortic valve malformations: implications for aortic dilatation. [Research Support, Non-U.S. Gov't]. J Thorac Cardiovasc Surg, 126(3), 797-806.

Fedak, P. W., Verma, S., David, T. E., Leask, R. L., Weisel, R. D., & Butany, J. (2002). Clinical and pathophysiological implications of a bicuspid aortic valve. [Case Reports Research Support, Non-U.S. Gov't]. Circulation, 106(8), 900-904.

Fenoglio, J. J., Jr., McAllister, H. A., Jr., DeCastro, C. M., Davia, J. E., & Cheitlin, M. D. (1977). Congenital bicuspid aortic valve after age 20. Am J Cardiol, 39(2), 164-169.

Fernandes, S. M., Khairy, P., Sanders, S. P., & Colan, S. D. (2007). Bicuspid aortic valve morphology and interventions in the young. [Comparative Study]. J Am Coll Cardiol, 49(22), 2211-2214. doi: 10.1016/j.jacc.2007.01.090.

Fernandes, S. M., Sanders, S. P., Khairy, P., Jenkins, K. J., Gauvreau, K., Lang, P., . . . Colan, S. D. (2004). Morphology of bicuspid aortic valve in children and adolescents. J Am Coll Cardiol, 44(8), 1648-1651. doi: 10.1016/j.jacc.2004.05.063.

Foffa, I., Ait Ali, L., Panesi, P., Mariani, M., Festa, P., Botto, N., . . . Andreassi, M. G. (2013). Sequencing of NOTCH1, GATA5, TGFBR1 and TGFBR2 genes in familial cases of bicuspid aortic valve. BMC Med Genet, 14, 44. doi: 10.1186/1471-2350-14-44.

Garg, V., Muth, A. N., Ransom, J. F., Schluterman, M. K., Barnes, R., King, I. N., . . . Srivastava, D. (2005). Mutations in NOTCH1 cause aortic valve disease. [Research Support, N.i.H., Extramural Research Support, Non-U.S. Gov't Research Support, U.S. Gov't, P.H.S.]. Nature, 437(7056), 270-274. doi: 10.1038/nature03940.

Gersony, W. M., Hayes, C. J., Driscoll, D. J., Keane, J. F., Kidd, L., O'Fallon, W. M., . . . Weidman, W. H. (1993). Bacterial endocarditis in patients with aortic stenosis, pulmonary stenosis, or ventricular septal defect. Circulation, 87(2 Suppl), I121-126.

Glick, B. N., & Roberts, W. C. (1994). Congenitally bicuspid aortic valve in multiple family members. Am J Cardiol, 73(5), 400-404.

Guntheroth, W. G. (2008). A critical review of the American College of Cardiology/American Heart Association practice guidelines on bicuspid aortic valve with dilated ascending aorta. [Review]. Am J Cardiol, 102(1), 107-110. doi: 10.1016/j.amjcard.2008.02.106.

Habashi, J. P., Judge, D. P., Holm, T. M., Cohn, R. D., Loeys, B. L., Cooper, T. K., . . . Dietz, H. C. (2006). Losartan, an AT1 antagonist, prevents aortic aneurysm in a mouse model of Marfan syndrome. [Research Support, N.I.H., Extramural Research Support, Non-U.S. Gov't]. Science, 312(5770), 117-121. doi: 10.1126/science.1124287.

Hayashida, K., Bouvier, E., Lefevre, T., Chevalier, B., Hovasse, T., Romano, M., . . . Morice, M. C. (2013). Transcatheter aortic valve implantation for patients with severe bicuspid aortic valve stenosis. Circ Cardiovasc Interv, 6(3), 284-291. doi: 10.1161/CIRCINTERVENTIONS.112.000084.

Hiratzka, L. F., Bakris, G. L., Beckman, J. A., Bersin, R. M., Carr, V. F., Casey, D. E., Jr., . . . Williams, D. M. (2010). 2010 ACCF/AHA/AATS/ACR/ASA/SCA/SCAI/SIR/STS/SVM Guidelines for the diagnosis and management of patients with thoracic aortic disease. A Report of the American College of Cardiology Foundation/American Heart Association Task Force on Practice Guidelines, American Association for Thoracic Surgery, American College of Radiology,American Stroke Association, Society of Cardiovascular Anesthesiologists, Society for Cardiovascular Angiography and Interventions, Society of Interventional Radiology, Society of Thoracic Surgeons,and Society for Vascular Medicine. [Practice Guideline]. J Am Coll Cardiol, 55(14), e27-e129. doi: 10.1016/j.jacc.2010.02.015.

Holmes, K. W., Lehmann, C. U., Dalal, D., Nasir, K., Dietz, H. C., Ravekes, W. J., . . . Spevak, P. J. (2007). Progressive dilation of the ascending aorta in children with isolated bicuspid aortic valve. Am J Cardiol, 99(7), 978-983. doi: 10.1016/j.amjcard.2006.10.065.

Hope, M. D., Hope, T. A., Crook, S. E., Ordovas, K. G., Urbania, T. H., Alley, M. T., & Higgins, C. B. (2011). 4D flow CMR in assessment of valve-related ascending aortic disease. [Research Support, Non-U.S. Gov't]. JACC Cardiovasc Imaging, 4(7), 781-787. doi: 10.1016/j.jcmg.2011.05.004.

Huang, F. Q., & Le Tan, J. (2013). Pattern of Aortic Dilatation in Different Bicuspid Aortic Valve Phenotypes and its Association with Aortic Valvular Dysfunction and Elasticity. Heart Lung Circ. doi: 10.1016/j.hlc.2013.05.644.

Huntington, K., Hunter, A. G., & Chan, K. L. (1997). A prospective study to assess the frequency of familial clustering of congenital bicuspid aortic valve. J Am Coll Cardiol, 30(7), 1809-1812.

Janatuinen, M. J., Vanttinen, E. A., Saraste, M. K., & Ingberg, M. V. (1989). Surgical management of congenital aortic stenosis in children and young adults. Scand J Thorac Cardiovasc Surg, 23(3), 219-224.

Joo, I., Park, E. A., Kim, K. H., Lee, W., Chung, J. W., & Park, J. H. (2012). MDCT differentiation between bicuspid and tricuspid aortic valves in patients with aortic valvular disease: correlation with surgical findings. Int J Cardiovasc Imaging, 28(1), 171-182. doi: 10.1007/s10554-010-9780-3.

Kang, J. W., Song, H. G., Yang, D. H., Baek, S., Kim, D. H., Song, J. M., . . . Song, J. K. (2013). Association between bicuspid aortic valve phenotype and patterns of valvular dysfunction and bicuspid aortopathy: comprehensive evaluation using MDCT and echocardiography. [Research Support, Non-U.S. Gov't]. JACC Cardiovasc Imaging, 6(2), 150-161. doi: 10.1016/j.jcmg.2012.11.007.

Keane, J. F., Driscoll, D. J., Gersony, W. M., Hayes, C. J., Kidd, L., O'Fallon, W. M., . . . Weidman, W. H. (1993). Second natural history study of congenital heart defects. Results of treatment of patients with aortic valvar stenosis. Circulation, 87(2 Suppl), I16-27.

Keane, M. G., Wiegers, S. E., Plappert, T., Pochettino, A., Bavaria, J. E., & Sutton, M. G. (2000). Bicuspid aortic valves are associated with aortic dilatation out of proportion to coexistent valvular lesions. Circulation, 102(19 Suppl 3), III35-39.

Kerstjens-Frederikse, W. S., Du Marchie Sarvaas, G. J., Ruiter, J. S., Van Den Akker, P. C., Temmerman, A. M., Van Melle, J. P., . . . Berger, R. M. (2011). Left ventricular outflow tract obstruction: should cardiac screening be offered to first-degree relatives? [Comparative Study]. Heart, 97(15), 1228-1232. doi: 10.1136/hrt.2010.211433.

Khoo, C., Cheung, C., & Jue, J. (2013). Patterns of Aortic Dilatation in Bicuspid Aortic Valve-Associated Aortopathy. J Am Soc Echocardiogr, 26(6), 600-605. doi: 10.1016/j.echo.2013.02.017.

Kochman, J., Huczek, Z., Koltowski, L., & Michalak, M. (2012). Transcatheter implantation of an aortic valve prosthesis in a female patient with severe bicuspid aortic stenosis. [Case Reports]. Eur Heart J, 33(1), 112. doi: 10.1093/eurheartj/ehr316.

Koh, T. W. (2013). Diagnosis of bicuspid aortic valve: role of three-dimensional transesophageal echocardiography and multiplane review analysis. [Case Reports]. Echocardiography, 30(3), 360-363. doi: 10.1111/echo.12068.

Ladouceur, M., Fermanian, C., Lupoglazoff, J. M., Edouard, T., Dulac, Y., Acar, P., . . . Jondeau, G. (2007). Effect of beta-blockade on ascending aortic dilatation in children with the Marfan syndrome. [Multicenter Study Research Support, Non-U.S. Gov't]. Am J Cardiol, 99(3), 406-409. doi: 10.1016/j.amjcard.2006.08.048.

Laforest, B., Andelfinger, G., & Nemer, M. (2011). Loss of Gata5 in mice leads to bicuspid aortic valve. [Research Support, Non-U.S. Gov't]. J Clin Invest, 121(7), 2876-2887. doi: 10.1172/JCI44555.

Larson, E. W., & Edwards, W. D. (1984). Risk factors for aortic dissection: a necropsy study of 161 cases. [Comparative Study]. Am J Cardiol, 53(6), 849-855.

Lee, S. C., Ko, S. M., Song, M. G., Shin, J. K., Chee, H. K., & Hwang, H. K. (2012). Morphological assessment of the aortic valve using coronary computed tomography angiography, cardiovascular magnetic resonance, and transthoracic echocardiography: comparison with intraoperative findings. [Comparative Study]. Int J Cardiovasc Imaging, 28 Suppl 1, 33-44. doi: 10.1007/s10554-012-0066-9.

Leone, O., Biagini, E., Pacini, D., Zagnoni, S., Ferlito, M., Graziosi, M., . . . Rapezzi, C. (2012). The elusive link between aortic wall histology and echocardiographic anatomy in bicuspid aortic valve: implications for prophylactic surgery. Eur J Cardiothorac Surg, 41(2), 322-327. doi: 10.1016/j.ejcts.2011.05.064.

Malaisrie, S. C., Carr, J., Mikati, I., Rigolin, V., Yip, B. K., Lapin, B., & McCarthy, P. M. (2012). Cardiac magnetic resonance imaging is more diagnostic than 2-dimensional echocardiography in determining the presence of bicuspid aortic valve. [Comparative Study]. J Thorac Cardiovasc Surg, 144(2), 370-376. doi: 10.1016/j.jtcvs.2011.09.068.

McKellar, S. H., Tester, D. J., Yagubyan, M., Majumdar, R., Ackerman, M. J., & Sundt, T. M., 3rd. (2007). Novel NOTCH1 mutations in patients with bicuspid aortic valve disease and thoracic aortic aneurysms. [Research Support, Non-U.S. Gov't]. J Thorac Cardiovasc Surg, 134(2), 290-296. doi: 10.1016/j.jtcvs.2007.02.041.

Michelena, H. I., Desjardins, V. A., Avierinos, J. F., Russo, A., Nkomo, V. T., Sundt, T. M., . . . Enriquez-Sarano, M. (2008). Natural history of asymptomatic patients with normally functioning or minimally dysfunctional bicuspid aortic valve in the community. Circulation, 117(21), 2776-2784. doi: 10.1161/CIRCULATIONAHA.107.740878.

Michelena, H. I., Khanna, A. D., Mahoney, D., Margaryan, E., Topilsky, Y., Suri, R. M., . . . Enriquez-Sarano, M. (2011). Incidence of aortic complications in patients with bicuspid aortic valves. [Research Support, Non-U.S. Gov't]. JAMA, 306(10), 1104-1112. doi: 10.1001/jama.2011.1286.

Mills, P., Leech, G., Davies, M., & Leathan, A. (1978). The natural history of a non-stenotic bicuspid aortic valve. Br Heart J, 40(9), 951-957.

Mohamed, S. A., Aherrahrou, Z., Liptau, H., Erasmi, A. W., Hagemann, C., Wrobel, S., . . . Erdmann, J. (2006). Novel missense mutations (p.T596M and p.P1797H) in NOTCH1 in patients with bicuspid aortic valve. [Research Support, Non-U.S. Gov't]. Biochem Biophys Res Commun, 345(4), 1460-1465. doi: 10.1016/j.bbrc.2006.05.046.

Mokhles, M. M., Rizopoulos, D., Andrinopoulou, E. R., Bekkers, J. A., Roos-Hesselink, J. W., Lesaffre, E., . . . Takkenberg, J. J. (2012). Autograft and pulmonary allograft performance in the second post-operative decade after the Ross procedure: insights from the Rotterdam Prospective Cohort Study. [Research Support, Non-U.S. Gov't]. Eur Heart J, 33(17), 2213-2224. doi: 10.1093/eurheartj/ehs173.

Mordi, I., & Tzemos, N. (2012). Bicuspid aortic valve disease: a comprehensive review. Cardiol Res Pract, 2012, 196037. doi: 10.1155/2012/196037.

Morgan-Hughes, G. J., Roobottom, C. A., Owens, P. E., & Marshall, A. J. (2004). Dilatation of the aorta in pure, severe, bicuspid aortic valve stenosis. [Research Support, Non-U.S. Gov't]. Am Heart J, 147(4), 736-740. doi: 10.1016/j.ahj.2003.10.044.

Nathan, D. P., Xu, C., Plappert, T., Desjardins, B., Gorman, J. H., 3rd, Bavaria, J. E., . . . Jackson, B. M. (2011). Increased ascending aortic wall stress in patients with bicuspid aortic valves. [Comparative Study Research Support, N.I.H., Extramural]. Ann Thorac Surg, 92(4), 1384-1389. doi: 10.1016/j.athoracsur.2011.04.118.

Nistri, S., Sorbo, M. D., Marin, M., Palisi, M., Scognamiglio, R., & Thiene, G. (1999). Aortic root dilatation in young men with normally functioning bicuspid aortic valves. Heart, 82(1), 19-22.

Niwa, K., Perloff, J. K., Bhuta, S. M., Laks, H., Drinkwater, D. C., Child, J. S., & Miner, P. D. (2001). Structural abnormalities of great arterial walls in congenital heart disease: light and electron microscopic analyses. [Comparative Study]. Circulation, 103(3), 393-400.

Novaro, G. M., Tiong, I. Y., Pearce, G. L., Grimm, R. A., Smedira, N., & Griffin, B. P. (2003). Features and predictors of ascending aortic dilatation in association with a congenital bicuspid aortic valve. Am J Cardiol, 92(1), 99-101.

Pachulski, R. T., Weinberg, A. L., & Chan, K. L. (1991). Aortic aneurysm in patients with functionally normal or minimally stenotic bicuspid aortic valve. Am J Cardiol, 67(8), 781-782.

Padang, R., Bagnall, R. D., Richmond, D. R., Bannon, P. G., & Semsarian, C. (2012). Rare non-synonymous variations in the transcriptional activation domains of GATA5 in bicuspid aortic valve disease. [Research Support, Non-U.S. Gov't]. J Mol Cell Cardiol, 53(2), 277-281. doi: 10.1016/j.yjmcc.2012.05.009.

Padang, R., Bannon, P. G., Jeremy, R., Richmond, D. R., Semsarian, C., Vallely, M., . . . Yan, T. D. (2013). The genetic and molecular basis of bicuspid aortic valve associated thoracic aortopathy: a link to phenotype heterogeneity. Ann Cardiothorac Surg, 2(1), 83-91. doi: 10.3978/j.issn.2225-319X.2012.11.17.

Parai, J. L., Masters, R. G., Walley, V. M., Stinson, W. A., & Veinot, J. P. (1999). Aortic medial changes associated with bicuspid aortic valve: myth or reality? [Comparative Study]. Can J Cardiol, 15(11), 1233-1238.

Pomerance, A. (1972). Pathogenesis of aortic stenosis and its relation to age. Br Heart J, 34(6), 569-574.

Presbitero, P., Demarie, D., Villani, M., Perinetto, E. A., Riva, G., Orzan, F., . . . Brusca, A. (1987). Long term results (15-30 years) of surgical repair of aortic coarctation. Br Heart J, 57(5), 462-467.

Radonic, T., de Witte, P., Baars, M. J., Zwinderman, A. H., Mulder, B. J., & Groenink, M. (2010). Losartan therapy in adults with Marfan syndrome: study protocol of the multi-center randomized controlled COMPARE trial. [Multicenter Study Randomized Controlled Trial Research Support, Non-U.S. Gov't]. Trials, 11, 3. doi: 10.1186/1745-6215-11-3.

Restivo, A., Piacentini, G., Placidi, S., Saffirio, C., & Marino, B. (2006). Cardiac outflow tract: a review of some embryogenetic aspects of the conotruncal region of the heart. [Review]. Anat Rec A Discov Mol Cell Evol Biol, 288(9), 936-943. doi: 10.1002/ar.a.20367.

Roberts, W. C. (1970). The congenitally bicuspid aortic valve. A study of 85 autopsy cases. Am J Cardiol, 26(1), 72-83.

Roberts, W. C. (1992). Morphologic aspects of cardiac valve dysfunction. [Review]. Am Heart J, 123(6), 1610-1632.

Robledo-Carmona, J., Rodriguez-Bailon, I., Carrasco-Chinchilla, F., Fernandez, B., Jimenez-Navarro, M., Porras-Martin, C., . . . De Teresa-Galvan, E. (2013). Hereditary patterns of bicuspid aortic valve in a hundred families. Int J Cardiol. doi: 10.1016/j.ijcard.2013.04.180.

Rosenfeld, H. M., Landzberg, M. J., Perry, S. B., Colan, S. D., Keane, J. F., & Lock, J. E. (1994). Balloon aortic valvuloplasty in the young adult with congenital aortic stenosis. Am J Cardiol, 73(15), 1112-1117.

Ross, D. N. (1962). Homograft replacement of the aortic valve. Lancet, 2(7254), 487.

Russo, C. F., Mazzetti, S., Garatti, A., Ribera, E., Milazzo, A., Bruschi, G., . . . Vitali, E. (2002). Aortic complications after bicuspid aortic valve replacement: long-term results. [Comparative Study]. Ann Thorac Surg, 74(5), S1773-1776; discussion S1792-1779.

Sabet, H. Y., Edwards, W. D., Tazelaar, H. D., & Daly, R. C. (1999) Congenitally bicuspid aortic valves: a surgical pathology study of 542 cases (1991 through 1996) and a literature review of 2,715 additional cases. Mayo Clin Proc, 74(1), 14-26. doi: 10.4065/74.1.14.

Sadee, A. S., Becker, A. E., Verheul, H. A., Bouma, B., & Hoedemaker, G. (1992). Aortic valve regurgitation and the congenitally bicuspid aortic valve: a clinico-pathological correlation. Br Heart J, 67(6), 439-441.

Sadron Blaye-Felice, M. A., Seguela, P. E., Arnaudis, B., Dulac, Y., Lepage, B., & Acar, P. (2012). Usefulness of three-dimensional transthoracic echocardiography for the classification of congenital bicuspid aortic valve in children. Eur Heart J Cardiovasc Imaging, 13(12), 1047-1052. doi: 10.1093/ehjci/jes089.

Santarpia, G., Scognamiglio, G., Di Salvo, G., D'Alto, M., Sarubbi, B., Romeo, E., . . . Calabro, R. (2012). Aortic and left ventricular remodeling in patients with bicuspid aortic valve without significant valvular dysfunction: a prospective study. [Comparative Study Randomized Controlled Trial Research Support, Non-U.S. Gov't]. Int J Cardiol, 158(3), 347-352. doi: 10.1016/j.ijcard.2011.01.046.

Schaefer, B. M., Lewin, M. B., Stout, K. K., Byers, P. H., & Otto, C. M. (2007). Usefulness of bicuspid aortic valve phenotype to predict elastic properties of the ascending aorta. [Research Support, Non-U.S. Gov't]. Am J Cardiol, 99(5), 686-690. doi: 10.1016/j.amjcard.2006.09.118.

Schaefer, B. M., Lewin, M. B., Stout, K. K., Gill, E., Prueitt, A., Byers, P. H., & Otto, C. M. (2008). The bicuspid aortic valve: an integrated phenotypic classification of leaflet morphology and aortic root shape. [Multicenter Study Research Support, Non-U.S. Gov't]. Heart, 94(12), 1634-1638. doi: 10.1136/hrt.2007.132092.

Schafers, H. J., Kunihara, T., Fries, P., Brittner, B., & Aicher, D. (2010). Valve-preserving root replacement in bicuspid aortic valves. J Thorac Cardiovasc Surg, 140(6 Suppl), S36-40; discussion S45-51. doi: 10.1016/j.jtcvs.2010.07.057.

Shores, J., Berger, K. R., Murphy, E. A., & Pyeritz, R. E. (1994). Progression of aortic dilatation and the benefit of long-term beta-adrenergic blockade in Marfan's syndrome. [Clinical Trial Randomized Controlled Trial Research Support, Non-U.S. Gov't Research Support, U.S. Gov't, P.H.S.]. N Engl J Med, 330(19), 1335-1341. doi: 10.1056/NEJM199405123301902.

Sievers, H. H., & Schmidtke, C. (2007). A classification system for the bicuspid aortic valve from 304 surgical specimens. J Thorac Cardiovasc Surg, 133(5), 1226-1233. doi: 10.1016/j.jtcvs.2007.01.039.

Siu, S. C., & Silversides, C. K. (2010). Bicuspid aortic valve disease. [Research Support, Non-U.S. Gov't Review]. J Am Coll Cardiol, 55(25), 2789-2800. doi: 10.1016/j.jacc.2009.12.068.

Stewart, A. B., Ahmed, R., Travill, C. M., & Newman, C. G. (1993). Coarctation of the aorta life and health 20-44 years after surgical repair. [Research Support, Non-U.S. Gov't]. Br Heart J, 69(1), 65-70.

Subramanian, R., Olson, L. J., & Edwards, W. D. (1984). Surgical pathology of pure aortic stenosis: a study of 374 cases. Mayo Clin Proc, 59(10), 683-690.

Tanaka, R., Yoshioka, K., Niinuma, H., Ohsawa, S., Okabayashi, H., & Ehara, S. (2010). Diagnostic value of cardiac CT in the evaluation of bicuspid aortic stenosis: comparison with echocardiography and operative findings. [Comparative Study Research Support, Non-U.S. Gov't]. AJR Am J Roentgenol, 195(4), 895-899. doi: 10.2214/AJR.09.3164.

Thanassoulis, G., Yip, J. W., Filion, K., Jamorski, M., Webb, G., Siu, S. C., & Therrien, J. (2008). Retrospective study to identify predictors of the presence and rapid progression of aortic dilatation in patients with bicuspid aortic valves. Nat Clin Pract Cardiovasc Med, 5(12), 821-828. doi: 10.1038/ncpcardio1369.

Tsai, S. F., Trivedi, M., & Daniels, C. J. (2012). Comparing imaging modalities for screening aortic complications in patients with bicuspid aortic valve. [Comparative Study]. Congenit Heart Dis, 7(4), 372-377. doi: 10.1111/j.1747-0803.2012.00683.x

Tutar, E., Ekici, F., Atalay, S., & Nacar, N. (2005). The prevalence of bicuspid aortic valve in newborns by echocardiographic screening. Am Heart J, 150(3), 513-515. doi: 10.1016/j.ahj.2004.10.036.

Tworetzky, W., Wilkins-Haug, L., Jennings, R. W., van der Velde, M. E., Marshall, A. C., Marx, G. R., . . . Perry, S. B. (2004). Balloon dilation of severe aortic stenosis in the fetus: potential for prevention of hypoplastic left heart syndrome: candidate selection, technique, and results of successful intervention. [Evaluation Studies Research Support, Non-U.S. Gov't]. Circulation, 110(15), 2125-2131. doi: 10.1161/01.CIR.0000144357.29279.54.

Tzemos, N., Lyseggen, E., Silversides, C., Jamorski, M., Tong, J. H., Harvey, P., . . . Siu, S. (2010). Endothelial function, carotid-femoral stiffness, and plasma matrix metalloproteinase-2 in men with bicuspid aortic valve and dilated aorta. [Research Support, Non-U.S. Gov't]. J Am Coll Cardiol, 55(7), 660-668. doi: 10.1016/j.jacc.2009.08.080.

Tzemos, N., Therrien, J., Yip, J., Thanassoulis, G., Tremblay, S., Jamorski, M. T., . . . Siu, S. C. (2008). Outcomes in adults with bicuspid aortic valves. [Research Support, Non-U.S. Gov't]. JAMA, 300(11), 1317-1325. doi: 10.1001/jama.300.11.1317.

Vahanian, A., Alfieri, O., Andreotti, F., Antunes, M. J., Baron-Esquivias, G., Baumgartner, H., . . . Zembala, M. (2012). Guidelines on the management of valvular heart disease (version 2012). [Practice Guideline]. Eur Heart J, 33(19), 2451-2496. doi: 10.1093/eurheartj/ehs109.

Vallely, M. P., Semsarian, C., & Bannon, P. G. (2008). Management of the ascending aorta in patients with bicuspid aortic valve disease. [Review]. Heart Lung Circ, 17(5), 357-363. doi: 10.1016/j.hlc.2008.01.007.

Wallby, L., Janerot-Sjoberg, B., Steffensen, T., & Broqvist, M. (2002). T lymphocyte infiltration in non-rheumatic aortic stenosis: a comparative descriptive study between tricuspid and bicuspid aortic valves. [Comparative Study]. Heart, 88(4), 348-351.

Ward, C. (2000). Clinical significance of the bicuspid aortic valve. [Review]. Heart, 83(1), 81-85.

Warnes, C. A., Williams, R. G., Bashore, T. M., Child, J. S., Connolly, H. M., Dearani, J. A., . . . Webb, G. D. (2008). ACC/AHA 2008 Guidelines for the Management of Adults with Congenital Heart Disease: a report of the American College of Cardiology/American Heart Association Task Force on Practice Guidelines (writing committee to develop guidelines on the management of adults with congenital heart disease). [Practice Guideline]. Circulation, 118(23), e714-833. doi: 10.1161/CIRCULATIONAHA.108.190690.

Warnes, C. A., Williams, R. G., Bashore, T. M., Child, J. S., Connolly, H. M., Dearani, J. A., . . . Yancy, C. W. (2008). ACC/AHA 2008 guidelines for the management of adults with congenital heart disease: a report of the American College of Cardiology/American Heart Association Task Force on Practice Guidelines (Writing Committee to Develop Guidelines on the Management of Adults With Congenital Heart Disease). Developed in Collaboration With the American Society of Echocardiography, Heart Rhythm Society, International Society for Adult Congenital Heart Disease, Society for Cardiovascular Angiography and Interventions, and Society of Thoracic Surgeons. [Practice Guideline]. J Am Coll Cardiol, 52(23), e143-263. doi: 10.1016/j.jacc.2008.10.001.

Yetman, A. T., Bornemeier, R. A., & McCrindle, B. W. (2005). Usefulness of enalapril versus propranolol or atenolol for prevention of aortic dilation in patients with the Marfan syndrome. [Clinical Trial Comparative Study Research Support, Non-U.S. Gov't]. Am J Cardiol, 95(9), 1125-1127. doi: 10.1016/j.amjcard.2005.01.032.

Yotsumoto, G., Moriyama, Y., Toyohira, H., Shimokawa, S., Iguro, Y., Watanabe, S., . . . Taira, A. (1998). Congenital bicuspid aortic valve: analysis of 63 surgical cases. J Heart Valve Dis, 7(5), 500-503.

Optimizing Myocardial Oxygen Delivery Clinical Impact of Coronary Retroperfusion Strategies

Frank Harig

Department of Cardiac Surgery
University Hospital Erlangen, Friedrich Alexander University,
Erlangen, Germany

Joachim Schmidt

Department of Anaesthesiology
University Hospital Erlangen, Friedrich Alexander University
Erlangen, Germany

Michael Weyand

Department of Cardiac Surgery
University Hospital Erlangen, Friedrich Alexander University
Erlangen, Germany

1   Treatment Strategies of Coronary Artery Disease

1.1   Historical Aspects

In healthy hearts, the coronary arteries deliver nourishing metabolites and oxygen to the myocardial tissue, so that ATP is generated in the mitochondria and the contractile apparatus built of actin and myosin filaments is enabled to perform the "power stroke", i.e. contractions called systole. In the case of coronary artery disease (CAD), oxygen supply does not fulfil the demands of the cardiomyocytes (coronary insufficiency) and the heart's contractility diminishes (hibernating myocardium) and the oxygen demands of the whole organism are no longer fulfilled (myocardial insufficiency).

Patients suffer from angina pectoris as a symptom of CAD, which was initially described by Wiliam Heberden in 1772. The underlying pathophysiology of obstructions of coronary arteries has been described by Herrick (1912) who published a landmark article in JAMA 1912 called "Modern concept of coronary thrombosis and myocardial infarction". Despite the knowledge of causality, treatment options were limited for a long time. As pharmacological treatment since 1840, nitroglycerin, a potent vasodilator, was applicated [C. Hering], and inhaled as amyl nitrate since 1867 (Sir T. Lauder Brunton).

Surgical options were not yet established in this time. Some milestones had to be passed. One of them has has been the first open cardiac operation in 1896 by Thomas Rehn in Frankfurt a.M., Germany. But because of obstacles of contemporary surgeons, surgical procedures had to wait until the 1960's. First, Alexis Carrel, a french Surgeon working at Rockefeller Institute in New York since 1906, had to establish anastomotic techniques and perfusion devices (this was awarded with the Nobel Prize 1912). Further, Werner Forssmann had to invent the catheterization of the heart in Berlin, Germany, 1929 (he received the Nobel Prize together with Cournad & Richards in 1956). The first coronary angiogram was performed by F. Mason Sones at the Cleveland Clinic, Ohio in 1958, when he spontenously pushed the catheter forward into the right coronary artery (RCA). The invention and clinical refinement of the heart-lung-machine by John Gibbon (first use in 1953 in Boston, MA) made it possible to work on the heart without placing the patients at the risk of circulatory collapse. With this knowledge and technical support, the preconditions for a solution of the underlying problem of CAD, the stenotic coronary vessels were given and surgeons began to patch the stenoses to place interpositions and finally to bypass the stenotic coronary artery. It is noteworthy that those pioneers had to work against the massive criticicsm from the medical collegues.

Coronary artery bypass grafting was experimentally and clinically evaluated in the 1960's (first clinical CABG was performed by the team of Robert Goetz in 1960 (New York, RITA- Bypass), David Saviston in 1962, then Vasili Kolessov in Russia (Feb 1964, St. Petersburg, LITA- Bypass). Garret, Dennis, DeBakey in the US in Nov 1964 (reported 1973). The first series were published by Rene Favaloro 1967 during his time at Cleveland Clinic, Ohio, prefering the vena saphena graft. The left internal thoracic artery (LITA, also called Mammarian artery, LIMA) with better long-term patency rates was used and promoted by George Green, New York. In 1967, CABG procedures were performed by Rene Favaloro in Cleveland, Dudley Johnson in Milwaki, Michael DeBakey in Houston and David Sabiston in Duke University. In Germany, the first CABG was performed in 1969 by Prof. Gerd Hegemann in Erlangen.

In 1977, the catheter-based techniques were clinically inaugurated by Andreas Gruntzig who performed in Zurich, Swiss, the first percutaneous transluminal catheter angioplasty (PTCA). Since then, the direct revascularization techniques like the non- invasive percutaneous catheter interventions (PCI) and the invasive coronary surgery (CABG) are in direct concurrence offering the best method for the treatment of CAD.

Nowadays, on the basis of several clinical trials (e.g. SYNTAX-study (Mohr *et al.*, 2013)) guidelines attempt to provide clinicians with some information on decision- making in CAD, i.e. when and how to apply the best method for any coronary morphology (i.e. left main stem stenosis, 1-, 2-, or 3 vessel disease) (Stephan, *et al.*, 2012). Nevertheless, large knowledge gaps and grey zones remain.

1.1 The Need for Alternatives to Established Techniques

Although being in the focus of investigators since 1898 (Pratt, 1898), this anatomical "back door" of the heart's perfusion, the coronary veins, have lost investigators interest.

This concept is based on the observations of Pratt more than 100 years ago (Pratt, 1898). In 1898, he could show in experiments with cats, that the blood supply via the coronary sinus could prevent myocardial infarction and stabilize the pumping heart. Since then, in the first half of the 19th century, observations and hypotheses were evaluated in animal models and technically refined. Basic aspects of pathophysiology and anatomy in retroperfusion techniques were investigated, so that the feasibility and protective effect of retroperfusion in experimental ischemia could be demonstrated (Pratt, 1898; Roberts *et al.*, 1943).

Nowadays, with better technical support and refined understanding of pathophysiology, a revival of this technique seems to be useful in order to have an additional treatment option for sick heart suffering from oxygen shortage. In today's daily surgical practice, coronary surgery often has to face coronary arteries with difficult conditions to perform bypass grafting. Patients become older (in 2009, more than 50% are older than 70 years and 12% of CABG are performed in pts. older than 80 years) and the number of redo operations is growing (2009: 8.7%) (Gummert *et al.*, 2009).

Thus technical considerations like obliterated vessels, intramural course and small vessel disease in a growing patient population suffering from diabetes demonstrates limitations to cardiac surgeons efforts. In this context, arterialization of of cardiac venous system may lead to an optimization of myocardial blood flow to ischemic regions.

1.2. Interventions on the Coronary Sinus in Animal Models

1.2.1. Global Permanent Retroperfusion

Investigators have used different animal models dealing with arterialization of the coronary sinus (CS). Roberts placed in an experiment with dogs an arterio-venous shunt between the Truncus brachiocephalicus and the CS using a canula made of glass. Later on, the carotid artery was used as an autologous bypass graft placed between aorta descendens and the CS (Roberts *et al.*, 1943).

On the basis of these experiments, Beck started a series of 350 operations in dogs anastomosing the carotid artery directly to the CS. The first use in humans was started in 1948. A segment of the saphenous vein (SVG, saphenous vein graft) was placed between the aorta and the CS. Two weeks later, in a second step called Beck II procedure, the CS was partially occluded in order to reduce the amount of blood flow shunting directly to the venous part instead of flowing to the myocardial capillary bed (Beck *et al.*, 1948a; 1948b; 1954). The wording "global retroperfusion" was used because of the fact that the arterial flow reached the complete venous system and not only the ischemic region. Some surgeons like Bakst could achieve relief from angina (Bakst *et al.*, 1956), and some pts. with severe CAD were offered this procedure. But due to an inacceptable high mortality rate, this procedure had to be abandoned. Histopathologically, the wall of the CS showed severe damage resulting in myocardial edema and hemorrhagia, signs of an reduced drainage of venous blood.

Thus, the technique of global retroperfusion (RP) had been given up. But the selective use of retroperfusion techniques was something special. Anatomical considerations support the idea of selective RP. Ludinghausen analyzed in 1987 the anatomical variance of the human coronary venous system in 350 heart specimen (Ludinghausen, 1987). He could show that in 13% the venous drainage of vast regions of the left ventricle is not directed into the coronary sinus directly. In the case of global retroperfusion these regions would not have been perfused and thus did not have had any benefit regarding additional oxygen supply. This anatomical characteristic could also be shown in animal studies of dogs by Hahn and Kim (1952). They found the Vena cordis magna (Anterior cardiac vein), draining directly into the Right Atrium in dogs. In the case of global RP, these vein did not show intimal proliferation, whereas veins that have been exposed to arterial pressure developed intimal proliferation.

Retroperfusion studies in dogs have to take into account the peculiarity of the canine coronary system of having a good collateral coronary supply, in contrast to the human and porcine coronary system having coronary end arteries.

1.2.2.   Direct Selective Retroperfusion

In the 1970's the technique of retroperfusion was refined on the basis of a better pathophysiolgical understanding. The arterio-venous connections/ anastomose were established more selectively, by creating connections between the veins of the ischemic myocardial regions and the IMA (internal mammary artery) or by interposing a segment of the SVG (saphenous vein graft). The technical feasibility could be proved by some working groups (Arealis et al., 1973; Bhayana et al., 1974; Park et al., 1975; Kay & Suzuki, 1975). Further pathophysiological investiagtions were undertaken. Hochberg (Hochberg, 1977) used radioactive microspheres (isotope [114]Cer) in order to quantify the flow quotient of subendocardial to epicardial flow. Longterm observation for 3 to 5 months were made in a canine model using 18 dogs. These encouraging results showed a late bypass flow that was nearly as high as it was initially, histological analyses showed that coronary venous bypasses did not show signs of sclerosis or thrombosis, nor signs of interstitial edema or myocardial hemorraghia (Hammond et al., 1967; Hochberg et al., 1979; Rhodes et al., 1978).

Despite these positive results of venous retroperfusion, the fast propagation and spreading of arterial revascularization techniques in the 1960's (CABG) and 1970's (PTCA) prevented retroperfusion techniques from achieving clinical relevance. The capacity for interventional cardiology rapidly increased (so that Germany today is international leader in PCI treatment of CAD). This led to the nowadays usual but often not guideline- conformed treatment of CAD by placement of stents, whereas the surgical treatment is reduced since some years (Bundesgeschäftsstelle Qualitätssicherung (BQS) Bundesauswertung, 2006; Gummert et al., 2009).

Discussions about the right choice of treatment is reactivated since the SYNTAX-Trial showed positive long tem survival and less collateral damage for patients choosing the initially more invasive but on the long way successful treatment. Both techniques CABG and PCI have their limits in treating patients with end stage coronary artery disease (CAD). Some studies quantify this cohort of patients by 15 -20% (Bundesgeschäftsstelle Qualitätssicherung (BQS) Bundesauswertung, 2006; Gummert et al., 2009), so that alternative methods will be of greater importance in the future.

2   Current Studies for Selective Retroperfusion of Cardiac Veins: Retrobypass in an Experimental Porcine Model

In ischemic hearts, venous retroperfusion is a potential myocardial revascularization strategy. The goal underlying retrograde coronary sinus (CS) perfusion is perfusion of the ischemic myocardium proximal to the occlusion or stenosis. The lack of suitable target vessels remains a challenge for aortocoronary bypass grafting in end stage coronary heart disease. This study aimed to investigate the arterialization of cardiac veins as an alternative myocardial revascularization strategy in an experimental long term model in pigs.

In 2.1, the technical and functional aspects of a pig model of acute myocardial infarction and retroperfusion was refined with respect to the azygos connection. Previous animal studies on interspecies anatomic differences in mammals have concentrated on the venous connections of the vessels draining the myocardium and have demonstrated a need for further feasibility studies of the pig model that focus on hemodynamic performance (Harig *et al.*, 2010). Global retroperfusion after ligation of the ramus interventricularis paraconalis (equivalent to the left anterior descending artery in humans) was performed. Hemodynamic performance was significantly better in pigs that underwent coronary sinus perfusion. For the first time, we showed that effective retrograde flow and thus hemodynamic stability was achieved by ligation of the azygos vein. Therefore, experiments focusing on global retroperfusion will benefit from effective inhibition of the blood flow through the azygos vein.

In 2.2 and following, selective retrograde perfusion of a coronary vein (aorta to coronary vein bypass, retrobypass) was studied in a pig model of myocardial ischemia. Retroperfusion (RP) of the concomitant vein of the LAD was performed after ligation of the ramus interventricularis paraconalis (equivalent to the left anterior descending artery (LAD) in humans).

Hemodynamic was significantly better in pigs that underwent selective retroperfusion with proximal ligation of vena cordis magna compared with all other animals. Long term survival was significant better in those pigs than in all other groups. Histological follow-up studies showed significant lower area of necrosis in all animals of the retroperfusion group. Venous retroperfusion can be an effective technique to achieve long term survival after acute LAD occlusion in a pig model. In this setting, proximal ligation of V. cordis magna is mandatory.

2.1   Methods: Anatomical preconditions of an adequate animal model

2.1.1   Anatomical studies of the Azygos system in pigs

Background: Retroperfusion using the venous system is of interest as a potential myocardial revascularization strategy in ischemic hearts. This study aimed to refine the technical and functional aspects of an acute pig model of myocardial infarction and retroperfusion with respect to the azygos connection.

Methods: Under anaesthesia and with hemodynamic monitoring of 16 male Landrace pigs (Sus scrofa domestica), median sternotomy and aorta-to-coronary sinus catheterization were performed. The animals were divided into 4 groups. For all groups, an acute infarction was simulated by ligation of the ramus paraconalis (equivalent to the left anterior descending artery, LAD), in groups 1 and 2 (n=8) without coronary sinus (CS) perfusion, in groups 3 and 4 (n=8) with CS perfusion for 1h. The azygos vein was left open in groups 1 and 3, and ligated in groups 2 and 4. Hemodynamic performance and intraoperative angiograms were analyzed.

Results: The presence of an azygos connection and great cardiac vein (vena cordis magna) was verified in all animals via intraoperative angiography (see Figure 1 and 2). Hemodynamic performance in group 4 (CO: 4.9 L/min) was significantly better than in groups 1, 2 or 3 (CO, 2.9, 3.2, 2.8 L/min respectively) (see Table 1).

Conclusions: Global retroperfusion was efficient in preventing hemodynamic deterioration after LAD occlusion, but ligation of an azygos connection was essential to achieving effective retrograde flow. Therefore, a basic requirement for long-term successful experiments focusing on global retroperfusion is to ensure effective inhibition of the blood flow via the azygos vein.

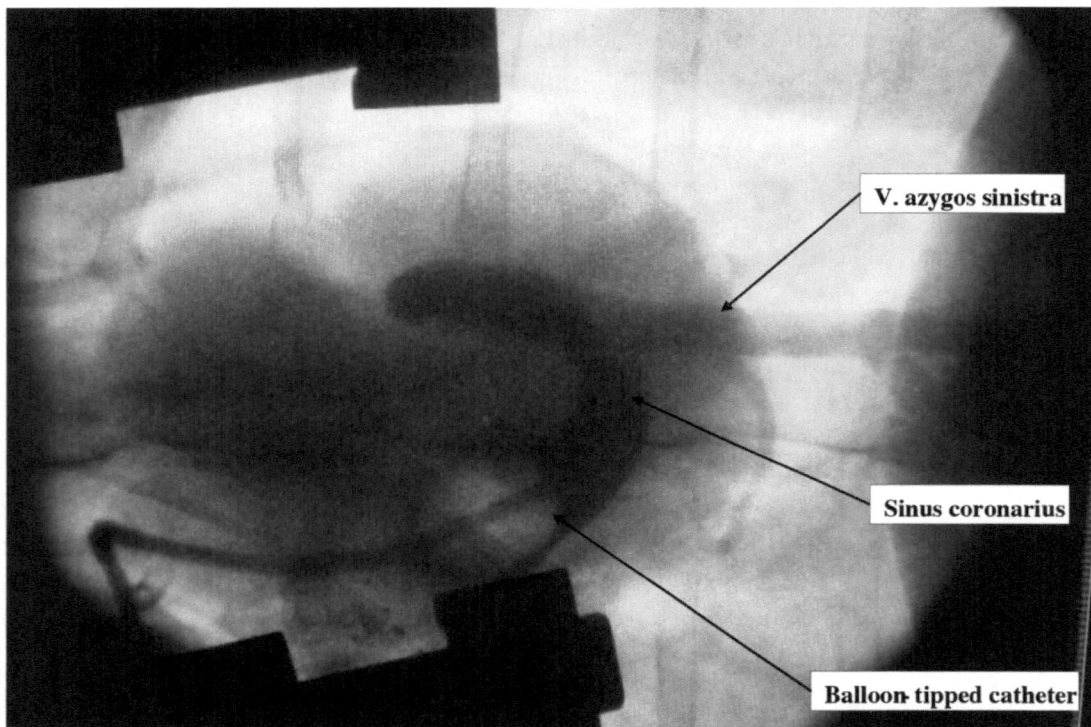

Figure 1: Anatomical studies of the cardiac venous system in pigs: Venogram after aplication of contrast medium into the V. azygos. Retrograde blood flow is indicated.

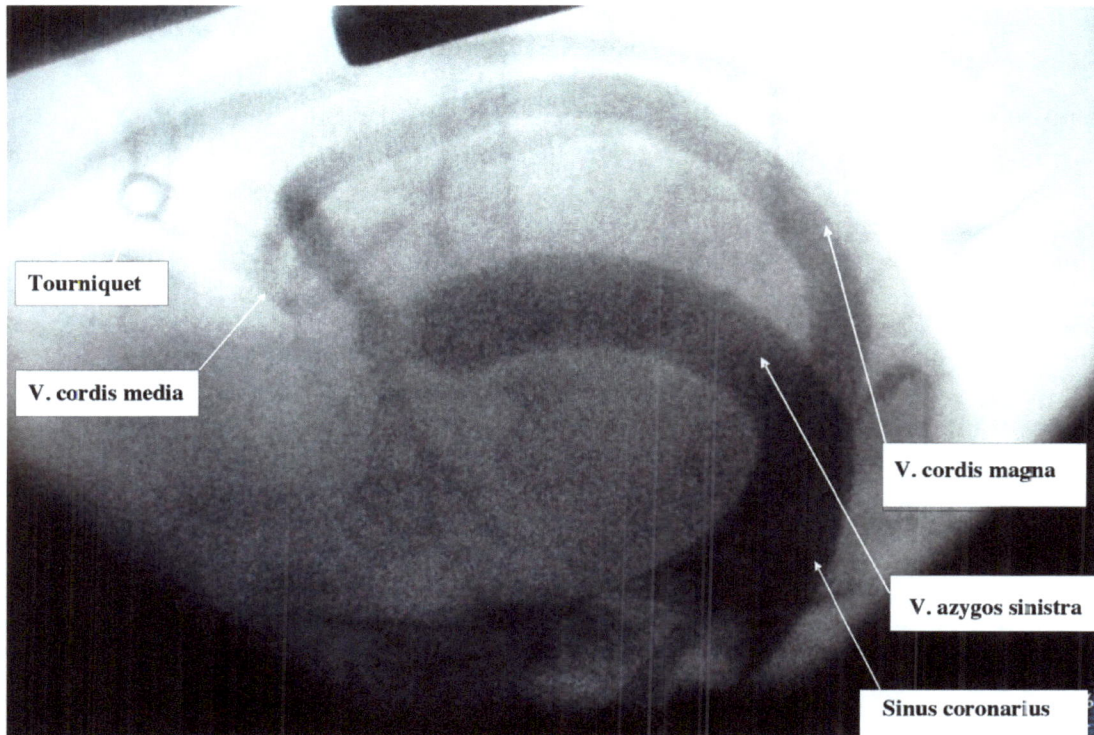

Figure 2: Anatomical study of the cardiac venous system in pigs. Venogram. After ligation of the V. azygos, contrast medium indicates the retrograde blood flow.

Parameter		preop.[0]	LAD ligation						
			without CS perfusion			**with** CS perfusion			
			azygos vein			azygos vein			
			open (group 1)	ligated (group 2)	p [1]vs.[2]	open (group 3)	ligated (group 4)	p [3]vs.[4]	p [0]vs.[4]
		n =16	n = 4	n = 4		n = 4	n = 4		
EF	[%][2]	60.5 ± 5	29.4 ± 8	28.2 ± 1	n.s.	32.3 ± 9	53.1 ± 1	< .05	n.s.
CO	[L/min][1]	5.6 ± 1.4	2.9 ± 1.1	3.2 ± .9	n.s.	2.7 ± .8	4.9 ± .8	n.s.	n.s.
HR	[1/min][4]	78.7 ± 12	86.8 ± 15	81.0 ± 1	n.s.	88.6 ± 17	80.0 ± 1	n.s.	n.s.
ST	[mm][4]	0.2 ± 1	11.5 ± 6	12.1 ± 4	n.s.	10.1 ± 3	2.1 ± 2	< .05	n.s.
MAP	[mmHg]	65.6 ± 5	44.4 ± 12	42.4 ± 1	n.s.	45.4 ± 11	59.5 ± 1	< .05	n.s.

Table 1: Hemodynamic values after LAD ligation. In groups 1 and 2, without coronary sinus (CS) perfusion, in groups 3 and 4, with CS perfusion, in groups 1 and 3, the azygos vein was left open, in groups 2 and 4 it was ligated. Abbreviations: LAD, left anterior descending artery; CS, coronary sinus; EF, ejection fraction; CO, cardiac output; HR, heart rate; ST, ST-segment elevation; MAP, mean arterial pressure; n.s. not significant. Methods used: 1: picco, 2: TEE, transesophageal echocardiography; 3: LAP, left atrial pressure; 4: ECG, electrocardiogram.

2.2   Histological Studies: Selective Coronary Venous Retroperfusion (Scvrp) Preserves Myocardium Effectively in Experimental Ischemia

Objectives: Cardiac veins are in the focus for myocardial revascularization strategies as alternatives for patients without suitable coronary target vessels. We studied retroperfusion techniques in a long term pig model and focused on histological examinations.

Methods: In 25 landrace pigs different retroperfusion models were performed. Acute infarction was simulated by LAD ligation. In group A (n=10), the left internal thoracic artery (LITA) was anastomosed to the Vena interventricularis anterior (selective RP) (Figure 3).

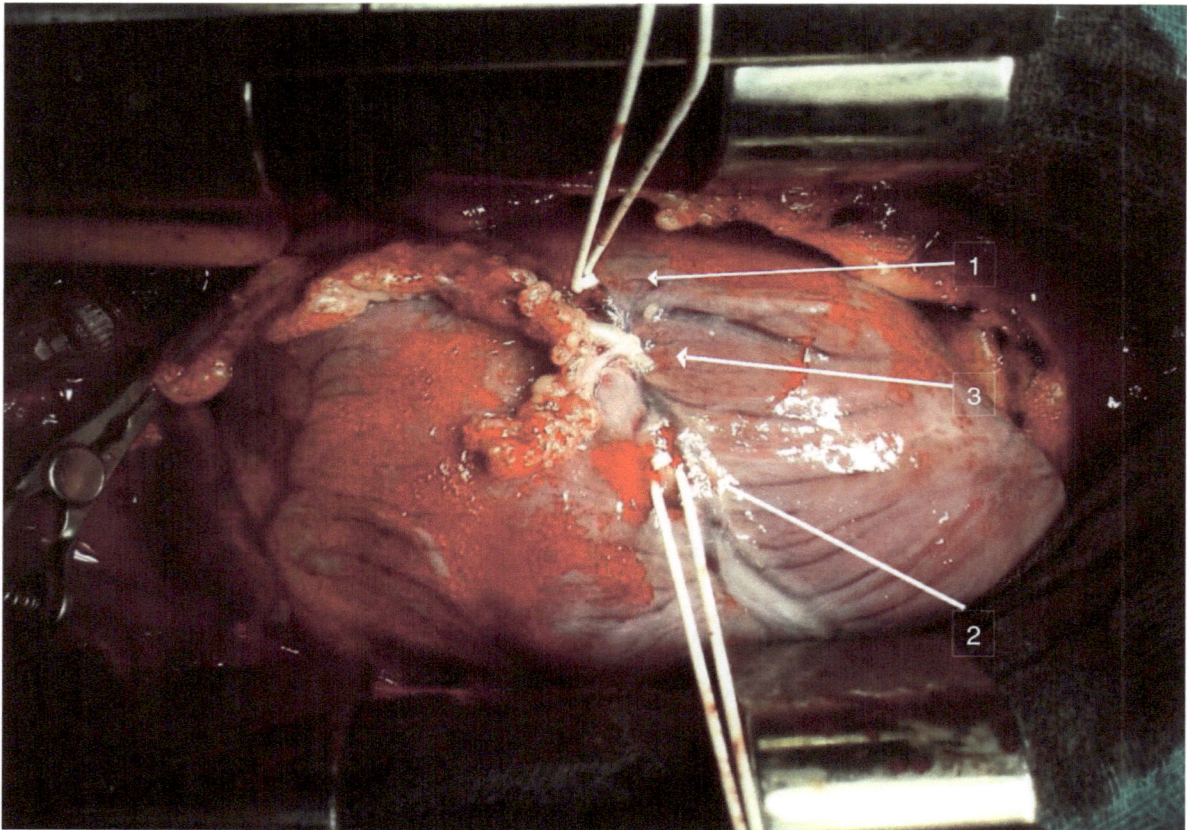

Figure 3: Intraoperative situs of a porcine heart after retrobypass using IMA graft. (1) The upper white tourniquet (at 12:00) ligates this vein and prevents central shunt via coronary sinus. (2) The downer (at 6:00) ligates the LAD. (3) Between the tourniquets, left internal thoracic artery (LITA) is anastomosed to the Vena interventricularis anterior, establishing retroperfusion.

In group B (n=5) coronary sinus (CS) perfusion (global RP) was established by an aorta-to-CS shunt with ligation of the V. azygos sinistra (P+L+). In group C (n=5) global RP was performed without ligation of the azygos vein (P+L-). In group D (n=5, control) LAD was ligated without RP and without ligation of the azygos connection (P-L-). After termination, all hearts were excised, cut into slices and histologically examined (Figure 4 and 5).

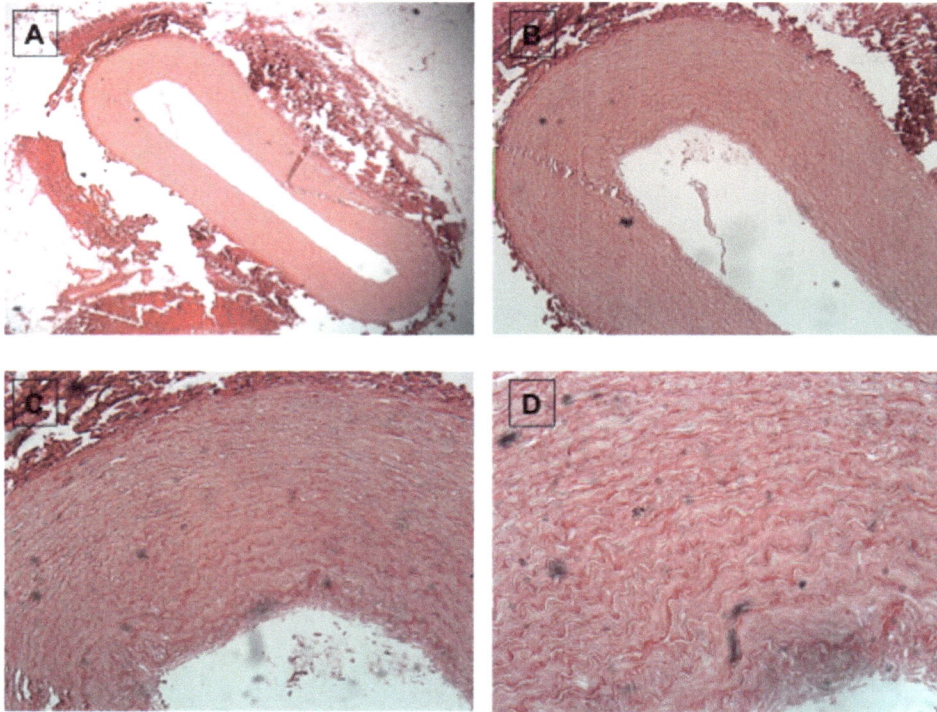

Figure 4: Histologic examination of the IMA bypass graft. Histologic slices (Sirius Red): LITA after 90d: magnification, A:40x, B:100x; C:200x, D:400x.

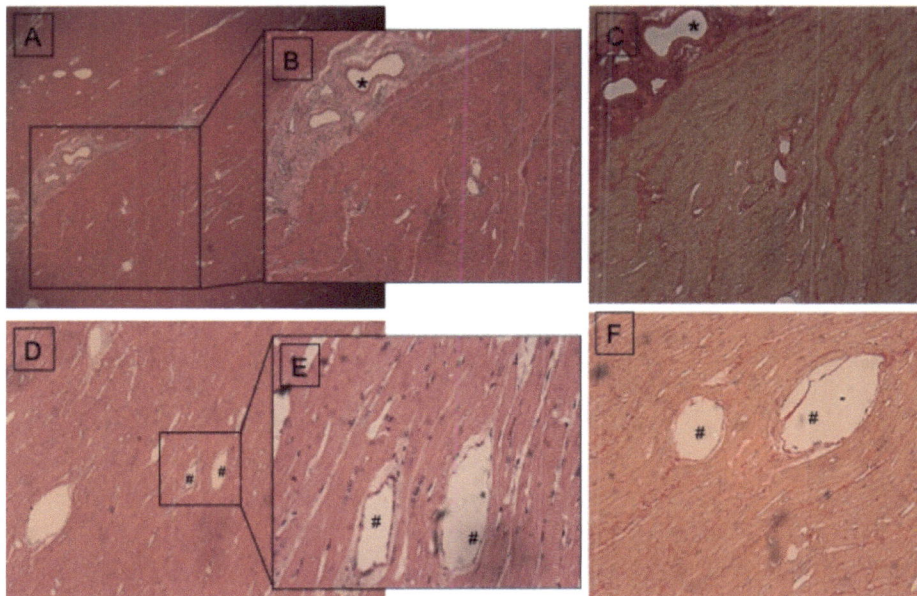

Figure 5: Histologic examination of the LV myocardium. Sirius Red staining. Histologic slices of left ventricular myocardium 90d after retroperfusion- above: basis of LV; down: apex of LV; magnification, A: 40x, B: 100x, D:100x, E: 400x, H.E. staining- magnification, C:100x, F:200x, Sirius Red staining.

Results: In group D (control), the hearts showed large infarcted areas (32.4% of the LV-Area) after LAD- ligation. With global RP in group C (P+L-), the infarcted area was reduced (19.8% of the LV) as was in group B (P+L+) (infarcted area, 10.9% of the LV). In group A (selective RP), the infarcted area was significantly reduced (1.1% of the LV). Subanalysis showed apical regions as most vulnerable (Figure 6).

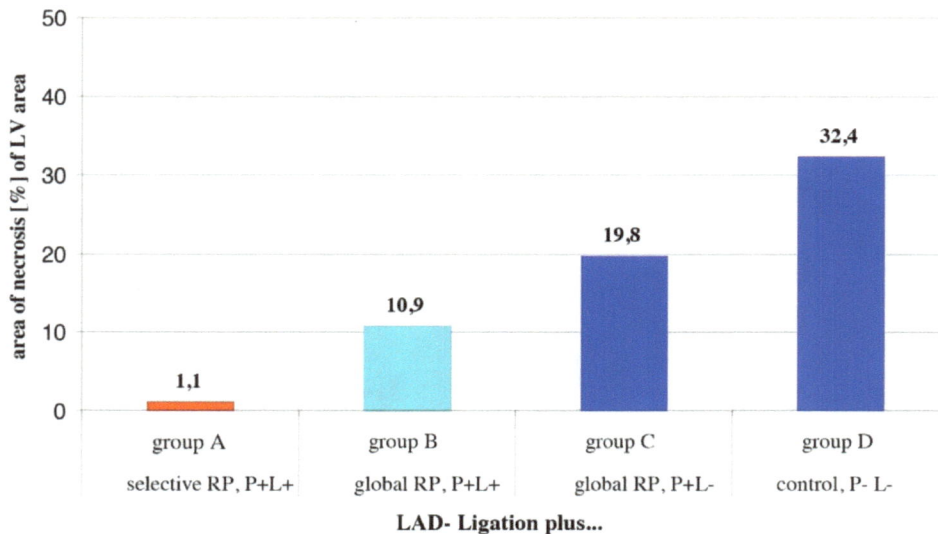

Figure 6: Histogram of the area of necrosis of LV area in different groups. In all groups, ischemia was induced by ligation of the left anterior descending artery (LAD); group A: selective retroperfusion (RP), with perfusion (P+) and ligation (L+) of the anterior descending vein (ADV); group B, global RP, with both, perfusion and ligation of the azygos vein; group C, global RP, only with perfusion of the ADV, without ligation of the azygos vein; group D, control, no perfusion, no ligation, as in all groups, LAD was ligated.

Conclusions: In global RP studies in pigs, ligation of the azygos connection is mandatory to save myocardium. Selective retroperfusion protects myocardium from infarction after experimental LAD occlusion. Apical regions of examined hearts seem to be at highest risk.

2.3   Pathophysiological Coronary Perfusion Studies: Influence of Flow & Pressure on Myocardial Contractility in Selective Coronary Venous Retroperfusion (Scvrp)

Background: Selective coronary venous retroperfusion is considered as an option for end stage coronary artery disease. As hyperperfusion of veins may cause damage to the endothelium and myocardial edema, the evaluation of flow and pressure conditions is important for further clinical application of selective retrograde perfusion therapy in humans.

Methods: After approval from the local veterinary office, retrobypass surgery was performed in 16 animals and left internal thoracic artery was anastomosed to the anterior cardiac vein (Figure 7). Complete hemodynamic monitoring was installed and myocardial contractility (dP/dt) was evaluated. For intracoronary flow measurements, Combo Map system (Volcano) was used. A correlation analysis (contractility - blood pressure; and contractility - blood flow) was performed.

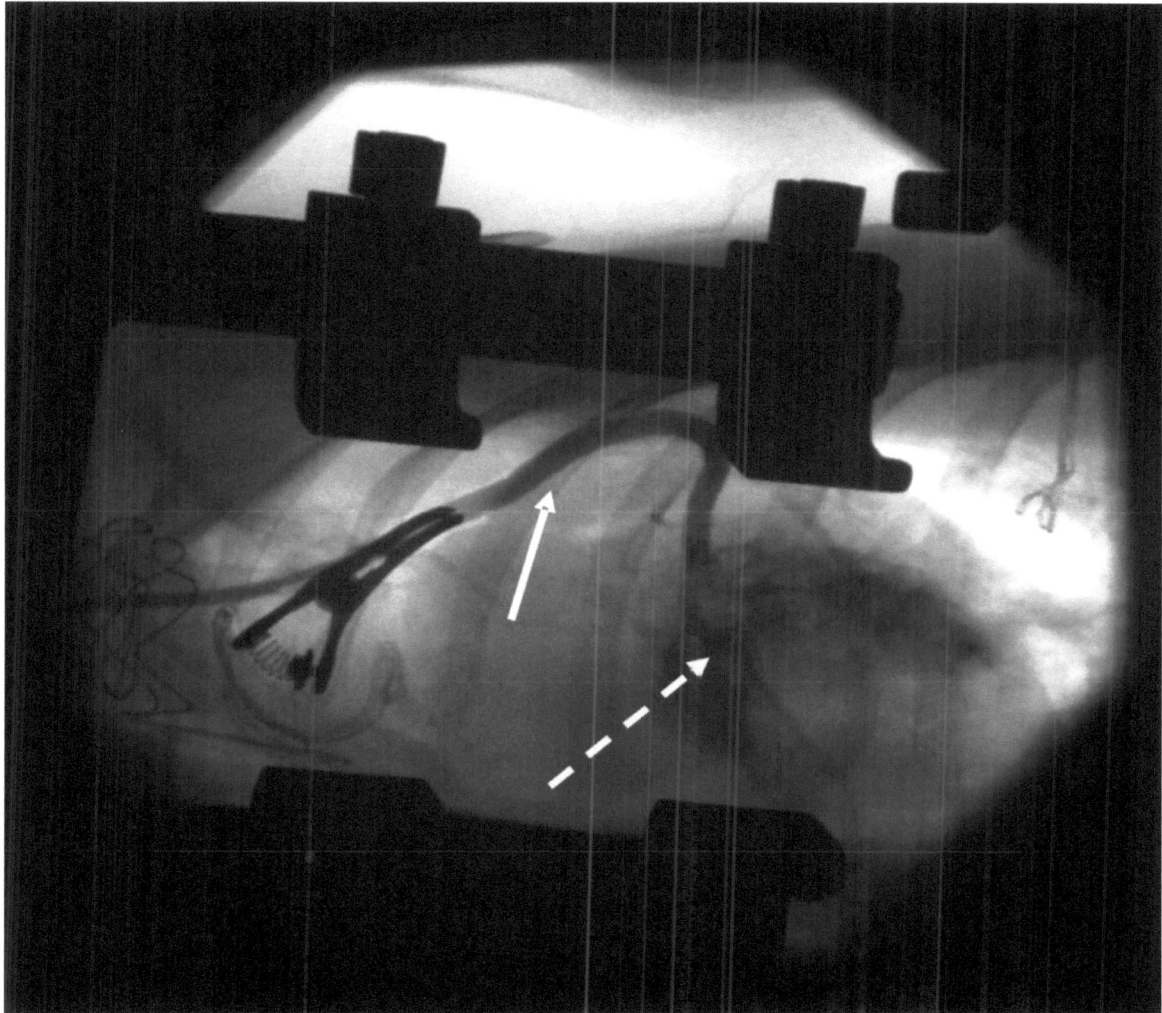

Figure 7: angiogram of retrobypass. Intraoperative angiogram of retroperfusion. Arrows indicate LITA graft (solid line) and blood flow in the anterior cardiac vein distal to the anastomosis (dotted line).

Results: Blood flow measurements showed values between 45 and 65ml/min in the anterior cardiac vein (VIVA). Intravasal blood pressure in the VIVA showed a mean venous pressure between 35mmHg (baseline) and maximum systolic value of 72mmHg. Correlation analysis (R^2=0.911) showed a maximum increase in pressure over time (1100mmHg/s) for blood pressure values in the VIVA between 65 and 75 mmHg. Below 60mmHg and above 80mmHg, contractility decreased below 900mmHg/s (Figure 8). Blood flow correlation analysis (R^2=0.602) showed an equivalent optimal range between 50ml/min and 70ml/min. Below 50ml/min and above 70ml/min, contractility dropped below 900mmHg/s (Figure 9).

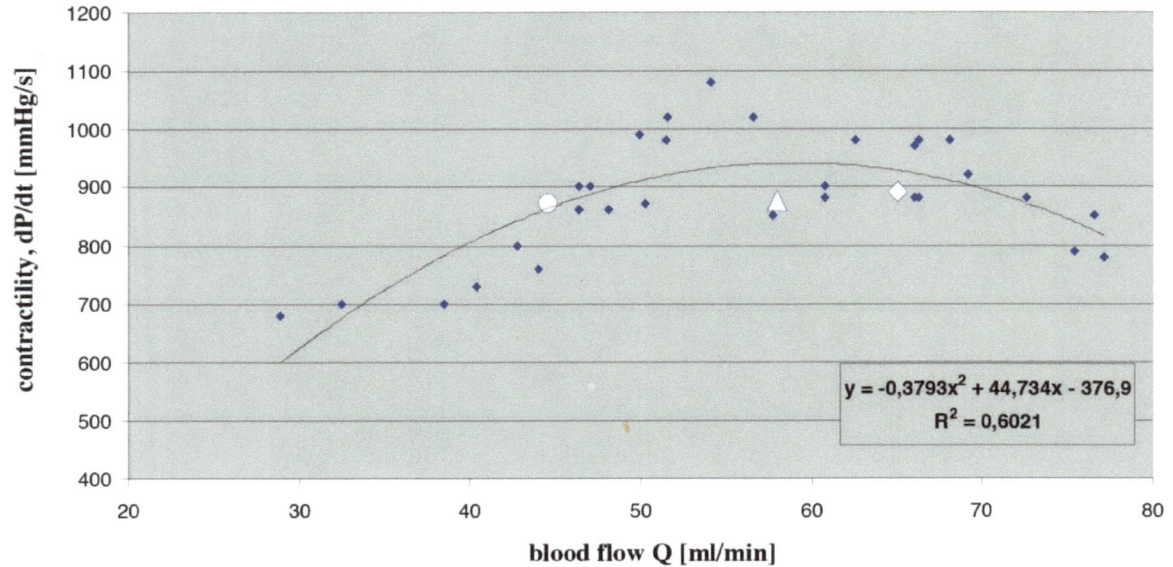

Figure 8: Analysis of contractility and blood flow. Myocardial contractility depends on blood flow: High values for contractility are observed in a range of blood flow between 50 and 70ml/min. Circle means baseline measurement, triangle: after 1h without vasodilation (no nitrotriglycerid), parallelogram: measurement after 1h with vasodilatating by application of nitrotriglyceride.

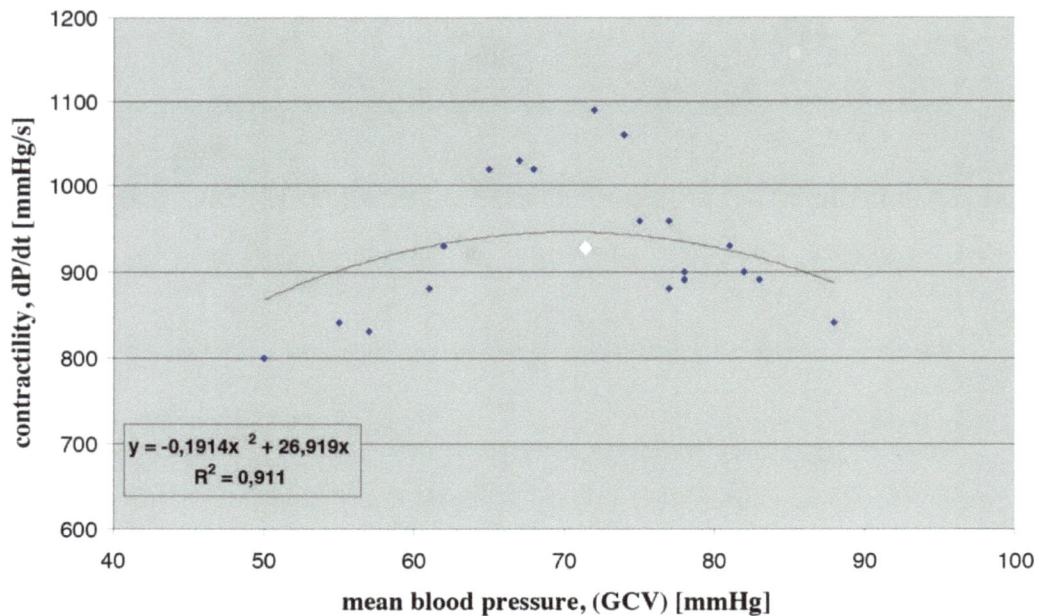

Figure 9: Perfusion studies. Correlation analysis of contractility and blood pressure. Myocardial contractility depends on blood pressure: High values for contractility are observed in a range of blood pressure around 70mmHg. Small white parallelogram means: mean value.

Conclusions: Myocardial contractility showed optimal performance within blood pressure ranges between 65 and 75mmHg and blood flow ranges between 50 and 70ml/min. These observations may serve as an early indirect sign of impaired myocardial integrity. Optimal pressure and flow patterns are preconditions for selective retroperfusion therapy.

2.4   Studies of Hemodynamics: Selective Arterialization of Vena Cordis Magna (Retrobypass) Prevents Hemodynamic Instability after LAD Occlusion

Objectives: The lack of eligible target vessels remains a challenge for aortocoronary bypass grafting in end stage coronary heart disease. Since the coronary sinus is a standardized access for retrograde cardioplegia, the arterialization of venous vessels is in the focus of research for alternative myocardial revascularisation strategies. Therefore the technical feasibility of this technique was investigated in a porcine long term model.

Methods: After anaesthesia, hemodynamic monitoring and median sternotomy of 16 landrace pigs, an aorta- to- coronary- vein (V. cordis magna, VCM) bypass (Retrobypass) was performed. Acute ischemia was simulated by LAD ligation. In group A.1 (in Figure 10 called RB+L+), LAD was ligated, a venous bypass performed and the VCM was proximally ligated. In group B.1, same procedure was performed without VCM ligation (in Figure 10 called RB+L-). Two control groups were added to the study design: group A.2 (in Figure 10 called RB-L+), in order to show effects of only ligating VCM, and group B.2 (in Figure 10 called RB-L-), in order to show effects of only performing LAD- ligation with no therapeutic intervention. Intraoperative angiograms, hemodynamic performance (Cardiac output, CO and stroke volume, SV) and survival time were analyzed.

Results: Hemodynamic performance in group A.1(RB+L+) was significantly better than in group B.1 (CO, 7.0ml/min vs. 3.2, p<.05; SV, 48ml vs. 29, p<.05). An open bypass could be verified angiographically in all animals of group A.1. Distal flow could only be established by proximal ligation of VCM. In all other groups, there was no long term survival after 4h. In group A.1, long term survival was 83% (10/12 animals) with a cumulative survival of 891 days, mean 99 d.

Conclusions: Retrobypass is an effective technique to achieve long term survival after acute LAD occlusion in a pig model. Proximal ligation of V. cordis magna is mandatory. Additional experiments will focus on structural and functional investigations.

2.5   Immunological Studies in Selective Retroperfusion: Cytokine Release after Retrobypass Surgery in Pigs

Background: This study aimed to analyze the effectiveness of selective retrograde perfusion of cardiac veins in pigs. Therefore we analyzed the cytokine release and typical parameters of cardiac ischemia during an acute infarction model. As the myocardium is a source of cytokines in ischemia/ reperfusion, it is interesting to get information about the cytokine release in retroperfusion.

Methods: In phase I of the study, 15 German landrace pigs (sus scrofa domestica) received cardiac bypass grafting under general anesthesia. After median sternotomy a retrobypass was established in off-pump cardiac surgery. A thirty minute period of ischemia by ligating the LAD was followed by retrograde reperfusion. Serial blood samples were taken to determine the concentration of lactate, troponin I, TNF-α, IL-6, IL-8 and IL-10. To assess the long-term effects of selective retroperfusion, troponin I was repeatedly measured three months after implanting the retrobypass. Furthermore, blood

Cardiac output

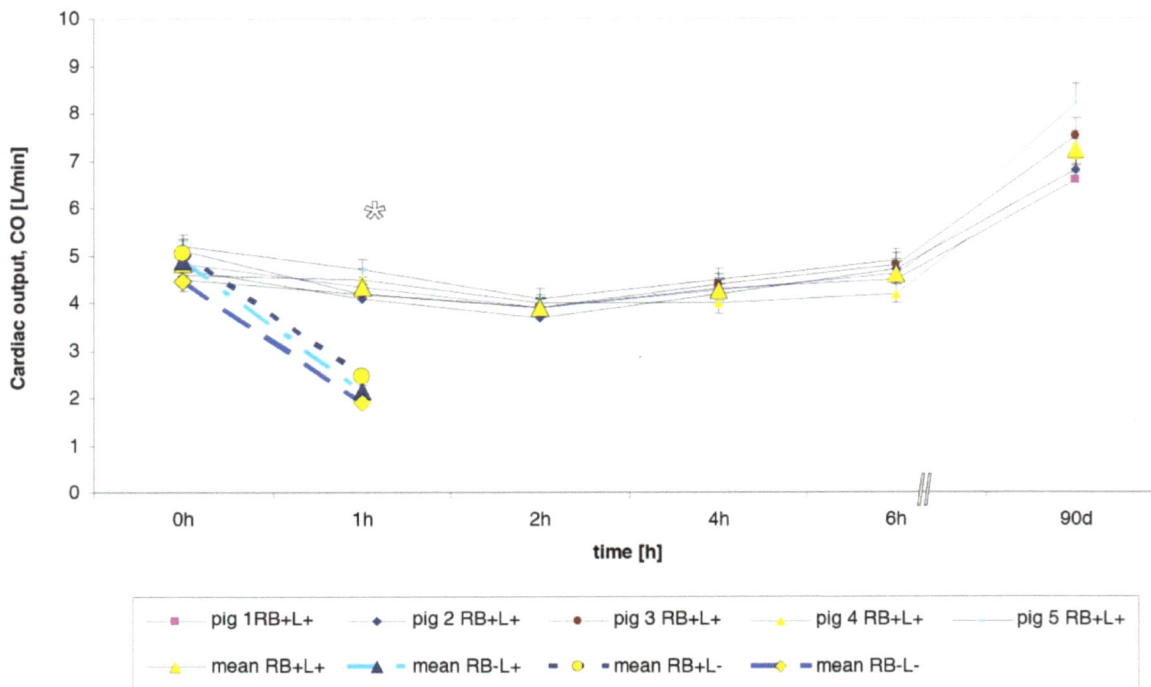

Figure 10: Hemodynamic effect of retroperfusion in ischemia. Studies on cardiac output were performed in different groups, all with myocardial ischemia induced by LAD ligation: The above thin lines represent cardiac output (CO) of animals with retrobypass (RB+) and ligation of the anterior cardiac vein, ACV (L+). The triangle indicates the mean value of this group. The dotted lines indicate the CO of animals without retrobypass and with ligation of the ACV (RB-L+); or with retrobypass but without ligation of the ACV (RB+L-); or without any intervention (RB-L-). Those animals did not survive myocardial ischemia longer than one hour.

samples for the determination of lactate and cytokine concentrations were collected three months after primary surgery.

Results: In the implantation period, the increase of troponin I (Figure 11a) suggests a myocardial ischemia, and therefore demonstrates this model of ischemia to be effective after LAD occlusion. The serum concentration of troponin I, the most specific blood parameter for myocardial damage, showed normal levels one month (data not shown) and three months (Figure 11b) after surgery. So were the lactate levels three month after the bypass grafting (data not shown). These findings were underlined by the analyzed cytokine concentrations, which were quantified by a porcine specific ELISA. An inter-individual variance in the determined cytokine release patterns was observed.

troponin I release

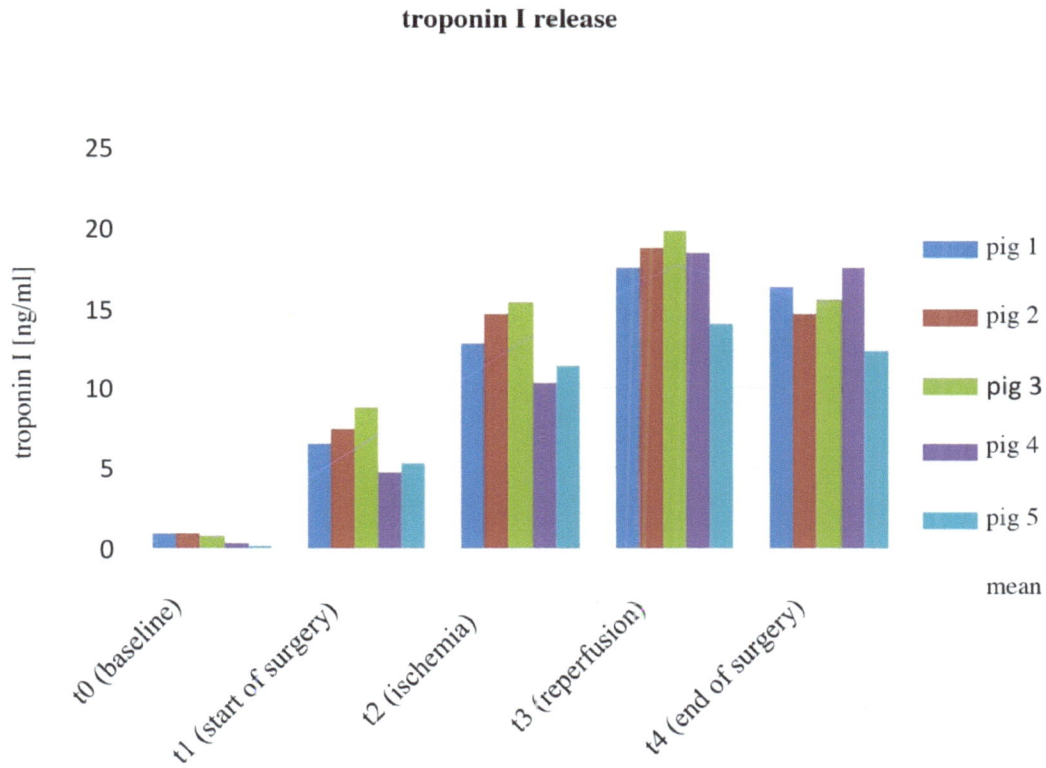

Figure 11a: Effect of selective retroperfusion on perioperative troponin I release.

troponin I release after 90d

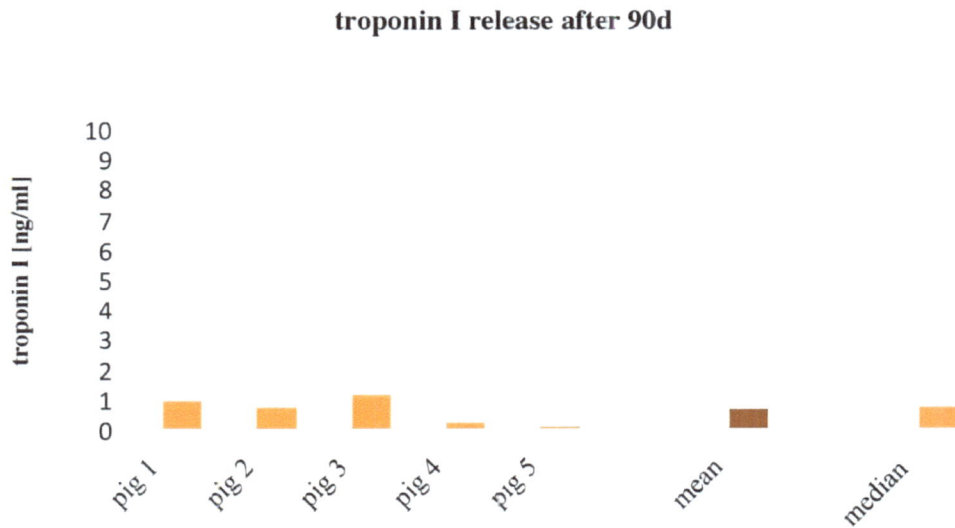

Figure 11b: Effect of selective retroperfusion on myocardial troponin I release after 90d.

The proinflammatory cytokines TNF-α (Figure 11c), IL-6 (Figure 11d), IL-8 (Figure 11e) showed a peak after the surgical trauma of median sternotomy. After the next trauma and possible trigger of cytokine release, the myocardial ischemia, a further cytokine peak could not be observed. During the observation period, plasma levels of the antiinflammatory cytokine IL-10 could not be detected (data not shown).

Conclusions: In this pig model of venous retroperfusion we could observe courses of myocardial metabolite (lactate) and enzyme parameters (troponin I). The analyzed cytokine trends showed a typical peak as an adequate answer to the surgical trauma. Ischemia and subsequent selective retroperfusion did not further increase cytokine levels. These findings encourage the hypothesis that selective retroperfusion may be an adequate and effective alternative method for myocardial revascularization. Cytokines underlie several potential influence factors, which limit their appropriateness as specific markers for cardiac ischemia.

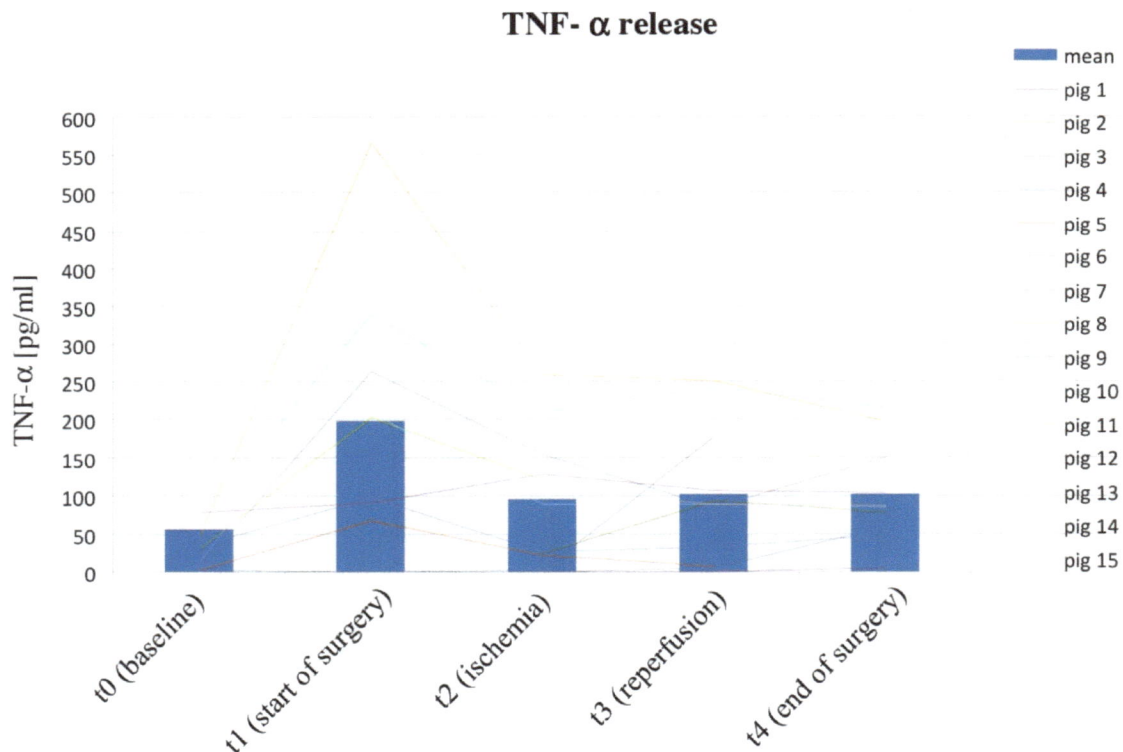

Figure 11c: Effect of selective retroperfusion on TNF-α release.

IL-6 release

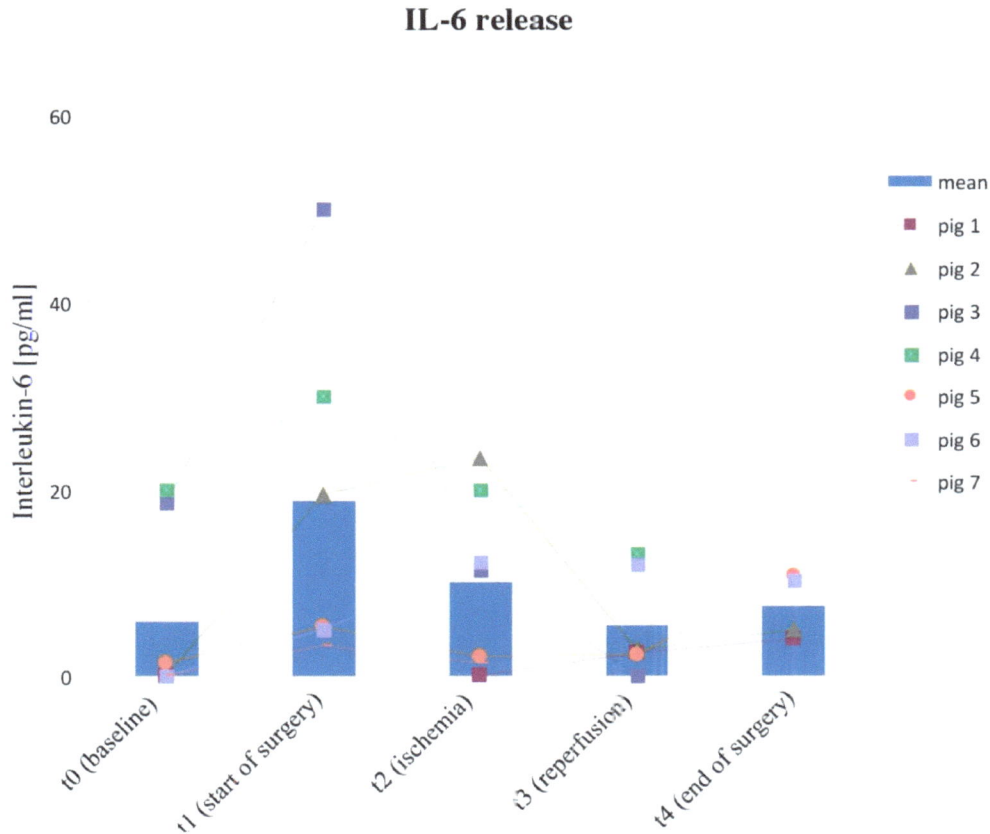

Figure 11d: Effect of selective retroperfusion on IL-6 release.

2.6   Discussion of Experimental Findings

In this study, pigs are used for experimental scientific research because they have a comparable cardiac anatomy and physiology to humans. The study was conducted in strict compliance with the Principles of Laboratory Animal Care formulated by the National Society for Medical Research and the Guide for the Care and Use of Laboratory Animals. All procedures were performed in accordance with the European Convention for the Protection of Vertebrate Animals Used for Experimental and Other Scientific Purposes and the German Animal Protection Law of 1998, and IACUC approval was obtained from the local Veterinary Office. In the following chapters the authors try to focus on special aspects of retroperfusion, the refinement of the methods and for the first time, it is shown that it is possible to perform a regional venous retrobypass (selective arterialization of the VIVA) in a long term pig model.

The importance of methods- Anatomical preconditions in an adequate animal model

In the methodical part of study, the clinical importance of the azygos connection in a pig model of retroperfusion was analyzed. During acute ischemia causing by LAD ligation, the impact of simultaneous

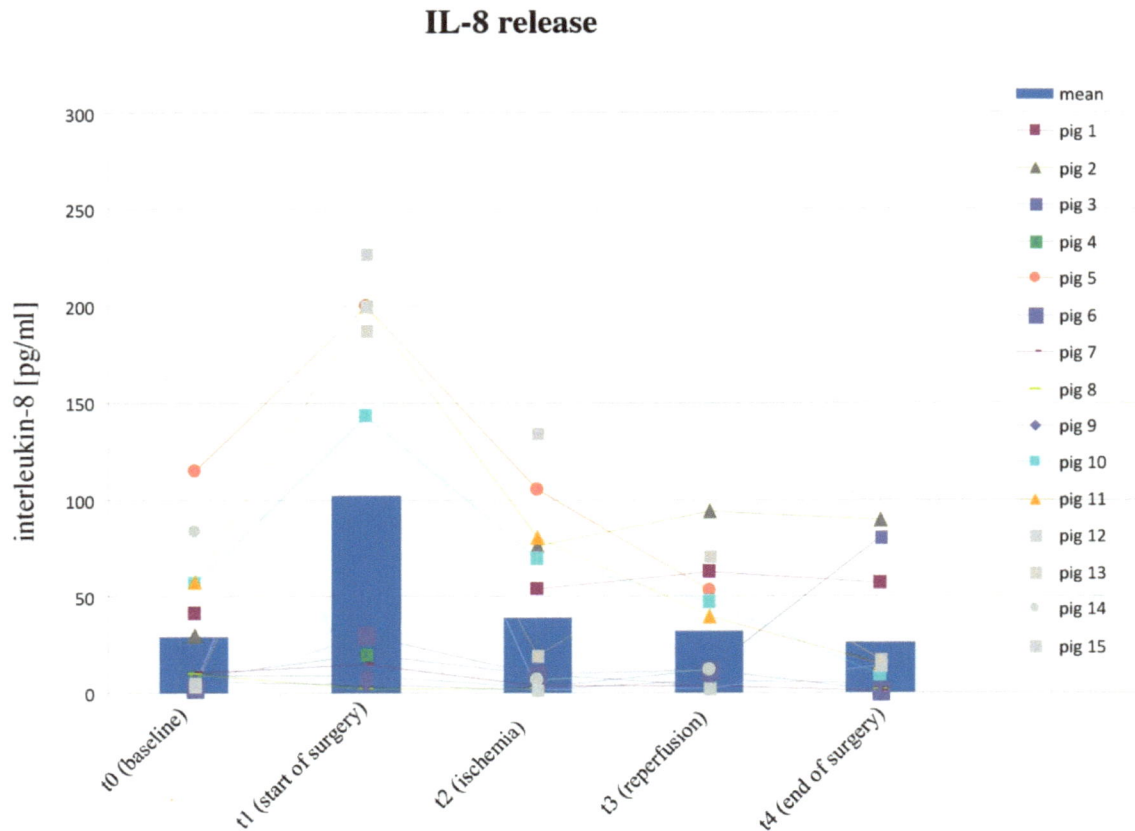

Figure 11e: Effect of selective retroperfusion on perioperative IL-8 release.

global retrograde perfusion of the CS by means of an aorta-to-coronary sinus (ACS) shunt was studied by analyzing hemodynamic parameters. As expected, it was found that mid- LAD occlusion reduced cardiac output and worsened cardiac and circulatory parameters. Previous studies using animal retroperfusion models in dogs, pigs and sheep did not focus on the potential obstacle created by anatomical variation. Global retroperfusion prevented hemodynamic deterioration only if it was used in combination with azygos ligation (Harig *et al.*, 2010).

Hemodynamical and histological studies- Selective coronary venous retroperfusion preserves myocardium effectively in experimental ischemia

In the clinical part of the study, we studied the impact of selective retrograde perfusion of the vena interventricularis anterior (VIVA) by means of a retrobypass (LITA to VIVA) by analyzing hemodynamic, histologic and other parameters.

As expected, we found that mid- LAD occlusion reduced cardiac output and worsened cardiac and circulatory parameters that were consistent with myocardial ischemia. Selective retroperfusion of the

VIVA prevented **hemodynamic** deterioration only when it was combined with proximal ligation of the LAD vein (vena cordis magna). When selective retroperfusion was performed in addition to proximal ligation of the VCM, arterialized blood was prevented from flowing into the CS (bypassing the heart) and was redirected to the ischemic myocardium (flow reversal). In this acute infarction model, selective retroperfusion led to improved hemodynamic stability, an indirect sign of sufficient myocardial oxygen supply.

These clinical parameters are consistent with the **histological** studies. The use of the retrobypass in combination with the ligation of the vena cordis magna reduced the area of necrosis significantly. In the histologic analysis of heart slices, the apical region showed a tendency towards higher percentage of histologically necrotic myocardium (5-8%) in contrast to mid ventricular and basal parts (1-3%). After ligation of the LAD the potential of retroperfusion seems to be a little bit limited. This is interpreted as a limited retrograde perfusion capability of the graft, but on the other side endothelial dysfunction due to high pressure and consecutive edema, swelling and capillary occlusion is also a possible explanation.

In global RP studies in pigs, ligation of the azygos connection is mandatory to save myocardium. Selective retroperfusion protects myocardium from infarction after experimental LAD occlusion.

Pathophysiological Coronary Perfusion Studies: Influence of Flow & Pressure on Myocardial Contractility in Selective Coronary Venous Retroperfusion

Optimal pressure and flow patterns are preconditions for selective retroperfusion therapy. In former experimental studies concerning retroperfusion, the modification of blood flow and blood pressure has been essential: The negative effect of high pressure on vascular endothelium was shown by Hammond *et al.* (1967). He could find histomorphological changes in the coronary sinuses of dogs beyond a pressure of 60mmHg. An interesting observation in studies on flow- dependent myocardial contractility in pigs could be made by Verdow, Serrhuys *et al.* (1988) They found an optimal myocardial contractility in a range of flow rates between 60ml and 80ml/min.

In our studies myocardial contractility showed optimal performance within blood pressure ranges between 65 and 75mmHg and blood flow ranges between 50 and 70ml/min. These observations may serve as an early indirect sign of impaired myocardial integrity. In the coronary sinuses of humans, flow rates of 120ml/min (with high interindividual ranges) could be measured at rest. In the V. interventricularis anterior, flow rates between 50 and 80ml/min could be measured (Swan *et al.* 1971).

Immunological Studies in Selective Retroperfusion: Retrobypass Does Not Further Increase Surgical Proinflammatory Cytokine Release in Pigs

In former studies on the cytokine response of patients after coronary artery bypass grafting, we could find an immediate peak of IL-10 and IL-8. The proinflammatory IL-6 followed some hours later as an indicator of *SIRS* (systemic inflammatory response syndrome) (Harig *et al.*, 1999a; 1999b; 2001).

In this pig model of venous retroperfusion the analyzed proinflammatory cytokine trends of TNF-α, IL-6 and IL-8 showed a typical peak as an adequate answer to the surgical trauma. Ischemia and subsequent selective retroperfusion did not further increase cytokine levels.

These findings encourage the hypothesis that selective retroperfusion may be an adequate and effective alternative method for myocardial revascularization. Cytokines underlie several potential influence factors, which limit their appropriateness as specific markers for cardiac ischemia.

2.7   Additional Aspects and Summary

Angiogenesis

Some investigators (Weigel *et al.*, 2007) analyzed the effect of pressure-controlled coronary sinus occlusion (PICSO) on the activation of proangiogenetic genes like HO-1 (Häm-Oxygenase 1) and VEGF (Vascular endothelial growth factor) by exerting pulsatile pressure on coronary venous endothelium. Mohl and coworkers hypothesized that neoangiogenesis may be the trigger for the positive effects of retroperfusion.

Staged procedure

Choy *et al.* (2006a; 2006b) introduced a novel strategy of ligating the vein of the target region in a first step, leading to an increasing wall thickness of coronary venules and then, in a second step, after remodeling of the coronary veins, creating the retrobypass as an alternative method of myocardial oxygen delivery. Resuming the broad spectrum of investigations concerning retroperfusion one can state that the impact of this method may lead to a broader clinical application for the treatment of end stage coronary disease.

References

Arealis, E.G., Volder, J.G.R. & Kolff, W.J. (1973). Arterialization of the coronary vein coming from an ischemic area. Chest, 63, 462

Bakst, A.A., Bailey, C.P. & Goldberg, H. (1956). Protection of the heart by arterialization of the coronary sinus in occlusive coronary artery disease. Journal of Thoracic Surgery, 31, 559-68

Beck, C.S. & Leighninger, D.S. (1954). Operations for coronary artery disease. JAMA, 13, 1226-1234

Beck, C.S. & Makao, A.E. (1948). Revascularization of the heart. Annals of Surgery, 128, 854

Beck, C.S., Stanton, E., & Batiuchok, W. (1948): Revascularization of the heart by graft of systemic artery into coronary sinus. JAMA, 137, 436-442

Beller, S.R. (2009). Retrograde myocardial perfusion via a new stent-based ventriculo- coronary-venous bypass (venous VPASS TM): Comparison to selective synchronized retroinfusion (SSR) in an experimental acute ischemia model. Doctorate Thesis, LMU Munich, Germany.

Bhayana, J.N., Olsen, D.B. & Byrne, J.P. (1974). Reversal of myocardial ischemia by arterialization of the coronary vein. Journal of Thoracic and Cardiovascular Surgery, 67, 125-132

Bundesgeschäftsstelle Qualitätssicherung (BQS) Bundesauswertung 2006, Koronarchirurgie, Abs. II 61, S. 2.32 (German Federal Office of Quality Assessment, Federal Data Analysis 2006, CABG, par.II61, p.2.32)

Chaikhouni, A. (2010). The magnificent century of cardiothoracic surgery. Heart Views, 11(1), 31–37.

Choy, J.S. & Kassab, G.S. (2006a). A novel strategy for increasing wall thickness of coronary venules prior to retroperfusion. American Journal of Physiology Heart and Circulatory Physiology, 291, 972-978

Choy, J.S., Dang, Q., Molloi, S. & Kassab, G.S. (2006b). Nonuniformity of axial and circumferential remodelling of large coronary veins in response to ligation. American Journal of Physiology Heart and Circulatory Physiology 2006, 290, 1558-1565.

Ganz, W., Tamura K.., Marcus H., Roberto Donoso, Shinji Yoshida, & Harold J. C. Swan. (1971a). Measurement of Coronary Sinus Blood Flow by Thermodilution in Man. Circulation;44:181-195

Ganz, W., Tamura,K., Marcus, H.S., Donoso, R., Yoshida, S. & Swan, H.J.C. (1971b). Measurement of Coronary Sinus Blood Flow by Thermodilution in Man. Circulation, 44, 181-195

Gummert, J.F., Funkat, A., Beckmann, A., Schiller, W., Hekmat. K., Ernst, M., & Beyersdorf, F. (2009). Cardiac Surgery in Germany during 2009. A report on behalf of the German Society of Thoracic and Cardiovascular Surgery. The Thoracic and Cardiovascular Surgeon, 58, 379-386

Hahn, R.S. & Kim, M. (1952). Revascularization of the heart: histologic changes after arterialization of the coronary sinus. Circulation, 5, 810

Hammond, G.L., Davies, A.L. & Austen, W.G. (1967). Retrograde coronary sinus perfusion: a method of myocardial protection in the dog during left coronary artery occlusion. Annals of Surgery, 166, 39-47.

Harig F, Cesnjevar R, Mahmoud FO & von der Emde J. (1999a). Perioperative factors influencing interleukin-10 release under cardiopulmonary bypass. Thorac Cardiovasc Surg. Dec;47(5):361-8.

Harig F, Feyrer R, Mahmoud FO, Blum U & von der Emde J (1999b). Reducing the post-pump syndrome by using heparin-coated circuits, steroids, or aprotinin. Thorac Cardiovasc Surg. Apr;47(2):111-8

Harig F, Hohenstein B, von der Emde J & Weyand M. (2001). Modulating IL-6 and IL-10 levels by pharmacologic strategies and the impact of different extracorporeal circulation parameters during cardiac surgery. Shock;16 Suppl 1:33-8.

Harig, F., Hoyer, E., Labahn, D., Schmidt, J., Weyand, M. & Ensminger, S.M. (2010). Refinement of pig retroperfusion technique: Global Retroperfusion with ligation of the Azygos Connection preserves hemodynamic function in an acute infarction model in pigs (sus scrofa domestica). Comparative Medicine, 60(1), 38-44

Harig, F., Schmidt, J., Hoyer, E., Eckl, S., Adamek, E., Ertel, D., Noch, E., Amann, K., Weyand, M. & Ensminger, S.M. (2011). Long-term evaluation of a selective retrograde coronary venous perfusion model in pigs (Sus scrofa domestica). Comparative Medicine, 61(2), 150-157

Herrick, J.B. (1912). A Modern concept of coronary thrombosis and myocardial infarction. JAMA 250, 13, 1757–65.

Hochberg, M. (1977). Hemodynamic evaluation of selective arterialization of the coronary venous system. Journal of Thoracic and Cardiovascular Surgery, 74, 774-783

Hochberg, M.S., Roberts, W.C. & Morrow, A.G. (1979): Selective arterialization of the coronary venous system: encouraging long- term flow evaluation utilizing radioactive microspheres Journal of Thoracic and Cardiovascular Surgery, 77, 1-12

Kay, E.B. & Suzuki, A. (1975). Coronary venous retroperfusion for myocardial revascularization. Annals of Thoracic Surgery, 19, 327-330

Ludinghausen, M.V. (1987). Clinical anatomy of cardiac veins, Vv. Cardiacae. Surgical and Radiology Anatomy, 9, 159-168

Mohr, F.W., Morice, M.C., Kappetein, P., Feldman, T.E., Staehle, E., Colombo, A., Mack, M.J., Holmes D., Morel, M.A., Van Dyck, N., Houle, V.M., Dawkins, K.D. & Serruys. P.W. (2013). Coronary artery bypass graft surgery versus percutaneous coronary intervention in patients with three-vessel disease and left main coronary disease: 5-year follow-up of the randomised, clinical SYNTAX trial. The Lancet, 381(9867), 629-638

Park, S.B., Magovern, G.I. & Liebler, G.A. (1975). Direct selective myocardial revascularization by internal mammary artery coronary vein anastomosis. Journal of Thoracic and Cardiovascular Surgery, 69, 63-72

Pratt, F.H. (1898). The nutrition of the heart through the vessels of thebesius and the coronary veins. American Journal of Physiology, 1, 86-103

Rhodes, G.R., Syracuse D.C. & MacIntosh, C.L. (1978). Evaluation of regional myocardial nutrient perfusion following selective retrograde arterialization of the coronary vein. Annals of Thoracic Surgery, 25, 329-335

Roberts, J.T., Jarvis, W.H. & Key, L. (1943). Nourishment of the myocardium by way of the coronary veins. Federal Proceedings, 2, 90

Stephan, D. et al. (2012). 2012 ACCF/AHA/ACP/AATS/PCNA/SCAI/STS Guideline for the Diagnosis and Management of Patients With Stable Ischemic Heart Disease: Executive Summary. Circulation, 126, 3097-3137

Verdouw, P.D., Beatt, K., Berk, L., Serrhuys, P.W. (1988). Does effective diastolic coronary venous retroperfusion depend on arterial-like blood pressure in the coronary sinus? The American Journal of Cardiology, 61, 1148-1149

Weigel, G., Kajgana, I., Bergmeister, H., Riedl, G., Glogar, H.D., Gyöngyösi, M., Blasnig, S., Heinze, G. & Mohl. G. (2007). Beck and back: A paradigm change in coronary sinus interventions- pulsatile stretch on intact venous endothelium. Journal of Thoracic and Cardiovascular Surgery, 133, 1581-1587

Implications of the Phosphate Regulatory FGF-23/Klotho System in Cardiovascular Disease

Javier Donate-Correa, Ernesto Martín-Núñez
Research Unit
University Hospital Nuestra Señora de Candelaria, Santa Cruz de Tenerife, Spain

Mercedes Muros-de-Fuentes
Clinical Analysis Service
University Hospital Nuestra Señora de Candelaria, Santa Cruz de Tenerife, Spain

Carmen Mora-Fernández
Research Unit
University Hospital Nuestra Señora de Candelaria, Santa Cruz de Tenerife, Spain

Juan F. Navarro-González
Research Unit and Nephrology Service
University Hospital Nuestra Señora de Candelaria, Santa Cruz de Tenerife, Spain

1   Introduction

Alterations in phosphorus homeostasis are involved in multiple physiopathologic mechanisms and clinical processes. These alterations are very frequent in chronic kidney disease (CKD) patients, in whom phosphorous retention and hyperphosphatemia are common features that contribute to explain the high cardiovascular morbidity and mortality in this population.

However, growing evidence in recent years demonstrated that not only variations in phosphate levels, but also in phosphate-regulatory factors are linked with morbidity and mortality (Kuro-o, 2010a; Block *et al.*, 2004; Foley, 2009; Kestenbaum *et al.*, 2005; Tonelli *et al.*, 2005a; Parker *et al.*, 2010; Mirza *et al.*, 2009a; Levin *et al.*, 2007). This suggests that both elements could be related to cardiovascular adverse risk factors and outcomes, including atherosclerosis, arterial calcification, vascular stiffness, and left ventricular hypertrophy (LVH) (Block *et al.*, 2004; Shuto *et al.*, 2009; Zisman *et al.*, 2010).

Classically, regulation of serum calcium and phosphate levels was believed to be achieved by a feedback between two main endocrine factors, calcitriol or 1,25-dihydroxyvitamin D3 (the active form of vitamin D) and parathyroid hormone (PTH) (Foley, 1998a; Foley, 1998b). However, in addition to PTH and calcitriol, recent studies have identified a novel regulator of phosphate levels: the fibroblast growth factor (FGF) 23 (Block *et al*, 2004; Shimada *et al.*, 2001) which is actually considered the as the principal regulator of phosphatemia inducing phosphaturia and inhibiting calcitriol synthesis in the kidney, therefore maintaining systemic phosphate homeostasis. Like other members of the endocrine FGFs group, FGF-23 requires a co-factor for bind and activate its cognate receptors (Itoh, 2010; Kuro-o, 2008). To exert its actions, FGF-23 requires Klotho, a single-pass transmembrane protein that is predominantly expressed in the kidney (Kurosu *et al.*, 2006; Yu *et al.*, 2005).

The appearing of this novel phosphatemic central regulator not only has changed our understanding about mineral metabolism regulation, but has also provided novel implications in the relationship between the phosphate imbalance and the increased cardiovascular risk. Thereby, diverse studies have showed the potential role of FGF-23 excess in cardiovascular disease (CVD) incidence in patients with and without kidney impairment, including increased mortality risk (Parker *et al.*, 2010; Gutiérrez *et al.*, 2008; Jean *et al.*, 2009), LVH (Mirza *et al.*, 2009b; Gutiérrez *et al.*, 2009), vascular dysfunction (Mirza *et al.*, 2009c), atherosclerosis (Mirza *et al.*, 2009c), and cardiovascular events (Kanbay *et al.*, 2010). Moreover, diverse studies have confirmed the role of Klotho in not FGF-23-related favourable effects over the vascular system, including calcitriol and nitric oxide synthesis, suppression of Wnt signalling, oxidative stress, and vascular calcifications (Kuro-o, 2009a). The recently described expression of Klotho in human vascular tissue and vascular smooth muscle cells (VSMCs) (Donate-Correa *et al.*, 2013; Lim *et al.*, 2012) may partially explain these effects of the FGF-23/Klotho axis over the cardiovascular system. Moreover, a soluble form of Klotho can be also detected in blood, urine, and cerebrospinal fluid, which appears to have diverse endocrine actions.

Currently, the potential utility of the mineral metabolism regulators, especially FGF-23 and Klotho, as clinical biomarkers is an area of intense investigation, especially focused in renal patients. However, there is a long way to go in which FGF-23 and Klotho will have to prove its usefulness in the early diagnosis and its prognostic value in CVD.

2 FGF-23/KLOTHO System: A Master Regulator of Phosphate Metabolism

The classic view of the regulation of serum calcium and phosphate levels is product of a feedback between calcitriol and PTH, by counterbalanced intestinal uptake, mobilization from bone, and renal excretion (Berndt & Kumar, 2003; Dusso *et al.*, 2005). Calcitriol is synthesized in the kidney and acts in the gut increasing the absorption of dietary calciumm and phosphate , and in the bone, promoting mobilization of these ions (Figure 1). As result, blood levels of both phosphate and calcium trend to increase. PTH is secreted from parathyroid glands in response to hypocalcemia, promoting bone resorption and stimulating calcitriol synthesis in the kidney. In addition, PTH induces phosphaturia by diminishing the reabsorption of phosphate in the kidney. Therefore, the final effect of PTH is an elevation of calcium without increase of phosphate blood levels (Berndt & Kumar, 2007).

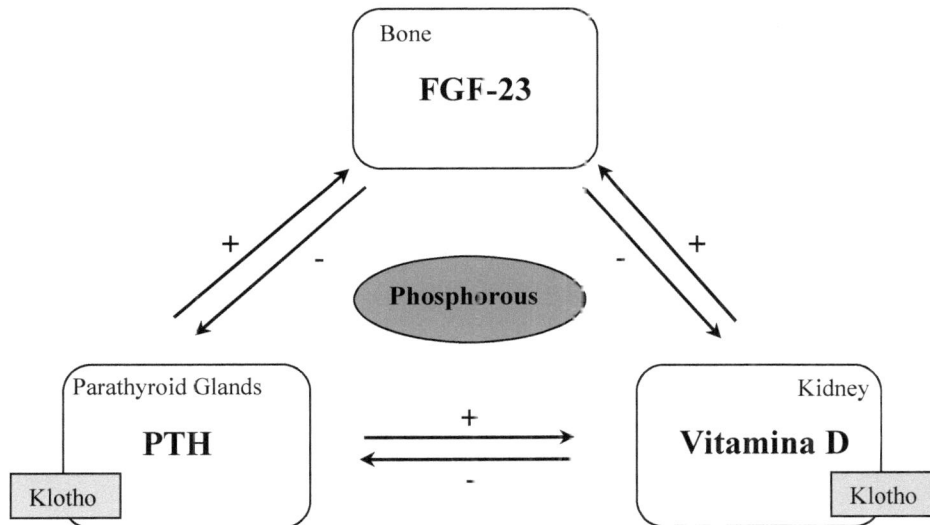

Figure 1: The physiological regulation of phosphorus serum levels is based on the interaction between vitamin D, PTH and FGF-23.

Thereby, variations in components of phosphate regulatory system traditionally associated with increased cardiovascular risk have been low calcitriol and high PTH levels (Foley, 1998a; Foley, 1998b). However, in addition to PTH and calcitriol, recent studies have identified a novel regulator of phosphate levels: FGF-23 (Block *et al*, 2004; Shimada *et al.*, 2001) which is actually considered the as the principal regulator of phosphatemia inducing phosphaturia and inhibiting calcitriol synthesis in the kidney, therefore maintaining systemic phosphate homeostasis. FGF-23 was first identified as the primary cause of two diseases characterized by phosphate-wasting syndromes originated by impaired renal phosphate reabsorption and low levels of calcitriol (Fukumoto *et al.*, 2007): autosomal dominant hypophosphatemic rickets (ADHR) (Consortium ADHR, 2000) and tumor-induced osteomalacia (TIO) (Shimada *et al.*, 2001), respectively. In contrast, low level of FGF-23 was identified as responsible of phosphate-retaining symptoms observed in patients with familial tumoral calcinosis (FTC) (Garringer *et al.*, 2006). These observations allowed the identification of FGF-23 as a critical factor in the physiological regulation of phosphate.

FGF-23, together with FGF-19 and FGF-21, belongs to the particular group of endocrine FGFs (Itoh, 2010), which are characterized by presenting low affinity for their FGF receptors (FGFRs), and the obligate requirement of a cofactor to bind and activate these receptors (Schlessinger *et al.*, 2000). Klotho protein is the cofactor implicated in the binding and activation of FGFRs by FGF-23. This explains why hyperphosphatemic phenotypes of Klotho-deficient mice are replicated in FGF-23-deficient mice (Razzaque & Lanske, 2006; Shimada *et al.*, 2004a). Organ-specific expression of Klotho restricts the activity of FGF-23 to few tissues including parathyroid glands, choroid plexus, renal distal tubules, and recently vascular tissue (Kuro-o *et al.*, 1997; Kuro-o, 2009a; Donate-Correa *et al.*, 2013; Lim *et al.*, 2012; Li *et al.*, 2004).

The *Klotho* gene was identified in a serendipitous experiment as a mutated gene in a mice strain that inherits a premature-ageing phenotypes including atherosclerosis, endothelial dysfunction, vascular calcification, hyperphosphatemia and shortened life span (Kuro-o *et al.*, 1997). The first clue to identify the putative cofactor required by FGF-23 for binding FGFRs came from verifying that the phenotypes of Klotho-deficient mice were replicated in FGF-23-deficient mice (Razzaque & Lanske, 2006), which not only were hyperphosphatemic, but also shared all the premature-ageing symptoms of Klotho-null mice (Shimada *et al.*, 2004a). This allowed to hypothesize a coordinated action of both factors to transmit the same signal pathway, explaining why mice lacking Klotho, FGF-23, or both exhibit identical phenotypes, as well as the insensibility of Klotho null mice to the high levels of FGF-23 present in this mutant (Nakatani *et al.*, 2009).

FGF-23 is secreted by osteocytes and osteoblasts in humans and mice in response to dietary phosphate intake to maintain phosphorus homeostasis (Kuro-o, 2009b; Antoniucci *et al.*, 2006). It acts increasing the renal phosphate excretion and inhibiting the calcitriol synthesis by reducing the traffic and/or expression of the sodium-phosphate cotransporters type 2 (Na/Pi-2a and Na/Pi-2c), responsible of phosphate reabsorption (Miyamoto *et al.*, 2004; Segawa *et al*, 2007; Segawa *et al.* 2003; Shimada *et al.*, 2004b; Kuro-o, 2010b), and decreasing renal activation of calcitriol, leading to a reduction in the intestinal absorption of phosphate (Liu *et al.*, 2006; Wang & Sun, 2009) (Figure 1).

GF-23 also inhibits the expression and production of PTH in parathyroid glands (Ben-Dov *et al.*, 2007; Krajisnik *et al.*, 2007). This results in lower PTH and calcitriol levels (since PTH also reduces renal calcitriol synthesis) and subsequently in a lesser phosphate absorption from gut and resorption from bone. The regulatory feedback loops among kidney, bone, and parathyroid glands is closed by the stimulatory effects exerted by calcitriol and PTH over FGF-23 expression and/or secretion in bone (Kuro-o, 2009a; Shimada *et al.*, 2004b; Saji *et al.*, 2009; Perwad *et al.*, 2005; López *et al.*, 2011) (Figure 1).

3   Emerging Role of Phosphorus as Predictor of Cardiorenal Progression Disease

Inorganic phosphate plays essential roles in every biological process since is an integral part of important compounds including nucleic acids, cyclic nucleotides, phospholipids, and the energy metabolism intermediates (Gaasbeek & Meinders, 2005). Although in humans almost all the phosphorous is found in bone and teeth, and only a low percentage exists as serum phosphate (Razzaque, 2009), the regulation of this percent is extremely important. This regulation is achieved balancing dietary absorption, bone formation, and renal excretion, as well as by equilibration with intracellular stores.

Disturbances in phosphorous homeostasis are involved in multiple physiopathologic mechanisms and clinical processes. Hypophosphatemia causes muscle weakness and circulatory collapse, whilst hyperphosphatemia is associated with endothelial apoptosis, vascular calcification and LVH, and constitutes a risk factor for cardiovascular mortality (Di Marco et al., 2008; Jono et al., 2000; Reynolds et al., 2004; Ellam & Chico, 2012; Ayus et al., 2005). Importantly, beyond those extreme pathological states, recent observational data have linked narrow variations in phosphate levels and, as will be discussed later, in phosphate-regulatory factors, with cardiovascular events and mortality (Kuro-o, 2010a; Block et al., 2004; Foley, 2009; Kestenbaum et al., 2005; Tonelli et al., 2005a; Parker et al., 2010; Mirza et al. 2009a,b,c; Adeney et al., 2009), suggesting a very intriguing link between phosphate and cardiovascular disease (Kuro-o, 2010a; Block et al., 2004; Shuto et al., 2009).

Although most of studies linking phosphate with cardiovascular risk and mortality have been carried out in CKD patients, in which phosphate overload and overt hyperphosphatemia are usual features (Palmer et al., 2011; Tentori et al., 2008; Block et al., 2004), increased serum phosphate within the normal range has also been associated with adverse clinical outcomes in individuals free of CKD and CVD in the community (Dhingra et al., 2007), in subjects with prior acute myocardial infarction and without impaired kidney function (Tonelli et al., 2005b), and in community-dwelling adults after adjusted for glomerular filtration rate (GFR) (Foley et al., 2008).

The pathophysiological basis of the increased cardiovascular risk linked to phosphorous is explained by subyacent vascular calcification (Shanahan et al., 2011), atherosclerosis (Ellam et al., 2011), endothelial dysfunction (Shuto et al., 2009), and LVH (Ayus et al., 2005).

In CKD patients, in whom hyperphosphatemia, low levels of calcitriol and secondary hyperparathiroidism (SHPT) are common features, FGF-23 serum levels are increased in early stages of CKD, even before serum phosphate, PTH concentrations or vitamin D levels had become abnormal (Isakova et al., 2011; Gutiérrez et al., 2005) (Figure 2).

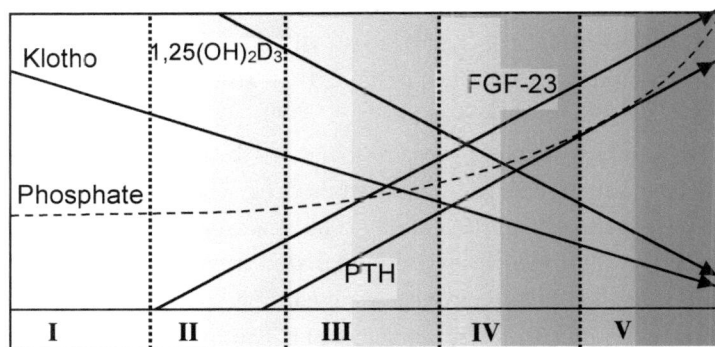

Figure 2: Variations in FGF-23, Klotho, PTH, Vitamin D, and phosphate levels during the progression of CKD. The first alteration is the decrease in Klotho expression, which provokes an increase in FGF-23 levels. FGF-23 lowers circulating vitamin D production in kidney which increases PTH expression. The resultant is an hyperphosphatemic, low calcitriol and high PTH state in late stages of CKD.

Diverse studies point to a progressive increase in FGF-23 as the renal function declines (Gutiérrez *et al.*, 2005; Larsson *et al.*, 2003). In dialysis patients, the raise can be up to 1000-fold higher than in healthy individuals (Larsson *et al.*, 2003). This elevation may reflect a compensatory response to maintain normal phosphatemia, which tend to increase when glomerular filtration rate (GFR) declines. An alternative hypothesis suggests that the increase of FGF-23 reflects an end-organ resistance to the phosphaturic stimulus of FGF-23 because of a deficiency in Klotho (Koh *et al.*, 2001). Similarly, it is also unknown if the raise in FGF-23 represents an increased secretion from bone, a decreased degradation, or both (Wolf, 2009).

4   Role of FGF-23 in Cardiorenal Disease as Biomarker. Findings from *in vitro/vivo* Studies and Observational Studies

Diverse association studies have revealed that FGF-23 is an independent predictor of survival and cardiovascular morbidity both in populations with (Gutiérrez *et al.*, 2008; Kanbay *et al.*, 2010; Isakova *et al.*, 2011) and without (Parker *et al.*, 2010; Mirza, Larsson *et al.*, 2009b; Mirza *et al.*, 2009c) kidney function impairment. It is noteworthy the stronger magnitude of the association between mortality and CVD with FGF-23 than that observed with serum phosphate. This has been reflected in several studies including the Heart and Soul Study, that comprises a cohort of heart disease patients with normal-kidney function (Parker *et al.*, 2010) which is not attenuated in early CKD patients when adjusting for serum phosphate (Gutiérrez *et al.*, 2008; Kanbay *et al.*, 2010; Isakova *et al.*, 2011).

These results have led to consider whether FGF-23 acts simply as a phosphate disarrangement biomarker or might directly targets the cardiovascular system. If this is true, it is plausible to think in FGF-23-mediated toxic actions in different organs, including the cardiovascular system.

Several clinical studies have determined the association between FGF-23 and the incidence of specific cardiovascular injuries and risk factors. A direct correlation between FGF-23 level and the presence of LVH has been reported in patients with advanced CKD (Gutiérrez *et al.*, 2009; Faul *et al.*, 2011) and in elderly population (Mirza *et al.*, 2009a). Likewise, other studies in CKD patients have reported the association between FGF-23 and vascular dysfunction (Mirza *et al.*, 2009b), atherosclerosis (Mirza *et al.*, 2009c), coronary artery calcifications (Morena *et al.*, 2012), and increased risk of mortality and cardiovascular events (Kanbay *et al.*, 2010; Kendrick *et al*, 2011) (Table 1).

A mechanism suggested to explain these associations by direct effects of FGF-23 is a Klotho-independent low-affinity binding to FGFRs, which would occur under conditions characterized by elevated FGF-23 concentrations, such as CKD (Yu *et al.*, 2005; Larsson *et al.*, 2003; Wang *et al.*, 2008). This possibility has been recently confirmed in experimental studies, where intravenous and intramyocardial administration of FGF-23 resulted in hypertrophy of rat cardiomyocites and LVH, demonstrating the role of FGF-23 in the pathogenesis of LVH (Faul *et al.*, 2011). These findings strongly suggests that a component of cardiovascular risk in CKD patients could be directly attributable to FGF-23 (Faul *et al.*, 2011), although this must be confirmed in further studies.

Variable	Study Population	Adverse outcome	References
Higher levels of FGF-23	General Population	Vascular dysfunction	Mirza et al., 2009b
	General Population	Atherosclerosis	Mirza et al., 2009c
	Elderly subjects	Increased risk for the presence of LVH	Mirza et al., 2009a
	CKD patients	Increased risk for the presence of LVH	Gutiérrez et al., 2009; Faul et al., 2011
	CKD patients	CAD extent	Kanbay et al., 2010; Morena et al., 2012
	CKD patients	Increased risk of mortality and cardiovascular events	Kendrick et al., 2011.
	Hemodialysis adult patients	Increased risk of mortality	Gutiérrez et al., 2008; Isakova et al., 2011
	Hemodialysis patients	Increased risk of mortality and vascular calcifications	Jean et al., 2009
	Patients with stable CAD	Increased risk of mortality and cardiovascular events	Parker et al., 2010
Klotho gene polymorphisms	General Population	Increased risk of coronary artery disease	Arking et al., 2003; Imamura et al., 2006; Jo et al., 2009; Rhee et al., 2006

Table 1: FGF-23 and KLOTHO human cardiovascular events related studies. CKD: Chronic kidney disease; LVH: left ventricular hypertrophy; CAD: coronary artery disease.

Concerning vascular damage, only a few studies have been designed to investigate the effects of FGF-23 on vessel integrity. The recent demonstration of the expression of FGFRs and Klotho in the human vascular wall (Donate-Correa et al., 2013; Lim et al., 2012), together with experimental studies showing that binding of FGF-23 to vascular wall FGFRs could, theoretically, generates adverse effects (Wolf, 2010), reinforce the possibility of a direct FGF-23 effect upon vascular wall.

Independently of the promiscuity of binding of FGF-23, effects on vascular tissue might include regulation of Na/P cotransporters PiT-1 and/or PiT-2 in a similar way to the inhibitory effect exerted over Na-Pi2a and 2c cotransporters in kidney. Even more, inhibitory effect on 1-alpha-hydroxylase, expressed by endothelial and VSMCs, might result in reduced local synthesis of vascular calcitriol, a hormone with a protective role against vascular diseases (Judd & Tangpricha, 2009).

Although additional research is needed to confirm the existence of this new action model on the vascular tissue and to examine its substantial clinical implications, strategies aimed to decrease elevated FGF-23 levels in CKD could emerge as a novel renal disease therapeutic approach. Proposed strategies would include phosphorus restriction (Saito et al., 2000), administration of phosphate binders (Oliveira et al., 2010; Koiwa et al, 2005), and even the use of specific antibodies directed against FGF-23 (Wolf, 2010).

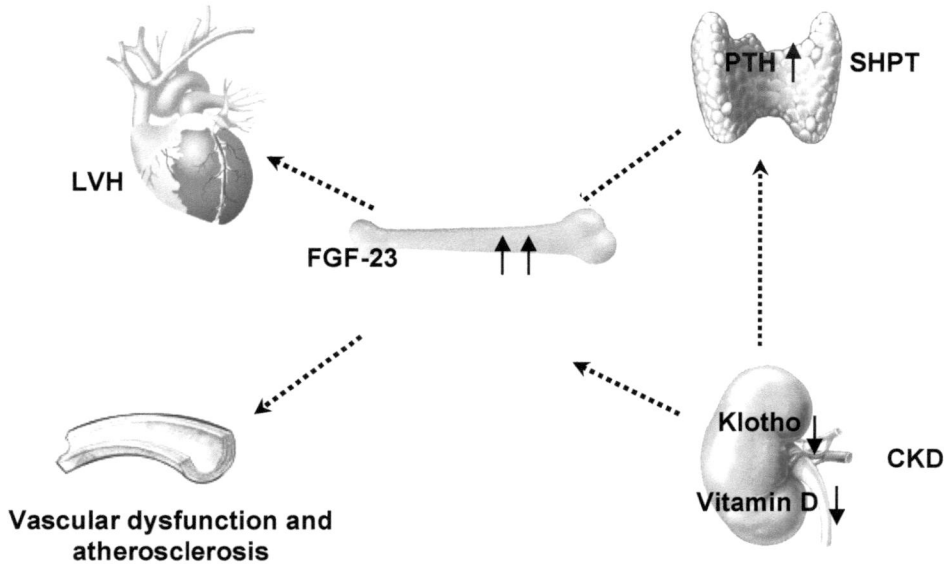

Figure 3: Under physiological conditions, the endocrine regulation of phosphate metabolism takes place by three different feedbacks: circulating vitamin D activates the FGF-23 promoter in bone. The secreted FGF-23 inactivates the production of vitamin D in kidney. On the contrary, PTH activates production of vitamin D. Finally, FGF-23 shuts off the PTH promoter in parathyroid glands. Pathologic processes derived from early-stage CKD are related with the increased secretion of FGF-23 from bone acting in the kidney, were Klotho is under-expressed, to maintain a neutral phosphate balance. This results in suppression of renal vitamin D production that triggers the early development of secondary hyperparathyroidism. The excess of FGF-23 is also associated to vascular dysfunctions, atherosclerosis and left ventricular hypertrophy (LVH).

5   Role of Circulating Klotho in Cardiorenal Disease as Biomarker and Therapeutic Factor

Research on Klotho has opened an extraordinary field because its implications in a multitude of biological processes, many of them related to human longevity. Klotho humam gene comprises 5 exons and encodes a single-pass transmembrane protein of 1012 amino acids with a large amino-terminal extracellular domain, consisting in two internal repeat sequences (KL1 and KL2), and two short membrane-spanning (21 amino acids) and intracellular carboxyl (11 amino acids) domains.

Soluble Klotho predominates in humans over the membrane form, declines with age (Xiao *et al.*, 2004) and can be generated through two different pathways: by an alternative Klotho mRNA splicing putatively encoding only the KL1 (Matsumura *et al.*, 1998) and by a proteolytic cleavage by membrane-anchored A Desintegrin and Metalloproteinases (ADAM)-17 and ADAM-10, that release the full-length extracellular domain into the extracellular space (Figure 4). This last processing could be important in the vessels since the gene expression level of ADAM-17 has been directly correlated with Klotho gene expression in human aortic thoracic samples (Donate-Correa *et al.*, 2013). Furthermore, the aminoacidic sequence between the repeats KL1 and KL2 (Lys-Lys-Arg-Lys) forms a potential site for proteolytic cleavage. Although these fragments are not detected in human serum and cerebrospinal fluid, the existence of the alternatively spliced KL1 transcript in urine should not be excluded and it would be interesting to determine whether these fragments have some biological properties.

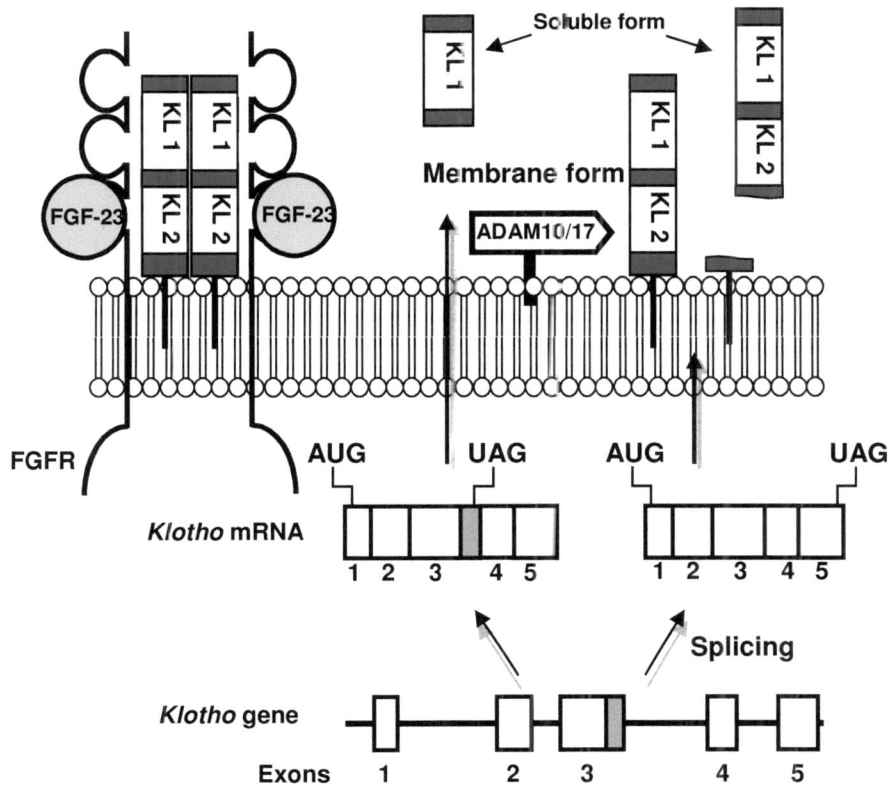

Figure 4: Representation of the complex formed by FGF-23, Klotho and the FGFRs in the cellular membrane. Alternative splicing of the mRNA generating the membrane and the soluble form (KL1) of Klotho and proteolytic cleavage by membrane proteinases that release the full-length extracellular domain into the extracellular space.

Although most part of the work with Klotho has been focused in its role as renal cofactor for the binding of FGF-23, the existence of a soluble form of Klotho and the expression of Klotho in the vascular tissue, allows consider this molecule as a novel circulating factor able to exert direct effects in multiple organs, including cardiovascular system. Klotho deficient-mice model shows a human-like aging syndrome that includes accelerated arteriosclerosis associated with extensive medial calcification of the aorta, and both medial calcification and intimal thickening of medium-sized muscular arteries (Saito et al, 2000). In addition, they exhibit impaired angiogenesis (Fukino *et al.*, 2002) and endothelial dysfunction (Saito *et al.*, 1998; Shiraki-Iida *et al.*, 2000) which can be ameliorated by in vivo gene delivery of the Klotho gene, by parabiosis with the Klotho wild type specimen (Saito *et al.*, 2000) or by administration of soluble Klotho which revert many age-related disorders (Chen *et al.*, 2013). Klotho deficient mice were also associated with higher phosphorous levels and severe calcification (Hu *et al.*, 2011).

Recent experimental studies confirm soluble Klotho protective effects upon vascular system. These effects include a role in maintaining endothelial wall homeostasis and in promoting the vascular health (Saito *et al.*, 2000; Saito *et al.*, 1998; Nagai *et al.*, 2000) triggering its absence endothelial dysfunction and vascular calcification in experimental models (Hu *et al.*, 2011; Nagai *et al.* 2000).

In addition, genetic variation studies have demonstrated that *Klotho* gene polymorphisms might be associated with longevity (Arking *et al.*, 2002) and coronary artery disease (CAD) (Arking *et al.*, 2003; Imamura *et al.,* 2006; Jo *et al.*, 2009; Rhee *et al.*, 2006) (Table 1). Although at least one of these variations influence to *Klotho* gene expression (Kawano *et al.*, 2002), the impact of serum levels of this protein on human coronary arteries remains to be clearly elucidated. Only one reported a decrease in the incidence of CAD with increasing tertile of plasma Klotho in older community-dwelling adults although this difference did not reach statistical significance (Semba *et al.*, 2011). CAD is mainly caused by established coronary arteriosclerosis derived from endothelial dysfunction which could be developed by low Klotho levels. Therefore, it has become evident the necessity to evaluate the contribution of endothelial protector serum Klotho to CAD risk.

Many vascular actions are proposed to explain Soluble Klotho vascular-protective activities. Endothelial protection could be due to a Klotho-mediated up-regulation of nitric oxide (NO) production in endothelial cells. This hormone besides acting as vasodilatador, prevents atherogenesis by suppressing VSMCs proliferation and by inhibiting adhesion molecules expression and platelet aggregation (Quyyumi *et al.*, 1998). *Klotho* gene deficiency reduces the capability of vasodilatation in aorta and arterioles of mice and attenuates the excretion of urinary nitric oxid metabolites (Saito *et al.*, 2000). This deficiency is reverted in parabiosis with wild-type mice and also by adenovirus-mediated Klotho gene delivery in the atherogenic model Otsuka Long-Evans Tokushima Fatty (OLETF) (Saito *et al.*, 1998), preventing adverse vascular remodelling.

Moreover, Klotho is also involved in the modulation of inflammation. In human umbilical vein endothelial cells (HUVECs), addition of recombinant Klotho suppresses TNFα-induced expression in the endothelium of adhesion molecules involved in the pathogenesis of vascular disease (Maekawa *et al.*, 2009).

On the other hand, it has been reported that soluble Klotho protein is able to binding to various Wnt family members, and that Wnt–Klotho interaction results in the suppression of Wnt biological activity (Liu *et al.*, 2007; Zhou *et al.*, 2013). This signal is essential for the proliferation and survival of stem cells, but continuous Wnt exposure may contribute to exhaustation and depletion, as well as accelerated cellular senescence (Kirstetter *et al.*, 2006). Klotho-mediated attenuation of Wnt signalling could contribute to the anti-ageing properties of Klotho by avoiding the continuous activation of Wnt signalling and the senescence of stem cells (Kuro-o, 2010b) and eliciting renoprotective effects (Zhou *et al.*, 2013).

Experimental studies show that calcitriol administration promotes expression of Klotho via the activation of vitamin D receptor (Tsujikawa *et al.*, 2003; Forster *et al.*, 2011). A recent work has demonstrated that administration of alfacalcidol, a vitamin D receptor activator, promoted an up regulation of Klotho gene expression in the kidney of nephrectomized spontaneously hypertensive rats (Fukui *et al.*, 2011). According this, Klotho variants associated with lower Klotho gene expression have been associated with a decrease in survival of dialysis patients, more pronounced among patients not treated with active forms of vitamin D (Friedman *et al.*, 2009).

Additionally, Klotho is also able to inhibit vascular calcification. As FGF-23 does in Kidney, soluble Klotho inhibits Na/Pi-2a and Na/Pi-2c, and also the Na/Pi cotransporters type 3 (Na/Pi-3 also known as Pit 1 and Pit 2) (Hu *et al.*, 2011; Hu *et al.*, 2010). These last two are widely expressed in tissues such as intestinal epithelium, liver, lung, heart and smooth muscle cells (Jono *et al.*, 2000; Kakita *et al.*, 2004; Okuda *et al.*, 2006). The addition of recombinant soluble Klotho protein to VSMCs cultures is able to decrease high Pi-induced calcification by diminishing expression of Na/Pi-3 cotransporters (Hu *et al.*, 2011). Secreted renal and/or vascular soluble Klotho might protect against vascular calcification through this inhibition of Na/Pi-3 expression.

Since soluble Klotho decreases at early CKD stages (Pavik *et al.*, 2013; Shimamura *et al.*, 2012), the utility of soluble Klotho as a biomarker CKD progression has been sugested. Diverse diverse observational studies that relate low circulating or urinary klotho levels with adverse kidney disease outcome (Kim *et al.*, 2013; Kitagawa *et al.*, 2013; Akimoto *et al.*, 2012; Satoh *et al.*, 2012). More data from larger prospective longitudinal studies are required to validate this possibility. Similarly, some studies suggest that administration of Klotho may have therapeutic possibilities in treating renal disease (Mitani *et al.*, 2002).

6   Utility of FGF-23 and Klotho as Biomarkers in the Clinical Practice

The recent discovery of the FGF-23/Klotho system has provided potentially reliable biomarkers with clinical utility especially in patients with kidney disease. But their potential utility seems to trascend the field of renal failure, and cover areas such as cardiovascular disease. However, several important obstacles must be overcome in order to include these molecules as reliable biomarkers in clinical practice.

Although several assay kits measure circulating FGF-23 in the intact form (iFGF-23) alone or both intact and the carboxi-terminal fragment (cFGF-23) product of degradation, it is unclear if all the assays provides comparable sensitivity for patients with different stages of renal function. Some studies suggest that measurements of iFGF-23 rather than cFGF-23 may be more physiologically relevant, whereas other works show significant associations only with cFGF-23. However, a recent clinical study has demostrated that virtually all detectable FGF-23 is in the active form, and thus, measurements obtained with iFGF-23 and cFGF-23 assays would reflect the same circulating moiety (Shimada *et al.*, 2010). Additional studies are needed to determine whether this occurs regardless of kidney function and if this value can be a marker of cardiovascular risk in the renal patient.

The potential use of this protein as a biomarker has originated a great interest in developing automated methods to improve the performance of the FGF-23 immunoassays overcoming the limitations of the ELISA kits. A new automated chemiluminiscence immunoassay has been recently developed to measure intact and cFGF-23 concentrations (Shimizu *et al.*, 2012). However, current assays should be evaluated and standardized more rigorously and further studies are also needed to establish clearly the influence of preanalytical factors. Moreover, population-based studies focused on defining clear cutoff values for clinical risk assessment are scarce. Furthermore, some are referred to specific assays and overlook variables which could alter the measures, so the utility is limited. Before its introduction in the clinical practice, we should get more robust reference values and establish and validate the recommended cutoff for treatment targets.

In contrast to FGF-23, studies that explore the relationships between human sKlotho levels and diverse cardiovascular clinical phenotypes are scarce due to the lack, until recently, of a reliable assay for measuring this protein (Yamazaki *et al.*, 2010). Paradoxically, although Klotho protein is expressed mainly in the kidney, renal investigators only have fixed their attention on this protein in recent years. Some of these works have been focused on the potential utilization of Klotho as a biomarker in CKD with prognostic and diagnostic capabilities.

Soluble Klotho is subjected to diurnal variations decreasing to their circadian nadir at midnight and a maximum in the early morning (Carpenter *et al.*, 2010). Although the physiological significance of this pattern is unknown, it should be taken into account for drawing blood and urine samples. Similarly, it has also been reported a negative relationships between Klotho levels and age in healthy volunteers (Yamazaki *et al.*, 2010) in patients with X-linked hypophasphataemia (Carpenter *et al.*, 2010), and in children with CKD (Wan *et al.*, 2013). There were no apparent differences regarding gender. However, much further research is needed to validate and standardize this biomarker in the translational arena, including studies to define reference values and measure its biological variability.

Currently, the human database for Klotho is scarce and is expected that the number of human studies will be increased in the very near future. Larger cohorts are needed and, more importantly, validate in different cardiovascular and renal injuries stages the ELISA kit currently employed by most of the studies.

7   Conclusion and Future Prospects

Nowadays, the major interest to the clinical application of FGF-23/Klotho research is related to CKD. Increased phosphate levels associated to reduced renal function in these patients has been related to progression of cardiovascular complications and enhanced morbi-mortality. However, serum phosphate level remains normal until advanced reduction in renal function, and in addition, the magnitude of its association with deleterious effects within the physiological range is very small (Kestenbaum *et al.*, 2005; Tonelli *et al.*, 2005a; Dhingra *et al.*, 2007) unlike increases in FGF-23 and decreases in Klotho, which have been linked with cardiovascular morbidity and mortality independently of phosphatemia (Kuro-o, 2010b; Block *et al.*, 2004; Kestenbaum *et al.*, 2005; Tonelli *et al.*, 2005a; Gaasbeek *et al.*, 2005; Razzaque, 2009). Importantly, these association remains in population without impaired kidney function.

Further studies are necessary to clarify the regulatory mechanisms controlling FGF-23 and Klotho expression and to evaluate the potential translation to the clinical setting. Another potential therapeutic option could be directed to elevation of Klotho levels. Although results depicted in this chapter clearly point to Klotho as a potential therapeutic agent in mineral-cardiovascular disorders, further studies are needed to evaluate the reliability and practical utility of this protein. In example, relationships between circulating Klotho and many clinical phenotypes in which this protein could be involved has not been extensively studied because of the scarce clinical studies measuring blood soluble Klotho in humans.

Finally, many questions about the direct effect of FGF-23 on CVD have emerged. For example, it is not clear if human hereditary hypophosphatemic rickets, caused by high FGF-23 systemic levels, is accompanied by increased atherosclerosis (Ellam *et al.*, 2012). Similarly, overexpression of FGF-23 in mice is not associated with adverse cardiovascular effects when hypophosphatemia is corrected through changes in diet (Ellam *et al.*, 2012; Liu *et al*, 2009). However, a possible explanation for this is the reported absence (Lim *et al.*, 2012), unlike humans, of Klotho expression in rat VSMCs.

Another open question is the elucidation of the contribution of soluble vascular Klotho in advanced stages of CKD, where low serum Klotho levels are frequent. It is unknown if vascular expression is also lowered in this states or remains physiologic levels. Anyway, it is probably that vascular derived Klotho plays a more important role in these patients since renal contribution is dramatically diminished.

FGF-23 and Klotho are emerging as unprecedented biomarkers for, but no exclusively, nephrologists. However, there is a long way to go in which FGF-23 and Klotho will have to prove its usefulness in the early diagnosis and its prognostic value.

References

Adeney K. L., Siscovick D. S., Ix J. H., Seliger S. L., Shlipak M. G., Jenny N. S. & Kestenbaum B.R. (2009). Association of serum phosphate with vascular and valvular calcification in moderate CKD. Journal of the American Society of Nephrology, 20, 381-387.

Akimoto T., Yoshizawa H., Watanabe Y., Numata A., Yamazaki T., Takeshima E., Iwazu K., Komada T., Otani N., Morishita Y., Ito C., Shiizaki K., Ando Y., Muto S., Kuro-o M. & Kusano E. (2012). Characteristics of urinary and serum soluble Klotho protein in patients with different degrees of chronic kidney disease. BMC Nephrology, 13, 155.

Antoniucci D. M. , Yamashita T. & Portale A. A. (2006). Dietary phosphorus regulates serum fibroblast growth factor-23 concentrations in healthy men. Journal of Clinical Endocrinology and Metabolism, 91, 3144-3149.

Arking D. E., Becker D. M., Yanek L. R., Fallin D., Judge D. P., Moy T. F., Becker L. C. & Dietz H. C. (2003). KLOTHO allele status and the risk of early-onset occult coronary artery disease. American Journal of Human Genetics, 72, 1154-1161.

Arking D. E., Krebsova A., Macek M. Sr., Macek M. Jr., Arking A., Mian I. S., Fried L., Hamosh A., Dey S., McIntosh I. & Dietz H. C. (2002). Association of human aging with a functional variant of klotho. Proceedings of the National Academy of Sciences of the United States of America, 99, 856-861

Ayus J. C., Mizani M. R., Achinger S. G., Thadhani R., Go A. S. & Lee S. (2005). Effects of short daily versus conventional hemodialysis on left ventricular hypertrophy and inflammatory markers: a prospective, controlled study. Journal of the American Society of Nephrology, 16, 2778-2788.

Ben-Dov I. Z., Galitzer H., Lavi-Moshayoff V., Goetz R., Kuro-o M., Mohammadi M., Sirkis R., Naveh-Many T. & Silver J. (2007). The parathyroid is a target organ for FGF23 in rats. Journal of Clinical Investigations, 117, 4003–4008.

Berndt T. & Kumar R. (2009). Novel mechanisms in the regulation of phosphorus homeostasis. Physiology, 24, 17–25.

Berndt T. & Kumar R. (2007). Phosphatonins and the regulation of phosphate homeostasis. Annual Review of Physiology, 69, 341–359.

Block G.A., Klassen P. S., Lazarus J. M., Ofsthun N., Lowrie E. G. & Chertow G. M. (2004). Mineral metabolism, mortality, and morbidity in maintenance hemodialysis. Journal of the American Society of Nephrology, 15, 2208–2218

Carpenter T. O., Insogna K. L., Zhang J. H., Ellis B., Niemen S., Simpson C., Olear E. & Gundberg C. M. (2010). Circulating levels of soluble klotho and FGF23 in X-linked hypophosphatemia: circadian variance, effects of treatment, and relationship to parathyroid status. The Journal of Clinical Endocrinology and Metabolism, 95, 352-357.

Chen C. D., Podvin S., Gillespie E., Leeman S. E. & Abrahem C. R. (2007). Insulin stimulates the cleavage and release of the extracellular domain of Klotho by ADAM10 and ADAM17. Proceedings of the National Academy of Sciences of the United States of America, 104, 19796–19801.

Chen T. H., Kuro-O M., Chen C. H., Sue Y. M., Chen Y. C., Wu H. H. & Cheng C. Y. (2013). The secreted Klotho protein restores phosphate retention and suppresses accelerated aging in Klotho mutant mice. European Journal of Pharmacology, 698, 67-73.

Consortium ADHR. Autosomal dominant hypophosphataemic rickets is associated with mutations in FGF23. (2000). Nature Genetics, 26, 345–348.

Dhingra R., Sullivan L. M., Fox C. S., Wang T. J., D'Agostino R. B. Sr., Gaziano J. M. & Vasan R. S. (2007). Relations of serum phosphorus and calcium levels to the incidence of cardiovascular disease in the community. Archives of Internal Medicine, 167, 879-885.

Di Marco G. S., Hausberg M., Hillebrand U., Rustemeyer P., Wittkowski W., Lang D. & Pavenstädt H. (2008). Increased inorganic phosphate induces human endothelial cell apoptosis in vitro. American Journal of Physiology. Renal Physiology, 294, 1381-1387.

Donate-Correa J., Mora-Fernández C., Martínez-Sanz R., Muros-de-Fuentes M., Pérez H., Meneses-Pérez B., Cazaña-Pérez V. & Navarro-González J. F. (2013). Expression of FGF23/KLOTHO system in human vascular tissue. International Journal of Cardiology, 165, 179–183.

Donate-Correa J., Muros-de-Fuentes M., Mora-Fernández C. & Navarro-González J. F. (2012). FGF23/Klotho axis: phosphorus, mineral metabolism and beyond. Cytokine and Growth Factor Reviews, 23, 37-46.

Dusso A. S., Brown A. J. & Slatopolsky E. (2005). Vitamin D. American Journal of Physiology. Renal Physiology, 289, 8–28.

Ellam T., Wilkie M., Chamberlain J., Crossman D., Eastell R., Francis S. & Chico T. J. (2011). Dietary phosphate modulates atherogenesis and insulin resistance in apolipoprotein E knockout mice--brief report. Arteriosclerosis Thrombosis and Vascular Biology, 31, 1988-1990.

Ellam T. J. & Chico T. J. (2012). Phosphate: the new cholesterol? The role of the phosphate axis in non-uremic vascular disease. Atherosclerosis, 220, 310-318.

Faul C., Amaral A. P., Oskouei B., Hu M. C., Sloan A., Isakova T., Gutiérrez O. M., Aguillon-Prada R., Lincoln J., Hare J. M., Mundel P., Morales A., Scialla J., Fischer M., Soliman E. Z., Chen J., Go A. S., Rosas S. E., Nessel L., Townsend R. R., Feldman H. I., St John Sutton M. , Ojo A., Gadegbeku C., Di Marco G. S., Reuter S., Kentrup D., Tiemann K., Brand M., Hill J. A., Moe O. W., Kuro-O M., Kusek J. W., Keane M. G. & Wolf M. (2011). FGF23 induces left ventricular hypertrophy. Journal of Clinical Investigations, 121, 4393–4408.

Foley R. N., Collins A. J., Ishani A. & Kalra P. A. (2008). Calcium-phosphate levels and cardiovascular disease in community-dwelling adults: the Atherosclerosis Risk in Communities (ARIC) Study. American Heart Journal, 156, 556-63.

Foley R. N., Parfrey P. S. & Sarnak M. J. (1998)a. Clinical epidemiology of cardiovascular disease in chronic renal disease. American Journal of Kidney Diseases, 32:112–119.

Foley R. N., Parfrey P. S. & Sarnak M. J. (1998)b. Epidemiology of cardiovascular disease in chronic renal disease. Journal of the American Society of Nephrology, 9, 16–23.

Foley R. N. (2009). Phosphate levels and cardiovascular disease in the general population. Clinical Journal of the American Society of Nephrology, 4, 1136–1139.

Forster R. E., Jurutka P. W., Hsieh J. C., Haussler C. A., Lowmiller C. L., Kaneko I., Haussler M. R. & Kerr Whitfield G. (2011). Vitamin D receptor controls expression of the anti-aging klotho gene in mouse and human renal cells. Biochemichal and Biophysical Research Communications, 414, 557–562.

Friedman D. J., Afkarian M., Tamez H., Bhan I., Isakova T., Wolf M., Ankers E., Ye J., Tonelli M., Zoccali C., Kuro-o M., Moe O., Karumanchi S. A. & Thadhani R. (2009). Klotho variants and chronic hemodialysis mortality. Journal of Bone Mineral Research, 24, 1847-1855.

Fukino K., Suzuki T., Saito Y., Shindo T., Amaki T., Kurabayashi M. & Nagai R. (2002). Regulation of angiogenesis by the aging suppressor gene klotho. Biochemichal and Biophysical Research Communications, 293, 332-337.

Fukui T., Munemura C., Maeta S., Ishida C. & Murawaki Y. (2011). The effects of olmesartan and alfacalcidol on renopro-

tection and klotho gene expression in 5/6 nephrectomized spontaneously hypertensive rats. Yonago Actamedica, 54, 49–58

Fukumoto S. & Yamashita T. (2007). FGF23 is a hormone-regulating phosphate metabolism—unique biological characteristics of FGF23. Bone, 40, 1190–1195.

Gaasbeek A. & Meinders A. E. (2005). Hypophosphatemia: an update on its etiology and treatment. American Journal of Medicine, 118, 1094–1101.

Garringer HJ, Fisher C, Larsson TE, et al. The role of mutant UDF-N-acetyl-alpha-D-galactosamine-polypeptide N-acetylgalactosaminyltransferase 3 in regulating serum intact fibroblast growth factor 23 and matrix extracellular phosphoglycoprotein in heritable tumoral calcinosis. The Journal of Clinical Endocrinology and Metabolism, 91, 4037–4042.

Garringer H. J., Fisher C., Larsson T. E., Davis S. I., Koller D. L., Cullen M. J., Draman M. S., Conlon N., Jain A., Fedarko N. S., Dasgupta B., White K. E. (2006). Fibroblast growth factor-23 mitigates hyperphosphatemia but accentuates calcitriol deficiency in chronic kidney disease. Journal of the American Society of Nephrology, 16, 2205–22015.

Gutiérrez O. M., Januzzi J. L., Isakova T., Laliberte K., Smith K., Collerone G., Sarwar A., Hoffmann U., Coglianese E., Christenson R., Wang T. J., deFilippi C. & Wolf M. (2009). Fibroblast growth factor 23 and left ventricular hypertrophy in chronic kidney disease. Circulation, 119, 2545-2452.

Gutiérrez O. M., Mannstadt M., Isakova T., Rauh-Hain J. A., Tamez H., Shah A., Smith K., Lee H., Thadhani R., Jüppner H. & Wolf M. (2008). Fibroblast growth factor 23 and mortality among patients undergoing hemodialysis. The New England Journal of Medicine, 359, 584-592.

Hu M. C., Shi M., Zhang J., Quiñones H., Griffith C., Kuro-o M. & Moe O. W. (2011). Klotho deficiency causes vascular calcification in chronic kidney disease. Journal of the American Society of Nephrology, 22:124-136.

Hu M. C., Shi M., Zhang J., Pastor J., Nakatani T., Lanske B., Razzaque M. S., Rosenblatt K. P., Baum M. G., Kuro-o M. & Moe O. W. (2010). Klotho: a novel phosphaturic substance acting as an autocrine enzyme in the renal proximal tubule. FASEB Journal, 24, 3438–3450.

Imamura A., Okumura K., Ogawa Y., Murakami R., Torigoe M., Numaguchi Y. & Murohara T. (2006). Klotho gene polymorphism may be a genetic risk factor for atherosclerotic coronary artery disease but not for vasospastic angina in Japanese. Clinica Chimica Acta, 371, 66-70.

Isakova T., Xie H., Yang W., Xie D., Anderson A. H., Scialla J., Wahl P., Gutiérrez O. M., Steigerwalt S., He J., Schwartz S., Lo J., Ojo A., Sondheimer J., Hsu C. Y., Lash J., Leonard M., Kusek J. W., Feldman H. I. & Wolf M; Chronic Renal Insufficiency Cohort (CRIC) Study Group. (2011). Fibroblast growth factor 23 and risks of mortality and end-stage renal disease in patients with chronic kidney disease. JAMA, 305, 2432-2439.

Itoh N. (2010) Hormone-like (endocrine) Fgfs: their evolutionary history and roles in development, metabolism, and disease. Cell Tissue Research, 342, 1–11.

Jean G., Terrat J. C., Vanel T., Hurot J. M., Lorriaux C., Mayor B. & Chazot C. (2009). High levels of serum fibroblast growth factor (FGF)-23 are associated with increased mortality in long haemodialysis patients. Nephrology, Dialysis, Transplantation, 24, 2792–2796.

Jo S. H., Kim S. G., Choi Y. J., Joo N. R., Cho G. Y., Choi S. R., Kim E. J., Kim H. S., Kim H. J., Rhim C. Y. (2009). KLOTHO gene polymorphism is associated with coronary artery stenosis but not with coronary calcification in a Korean population. Interantional Heart Journal, 50, 23-32.

Jono S., McKee M. D., Murry C. E., Shioi A., Nishizawa Y., Mori K., Morii H. & Giachelli C. M. (2000). Phosphate regulation of vascular smooth muscle cell calcification. Circulation Research, 87, 10–17.

Judd S. E. & Tangpricha V. (2009). Vitamin D deficiency and risk for cardiovascular disease. The American Journal of Medical Sciences, 338, 40–44.

Kakita A., Suzuki A., Nishiwaki K., Ono Y., Kotake M., Ariyoshi Y., Miura Y., Ltoh M. & Oiso Y. (2004). Stimulation of Na-dependent phosphate transport by platelet-derived growth factor in rat aortic smooth muscle cells. Atherosclerosis,

174, 17–24.

Kanbay M., Nicoleta M., Selcoki Y., Ikizek M., Aydin M., Eryonucu B., Duranay M., Akcay A., Armutcu F. & Covic A. (2010). Fibroblast growth factor 23 and fetuin A are independent predictors for the coronary artery disease extent in mild chronic kidney disease. Clinical Journal of the American Society of Nephrology, 5, 1780–1786.

Kawano K., Ogata N., Chiano M., Molloy H., Kleyn P., Spector T. D., Uchida M., Hosoi T., Suzuki T., Orimo H., Inoue S., Nabeshima Y., Nakamura K., Kuro-o M. & Kawaguchi H. (2002). Klotho gene polymorphisms associated with bone density of aged postmenopausal women. Journal of Bone and Mineral Research, 17, 1744-1751.

Kendrick J., Cheung A. K., Kaufman J. S., Greene T., Roberts W. L., Smits G., Chonchol M. & HOST Investigators. (2011). FGF-23 associates with death, cardiovascular events, and initiation of chronic dialysis. Journal of the American Society of Nephrology, 22, 1913–1922.

Kestenbaum B., Sampson J. N., Rudser K. D., Patterson D. J., Seliger S. L., Young B., Sherrard D. J. & Andress D. L. (2005). Serum phosphate levels and mortality risk among people with chronic kidney disease. Journal of the American Society of Nephrology, 16, 520–528.

Kim H. R., Nam B. Y., Kim D. W., Kang M. W., Han J. H., Lee M. J., Shin D. H., Doh F. M., Koo H. M., Ko K. I., Kim C. H., Oh H. J., Yoo T. H., Kang S. W., Han D. S. & Han S. H. (2013). Circulating α-klotho levels in CKD and relationship to progression. American Journal of Kidney Disease, 61, 899-909.

Kirstetter P., Anderson K., Porse B. T., Jacobsen S. E. & Nerlov C. (2006). Activation of the canonicalWnt pathway leads to loss of hematopoietic stem cell repopulation and multilineage differentiation block. Nature Immunology, 7, 1048–1056.

Kitagawa M., Sugiyama H., Morinaga H., Inoue T., Takiue K., Ogawa A., Yamanari T., Kikumoto Y., Uchida H. A., Kitamura S., Maeshima Y., Nakamura K., Ito H. & Makino H. (2013). A decreased level of serum soluble Klotho is an independent biomarker associated with arterial stiffness in patients with chronic kidney disease. PLoS One, 8, e56695.

Koh N., Fujimori T., Nishiguchi S., Tamori A., Shiomi S., Nakatani T., Sugimura K., Kishimoto T., Kinoshita S., Kuroki T., Nabeshima Y. (2001). Severely reduced production of klotho in human chronic renal failure kidney. Biochemical and Biophysical Research Communications, 280, 1015–1020.

Koiwa F., Kazama J. J., Tokumoto A., Onoda N., Kato H., Okada T., Nii-Kono T., Fukagawa M., Shigematsu T. & ROD21 Clinical Research Group. (2005). Sevelamer hydrochloride and calcium bicarbonate reduce serum fibroblast growth factor 23 levels in dialysis patients. Therapeutic Apheresis and Dialysis, 9, 336–339.

Krajisnik T., Björklund P., Marsell R., Ljunggren O., Akerström G., Jonsson K. B., Westin G. & Larsson T. E. (2007). Fibroblast growth factor-23 regulates parathyroid hormone and 1alphahydroxylase expression in cultured bovine parathyroid cells. The Journal of Endocrinology, 195, 125–131.

Kuro- o M. (2010)a. Phosphate and Klotho. Kidney International Supplement, 121, 20–233.

Kuro-o M., Matsumura Y., Aizawa H., Kawaguchi H., Suga T., Utsugi T., Ohyama Y., Kurabayashi M., Kaname T., Kume E., Iwasaki H., Iida A., Shiraki-Iida T., Nishikawa S., Nagai R. & Nabeshima YI. (1997). Mutation of the mouse klotho gene leads to a syndrome resembling ageing. Nature, 390, 45–51.

Kuro-o M. (2010)b. A potential link between phosphate and aging—lessons from Klotho-deficient mice. Mechanisms of Ageing and Development, 131, 270–275.

Kuro-o M. (2008). Endocrine FGFs and Klothos: emerging concepts. Trends in Endocrinology and Metabolism, 19, 239–245.

Kuro-o M. (2009)a. Klotho and aging. Biochimica et Biophysica Acta, 1790, 1049–1058.

Kuro-o M. (2009)b Klotho in chronic kidney disease—what's new? Nephrology, Dialysis and Transplantation, 24, 1705–1708.

Kuro-o M. (2010)c Klotho. Pflugers Archives, 459, 333–343.

Kurosu H., Ogawa Y., Miyoshi M., Yamamoto M., Nandi A., Rosenblatt K. P., Baum M. G., Schiavi S., Hu M. C., Moe O. W. & Kuro-o M. (2006). Regulation of fibroblast growth factor-23 signaling by klotho. The Journal of Biological Chemistry, 281, 6120–6123.

Kurosu H., Yamamoto M., Clark J. D., Pastor J. V., Nandi A., Gurnani P., McGuinness O. P., Chikuda H., Yamaguchi M., Kawaguchi H., Shimomura I., Takayama Y., Herz J., Kahn C. R., Rosenblatt K. P. & Kuro-o M. (2005). Suppression of aging in mice by the hormone Klotho. Science, 309, 1829–1833.

Larsson T., Nisbeth U., Ljunggren O., Juppner H. & Jonsson K. B. (2003). Circulating concentration of FGF-23 increases as renal function declines in patients with chronic kidney disease, but does not change in response to variation in phosphate intake in healthy volunteers. Kidney International, 64, 2272–2279.

Levin A., Bakris G.L., Molitch M., Smulders M., Tian J., Williams L. A. & Andress D. L. (2007). Prevalence of abnormal serum vitamin D PTH, calcium, and phosphorus in patients with chronic kidney disease: results of the study to evaluate early kidney disease. Kidney International, 71, 31–38.

Li SA, Watanabe M., Yamada H., Nagai A., Kinuta M.& Takei K. (2004). Immunohistochemical localization of Klotho protein in brain, kidney, and reproductive organs of mice Cell Structure and Function, 29, 91–99.

Lim K., Lu T. S., Molostvov G., Lee C., Lam F. T., Zehnder D & Hsiao L.L. (2012). Vascular Klotho Deficiency Potentiates the Development of Human Artery Calcification and Mediates Resistance to FGF-23. Circulation, 125. 2243-2255.

Liu H., Fergusson M. M., Castilho R. M., Liu J., Cao L., Chen J., Malide D., Rovira I. I., Schimel D., Kuo C. J., Gutkind J. S., Hwang P. M. & Finkel T. (2007). Augmented Wnt signaling in a mammalian model of accelerated aging. Science, 317, 803–806.

Liu P, Bai X, Wang H, Karaplis A, Goltzman D, Miao D. Hypophosphatemia-mediated hypotension in transgenic mice overexpressing human FGF-23. Am J Physiol Heart Circ Physiol 2009;297:1514-20.

Liu S., Tang W., Zhou J., Stubbs J. R., Luo Q., Pi M. & Quarles L. D. (2006). Fibroblast growth factor 23 is a counter-regulatory phosphaturic hormone for vitamin D. Journal of the American Society of Nephrology, 17, 1305–1315.

López I., Rodríguez-Ortiz M. E., Almadén Y., Guerrero F., de Oca A. M. Pineda C., Shalhoub V., Rodríguez M. & Aguilera-Tejero E. (2011). Direct and indirect effects of parathyroid hormone on circulating levels of fibroblast growth factor 23 in vivo. Kidney International, 80, 475–482.

Maekawa Y., Ishikawa K., Yasuda O., Oguro R., Hanasaki H., Kida I., Takemura Y., Ohishi M., Katsuya T. & Rakugi H. (2009). Klotho suppresses TNF-alpha-induced expression of adhesion molecules in the endothelium and attenuates NF-kappaB activation. Endocrine, 35, 341-346.

Matsumura Y., Aizawa H., Shiraki-Iida T., Nagai R., Kuro-o M. & Nabeshima Y. (1998). Identification of the human klotho gene and its two transcripts encoding membrane and Soluble klotho protein. Biochemical and Biophysical Research Communications, 242, 626–630.

Mirza M. A., Hansen T., Johansson L., Ahlström H., Larsson A., Lind L., Larsson T. E. (2009)c. Relationship between circulating FGF23 and total body atherosclerosis in the community. Nephrology, Dialysis, Transplantation, 24, 3125–3131.

Mirza M. A., Larsson A., Lind L., Larsson T. E. (2009)b. Circulating fibroblast growth factor- 23 is associated with vascular dysfunction in the community. Atherosclerosis, 205, 385–390.

Mirza M. A., Larsson A., Melhus H., Lind L., Larsson T. E. (2009)a. Serum intact FGF23 associate with left ventricular mass, hypertrophy and geometry in an elderly population. Atherosclerosis, 207, 546–551.

Mitani H., Ishizaka N., Aizawa T., Ohno M., Usui S., Suzuki T., Amaki T., Mori I., Nakamura Y., Sato M., Nangaku M., Hirata Y. & Nagai R. (2002). In vivo klotho gene transfer ameliorates angiotensin II-induced renal damage. Hypertension, 39, 838-3843.

Miyamoto K., Segawa H., Ito M. & Kuwahata M. (2004). Physiological regulation of renal sodium-dependent phosphate cotransporters. The Japanese Jurnal of Physiology, 54, 93–102.

Morena M., Jaussent I., Halkovich A., Dupuy A. M., Bargnoux A. S., Chenine L., Leray-Moragues H., Klouche K., Vernhet H., Canaud B. & Cristol J. P. (2012). Bone biomarkers help grading severity of coronary calcifications in non dialysis chronic kidney disease patients. PLoS One, 7, e36175.

Moreno J.A., Izquierdo M. C., Sanchez-Niño M. D., Suárez-Alvarez B., Lopez-Larrea C., Jakubowski A., Blanco J., Ramirez R., Selgas R., Ruiz-Ortega M., Egido J., Ortiz A. & Sanz A. B. (2011). The inflammatory cytokines TWEAK and TNFα reduce renal klotho expression through NFκB. Journal of the American Society of Nephrology, 22, 1315-1325

Nagai R., Saito Y., Ohyama Y., Aizawa H., Suga T., Nakamura T., Kurabayashi M. & Kuroo M. (2000). Endothelial dysfunction in the klotho mouse and downregulation of klotho gene expression in various animal models of vascular and metabolic diseases. Cellular and Mollecular Life Sciences, 57, 738-746.

Nakanishi S., Kazama J. J., Nii-Kono T., Omori K., Yamashita T., Fukumoto S., Gejyo F., Shigematsu T. & Fukagawa M. (2005). Serum fibroblast growth factor-23 levels predict the future refractory hyperparathyroidism in dialysis patients. Kidney International, 67, 1171–1178

Nakatani T., Sarraj B., Ohnishi M., Densmore M. J., Taguchi T., Goetz R., Mohammadi M., Lanske B., & Razzaque M. S. (2009). In vivo genetic evidence for klotho-dependent, fibroblast growth factor 23 (Fgf23)-mediated regulation of systemic phosphate homeostasis. FASEB Journal, 23, 433–441.

Okuda I., Maruno H., Kohno T., Yamase H., Mori K. & Kokubo T. (2006). Evaluation of imaging before lung volume reduction surgery for pulmonary emphysema; fused image of multi-detector row computed tomography and scintigram. Kyobu Geka, 59, 197–203.

Oliveira R. B., Cancela A. L., Graciolli F. G., Dos Reis L. M., Draibe S. A., Cuppari L., Carvalho A. B., Jorgetti V., Canziani M. E. & Moysés R. M. (2010). Early control of PTH and FGF23 in normophosphatemic CKD patients: a new target in CKD-MBD therapy? Clinicla Journal of the American Society of Nephrology, 5, 286–291.

Palmer S. C., Hayen A., Macaskill P., Pellegrini F., Craig J. C., Elder G. J. & Strippoli G. F. (2011). Serum levels of phosphorus, parathyroid hormone, and calcium and risks of death and cardiovascular disease in individuals with chronic kidney disease: a systematic review and meta-analysis. JAMA, 305, 1119-1127.

Parker B. D., Schurgers L. J., Brandenburg V. M., Christenson R. H., Vermeer C., Ketteler M., Shlipak M. G., Whooley M. A. & Ix J. H. (2010). The associations of fibroblast growth factor 23 and uncarboxylated matrix Gla protein with mortality in coronary artery disease: the Heart and Soul Study. Annals of Internal Medicine, 152, 640–648.

Pavik I., Jaeger P., Ebner L., Wagner C. A., Petzold K., Spichtig D., Poster D., Wüthrich R. P., Russmann S. & Serra A. L. (2013). Secreted Klotho and FGF23 in chronic kidney disease Stage 1 to 5: a sequence suggested from a cross-sectional study. Nephrology, Dialysis, Transplantation, 28, 352-359.

Perwad F., Azam N., Zhang M. Y., Yamashita T., Tenenhouse H. S. & Portale A. A. (2005). Dietary and serum phosphorus regulate fibroblast growth factor 23 expression and 1,25-dihydroxyvitamin D metabolism in mice. Endocrinology, 146, 5358–5364.

Quyyumi A. A. (1998). Endothelial function in health and disease: new insights into the genesis of cardiovascular disease. The American Journal of Medicine, 105, 32-39.

Razzaque M. S. & Lanske B. (2006). Hypervitaminosis D and premature aging: lessons learned from Fgf23 and Klotho mutant mice. Trends in Mollecular Medicine, 12, 298–305.

Razzaque M. S. (2009). FGF23-mediated regulation of systemic phosphate homeostasis: is Klotho an essential player? American Journal of Physiology. Renal Physiology, 296, 470–476.

Reynolds J. L., Joannides A. J., Skepper J. N., McNair R., Schurgers L. J., Proudfoot D., Jahnen-Dechent W., Weissberg P. L. & Shanahan C. M. (2004). Human vascular smooth muscle cells undergo vesicle-mediated calcification in response to changes in extracellular calcium and phosphate concentrations: a potential mechanism for accelerated vascular calcification in ESRD. Journal of the American Society of Nephrology, 15,2857-2867.

Rhee E. J., Oh K. W., Lee W. Y., Kim S. Y., Jung C. H., Kim B. J., Sung K. C., Kim B. S., Kang J. H., Lee M. H., Kim S. W. & Park J. R. (2006). The differential effects of age on the association of KLOTHO gene polymorphisms with coro-

nary artery disease. Metabolism, 55, 1344-1351.

Saito Y., Nakamura T., Ohyama Y., Suzuki T., Iida A., Shiraki-Iida T., Kuro-o M., Nabeshima Y., Kurabayashi M. & Nagai R. (2000). *In vivo klotho gene delivery protects against endothelial dysfunction in multiple risk factor syndrome. Biochemical and Biophysical Research Communications, 276, 767–772.*

Saito Y., Yamagishi T., Nakamura T., Ohyama Y., Aizawa H., Suga T., Matsumura Y., Masuda H., Kurabayashi M., Kuro-o M., Nabeshima Y. & Nagai R. (1998). *Klotho protein protects against endothelial dysfunction. Biochemical and Biophysical Research Communications, 248, 324–329.*

Saji F., Shiizaki K., Shimada S., Okada T., Kunimoto K., Sakaguchi T., Hotamura I. & Shigematsu T. (2009). *Regulation of fibroblast growth factor 23 production in bone in uremic rats. Nephron Physiology, 111, 59–66.*

Satoh M., Nagasu H., Morita Y., Yamaguchi T. P., Kanwar Y. S. & Kashihara N. (2012). *Klotho protects against mouse renal fibrosis by inhibiting Wnt signaling. American Journal of Physiology Renal Physiology, 303, 1641-1651.*

Schlessinger J., Plotnikov A. N., Ibrahimi O. A., Eliseenkova A. V., Yeh B. K., Yayon A., Linhardt R. J. & Mohammadi M. (2006). *Crystal structure of a ternary FGF-FGFR-heparin complex reveals a dual role for heparin in FGFR binding and dimerization. Molecular Cell, 6, 743–750.*

Segawa H., Kawakami E., Kaneko I., Kuwahata M., Ito M., Kusano K., Saito H., Fukushima N. & Miyamoto K. (2003). *Effect of hydrolysis-resistant FGF23-R179Q on dietary phosphate regulation of the renal type-II Na/Pi transporter. Pflügers Archives, 446, 585–592.*

Segawa H., Yamanaka S., Ohno Y., Onitsuka A., Shiozawa K., Aranami F., Furutani J., Tomoe Y., Ito M., Kuwahata M., Imura A., Nabeshima Y. & Miyamoto K. (2007).*Correlation between hyperphosphatemia and type II Na–Pi cotransporter activity in klotho mice. American Journal of Physiology. Renal Physiology, 292, 769–779.*

Semba R. D., Cappola A. R., Sun K., Bandinelli S., Dalal M., Crasto C., Guralnik J. M. & Ferrucci L. (2011). *Plasma klotho and mortality risk in older community-dwelling adults. The Journals of Gerontology. Seires A, Biological Sciences and Medical Sciences, 66, 794-800.*

Shanahan C. M., Crouthamel M. H., Kapustin A. & Giachelli C. M. (2011). *Arterial calcification in chronic kidney disease: key roles for calcium and phosphate. Circulation Research, 109, 697-711.*

Shimada T., Hasegawa H., Yamazaki Y., Muto T., Hino R., Takeuchi Y., Fujita T., Nakahara K., Fukumoto S. & Yamashita T. (2004)c. *FGF-23 is a potent regulator of vitamin D metabolism and phosphate homeostasis. Journal of Bone and Mineral Research, 19, 429–435.*

Shimada T., Kakitani M., Yamazaki Y., Hasegawa H., Takeuchi Y., Fujita T., Fukumoto S., Tomizuka K. & Yamashita T. (2004)a. *Targeted ablation of Fgf23 demonstrates an essential physiological role of FGF23 in phosphate and vitamin D metabolism. The Journal of Clinical Investigations, 113, 561–568.*

Shimada T., Mizutani S., Muto T., Yoneya T., Hino R., Takeda S., Takeuchi Y., Fujita T., Fukumoto S. & Yamashita T. (2001). *Cloning and characterization of FGF23 as a causative factor of tumor-induced osteomalacia. Proceedings of the National Academy of Sciences of the United States of America, 98, 6500–3505.*

Shimada T., Urakawa I., Isakova T., Yamazaki Y., Epstein M., Wesseling-Perry K., Wolf M., Salusky I. B. & Jüppner H. (2010). *Circulating fibroblast growth factor 23 in patients with end-stage renal disease treated by peritoneal dialysis is intact and biologically active. The Journal of Clinical Endocrinology and Metabolism, 95, 578-585*

Shimada T., Urakawa I., Yamazaki Y., Hasegawa H., Hino R., Yoneya T., Takeuchi Y., Fujita T., Fukumoto S. & Yamashita T. (2004)b .*FGF-23 transgenic mice demonstrate hypophosphatemic rickets with reduced expression of sodium phosphate cotransporter type IIa. Biochemical and Biophysical Research Communications314, 409–414.*

Shimamura Y., Hamada K., Inoue K., Ogata K., Ishihara M., Kagawa T., Inoue M., Fujimoto S., Ikebe M., Yuasa K., Yamanaka S., Sugiura T. & Terada Y. (2012). *Serum levels of soluble secreted α-Klotho are decreased in the early stages of chronic kidney disease, making it a probable novel biomarker for early diagnosis. Clinical and Experimental Nephrology, 16, 722-729.*

Shimizu Y., Fukumoto S. & Fujita T. (2012). *Evaluation of a new automated chemiluminescence immunoassay for FGF23.*

Journal of Bone and Mineral Metabolism, 30:217-21.

Shiraki-Iida T., Aizawa H., Matsumura Y., Sekine S., Iida A., Anazawa H., Nagai R., Kuro-o M. & Nabeshima Y. (1998). Structure of the mouse klotho gene and its two transcripts encoding membrane and Soluble protein. FEBS Letters, 424, 6–10.

Shiraki-Iida T., Iida A., Nabeshima Y., Anazawa H., Nishikawa S., Noda M., Kuro-o M. & Nabeshima Y. (2000) Improvement of multiple pathophysiological phenotypes of klotho (kl/kl) mice by adenovirus-mediated expression of the klotho gene. The Journal of Gene Medicine, 2, 233-242.

Shuto E., Taketani Y., Tanaka R., Harada N., Isshiki M., Sato M., Nashiki K., Amo K., Yamamoto H., Higashi Y., Nakaya Y. & Takeda E. (2009). Dietary phosphorus acutely impairs endothelial function. Journal of the American Society of Nephrology, 20, 1504–1512.

Tentori F., Blayney M. J., Albert J. M., Gillespie B. W., Kerr P. G., Bommer J., Young E. W., Akizawa T., Akiba T., Pisoni R. L., Robinson B. M. & Port F. K. (2008). Mortality risk for dialysis patients with different levels of serum calcium, phosphorus, and PTH: the Dialysis Outcomes and Practice Patterns Study (DOPPS). American Journal of Kidney Diseases, 52, 519–530.

Tonelli M., Sacks F., Pfeffer M., Gao Z. & Curhan G. (2005)b. Cholesterol And Recurrent Events Trial Investigators. Circulation, 112, 2627-2633.

Tonelli M., Sacks F., Pfeffer M., Gao Z. & Curhan G. (2005)a. Relation between serum phosphate level and cardiovascular event rate in people with coronary disease. Circulation, 112, 2627–2633.

Tsujikawa H., Kurotaki Y., Fujimori T., Fukuda K. & Nabeshima Y. (2003). Klotho a gene related to a syndrome resembling human premature aging, functions in a negative regulatory circuit of vitamin D endocrine system. Molecular Endocrinology, 17, 2393–2403.

Wan M., Smith C., Shah V., Gullet A., Wells D., Rees L. & Shroff R. (2013). Fibroblast growth factor 23 and soluble klotho in children with chronic kidney disease. Nephrology, Dialysis, Transplantation, 28, 153-161.

Wang H., Yoshiko Y., Yamamoto R., Minamizaki T., Kozai K., Tanne K., Aubin J. E. & Maeda N. (2008). Overexpression of fibroblast growth factor 23 suppresses osteoblast differentiation and matrix mineralization in vitro. Journal of Bone and Mineral Research, 23, 939–948.

Wang Y. & Sun Z. (2009). Current understanding of klotho. Ageing Research Reviews, 8, 43–51.

Wolf M. (2009). Fibroblast growth factor 23 and the future of phosphorus management. Current Opinnion in Nephrology and Hypertension, 18, 463–468.

Wolf M. (2010). Forging forward with 10 burning questions on FGF23 in kidney disease. Journal American Society of Nephrology, 21, 1427–1435.

Xiao N. M., Zhang Y. M., Zheng Q. & Gu J. (2004). Klotho is a serum factor related to human aging. Chinese Medical Journal, 117, 742-747.

Yamazaki Y., Imura A., Urakawa I., et al. Establishment of sandwich ELISA for soluble alpha-Klotho measurement: age-dependent change of soluble alpha-Klotho levels in healthy subjects. (2010). Biochemical and Biophysical Research Communications, 398, 513–518.

Yu X., Ibrahimi O. A., Goetz R., Zhang F., Davis S. I., Garringer H. J., Linhardt R. J., Ornitz D. M., Mohammadi M. & White K. E. (2005). Analysis of the biochemical mechanisms for the endocrine actions of fibroblast growth factor-23. Endocrinology, 146:4647–4656.

Zhou L., Li Y., Zhou D., Tan R. J. & Liu Y. (2013). Loss of Klotho contributes to kidney injury by derepression of Wnt/β-catenin signaling. Journal of the American Society of Nephrology, 24, 771-785.

Zisman A. L. & Wolf M. (2010). Recent advances in the rapidly evolving field of fibroblast growth factor 23 in chronic kidney disease. Current Opinion in Nephrology and Hypertension, 19, 335-342.

The Acute Effect of Continuous and Intermittent Exercise on the Exercise Efficiency and Physiological Responses of Ischemic Heart Disease Patients

James Faulkner, Michael Mann, Rebecca Grigg, Danielle Lambrick
School of Sport & Exercise
Massey University, Wellington, New Zealand

1   Introduction

Continuous (Dimopoulos *et al.*, 2006; Hambrecht *et al.*, 2004; Roditis *et al.*, 2007) and high-intensity intermittent exercise (Helgerud *et al.*, 2010; Rognmo *et al.*, 2004; Wisløff *et al.*, 2007) have been advocated to be an appropriate training stimulus for patients with elevated cardiovascular risk, coronary artery disease (CAD) and heart failure. Continuous exercise training has been shown to improve peak stroke volume and left ventricular function in CAD patients (Hagberg 1991; Hambrecht *et al.*, 2000), and improve oxygen uptake kinetics (Roditis *et al.*, 2007) and heart rate recovery in chronic heart failure patients (Dimopoulos *et al.*, 2006). High-intensity interval training, which is a well tolerated method of exercise for these population groups (Guiraud *et al.*, 2010; Meyer *et al.*, 2012), is generally associated with improvements in peak oxygen consumption, cardiovascular and muscular function, and quality of life in cardiac and non-cardiac subjects alike (Helgerud *et al.*, 2010, 2007; Guiraud *et al.*, 2010; Karlsen *et al.*, 2008; Rognmo *et al.*, 2004; Warburton *et al.*, 2005; Wisløff *et al.*, 2007). For example, two to four minutes of high-intensity walking, interspersed with an active recovery period, has been shown to be an effective training protocol for CAD patients (Rognmo *et al.*, 2004; Warburton *et al.*, 2005; Wisløff *et al.*, 2007). More recently, repeated short-bouts of high-intensity cycling (15 to 30 s) has been advocated to be an alternative and appropriate training stimulus for CAD and heart failure patients (Guiraud *et al.*, 2010; Meyer *et al.*, 2012; Normandin *et al.*, 2013).

Four key parameters have been identified for the assessment of an individual's aerobic fitness: maximal or peak oxygen uptake ($\dot{V}O_2$ max / $\dot{V}O_2$ peak), the gas exchange threshold (GET), exercise economy/efficiency and $\dot{V}O_2$ kinetics. Exercise efficiency is used to examine the ratio between useful work produced and the energy expended during the work. Improvements in exercise efficiency are often represented by a decrease in the $\dot{V}O_2$ required to sustain a given mechanical work output (Faria *et al.*, 2005; Lucia *et al.*, 2002). In healthy populations, it has been reported to be in the range of 8–25% (Gaesser & Brooks, 1975; Moseley & Jeukendrup, 2001), implying that ~75-92% of all the energy obtained from ATP hydrolysis is used to maintain homeostasis or is wasted as heat (Moseley & Jeukendrup, 2001). Although exercise efficiency has been suggested to be pertinent in reducing obesity (Schrauwen *et al.*,, 1999), promoting weight loss (Lammert & Hansen, 1982; Poole & Henson, 1988) and improving exercise performance (Horowitz *et al.*, 1994), for the cardiac disease population, exercise *in*efficiency may be a more important factor. It is plausible that the more inefficient one is, the greater the energy expenditure (as demonstrated by a higher $\dot{V}O_2$) for a given exercise intensity and therefore the greater the impact there may be on improving cardiovascular risk factors (*i.e.*, blood pressure, blood lipids, bodyweight) and overall health (Aggarwal et al., 2012). This in turn may reduce morbidity and mortality rates (Rognmo et al., 2004). However, the exercise efficiency of ischemic heart disease patients is yet to be investigated. To our knowledge, only one study has examined the effect of moderate-intensity continuous exercise and high-intensity interval exercise on exercise efficiency (Normandin et al, 2013), but this was in the more severe case of heart failure patients. In their study, Normandin *et al.*, demonstrated that patients were more efficient during high-intensity interval exercise (by ~3%) compared to moderate-intensity cycle exercise. It is important to assess the influence of continuous and intermittent exercise protocols on both the exercise (in) efficiency and physiological responses of ischemic heart disease patients as this may allow us to identify which exercise protocols and training stimuli should be implemented within the rehabilitation setting to improve an individual's recovery and quality of life.

The purpose of this study was therefore to determine whether ischemic heart disease patients were more (in)efficient during continuous exercise at either a moderate or high-intensity, or during high-intensity, intermittent exercise. In accordance with Normandin *et al.* (2013), it was hypothesised that participants would demonstrate superior (*i.e.*, better) efficiency during high-intensity intermittent exercise.

2   Methods

2.1   Participants

Fourteen men with ischemic heart disease volunteered to participate in this study. Demographic and baseline characteristics are presented in Table 1. All participants had recently completed a 12-week, phase II CR programme (3 × 75 minute exercise sessions per week), undertaken a CAD risk factor assessment, health-history questionnaire and a peak and/or symptom limited exercise ECG stress test using the modified-Bruce Protocol (ACSM's guidelines for exercise testing and prescription, 2013). Each exercise session within the 12-week exercise programme consisted of 30 minutes of aerobic exercise and 45 minutes of resistance training and postural, co-ordination and flexibility exercises. During the aerobic exercise, a continuous exercise programme was implemented for the first 6-weeks. Thereafter, participants' exercise sessions alternated between 30 minutes of continuous exercise and 30 minutes of high-intensity intermittent interval training.

Participants provided written consent prior to participation. Inclusion criteria included stable CAD and completion of a 12-week CR programme. Exclusion criteria included unstable angina pectoris, myocardial infarction or PCI one month prior to the research trial, complex ventricular arrhythmias, atrial fibrillation and orthopaedic limitations to exercise. None of the patients had an artificial cardiac pacemaker. Patients remained on their standard medication throughout the study (Table 1).

Emergency procedures and an automated defibrillator were in place during each exercise test to ensure that appropriate care was available if any adverse events were encountered during testing. Testing took place during the southern hemisphere summer and commenced following ethical approval from New Zealand's central regional health and disability ethics committee.

2.2   Procedures

All exercise tests were performed on a cycle ergometer (Velotron, RacerMate Inc, Seattle, USA) in a controlled thermo-neutral laboratory environment (temperature, 23.2 ± 1.5 °C; Humidity 43.2 ± 6.3 %; air pressure 1005 ± 10 N·m2). As a consequence of the moderate to high exercise intensities elicited during each exercise test, for safety reasons, a 12-lead ECG was worn throughout each test. Following completion if a graded-exercise test to 85 % HRmax (Gellish *et al.*, 2007), participants completed three experimental tests in a randomised order. This included a moderate-intensity continuous exercise test (MICE), a high-intensity continuous exercise test (HICE), and an intermittent exercise test incorporating both moderate (IE-M) and high (IE-H) intensities. Participants were familiar with these exercise protocols as a result of participating in their local phase II CR programme. Participants had a 48-72 hour recovery period between tests. Physiological data (heart rate [HR], $\dot{V}O_2$, minute ventilation [$\dot{V}_E$]) was continuously recorded before, during and post-exercise. On-line respiratory gas analysis occurred every 10-s via a breath-by-breath automatic gas exchange system (Sensormedic, AEI Technologies, Pittsburgh,

USA). Expired air was collected continuously using a facemask (Hans Rudolph Inc, Shawnee, USA). HR was monitored using a wireless chest strap telemetry system (Polar Electro T31, Kempele, Finland) and 12-lead ECG (Schiller, Baar, Switzerland). The ECG was used as a monitoring tool throughout each exercise test. All physical and physiological outputs were concealed from the participants.

Clinical Variables	Mean ± SD (%)
Age (y)	53.9 ± 10.3
Men (n)	14 (100 %)
Height (m)	1.74 ± 0.04
Weight (kg)	85.5 ± 12.6
BMI (kg·m^2)	28.0 ± 3.8
Medical History	81 ±13
Previous MI	4 (29 %)
Previous CABG	8 (57%)
Previous PCI	6 (43 %)
CVD risk factors	
Diabetes Mellitus	4 (29 %)
Hypertension (> 140/90mmHg)	6 (43 %)
Previous smoker	7 (50 %)
Current smoker	0 (0 %)
Obesity (BMI > 30 kg·m^2)	4 (29 %)
Medications	
B blockers (metropolol)	14 (100 %)
Anti-coagulants (aspirin, clopidogrel)	14 (100 %)
Statins (simvastatin, atorvastatin)	13 (93 %)
ACE inhibitors	5 (36 %)
Diuretic (furosemide)	2 (14 %)

ACE: angiotensin-converting enzyme; BMI: body mass index;
CABG: coronary artery bypass graft; CVD: cardiovascular disease;
MI: Myocardial infarction; PCI: percutaneous coronary intervention.

Table 1: Demographic and baseline characteristics of patients with ischemic heart disease. Values are reported as means ± SD or numbers of patients (%).

2.3   Measures

2.3.1   Graded-exercise Test (GXT)

The GXT was a continuous exercise test, commencing at 60 W and increasing by 1 W every 6-s until the attainment of 85% HRmax. The test was terminated at a sub-maximal intensity as maximal exercise constitutes a physiologic stress that may pose a great risk for people with previous cardiac diagnoses (Heyward, 2006; Ehrman *et al.*, 2009). For the purpose of this study, the termination of the exercise test will be referred to as $\dot{V}O_2$ peak. HR, $\dot{V}O_2$, $\dot{V}_E$ and blood pressure were monitored throughout the test.

2.3.2   Calculating Moderate & High Exercise Intensities

The V-slope method was used to analyse the slopes of $\dot{V}O_2$ and $\dot{V}CO_2$ volume curves from the initial GXT (Beaver et al., 1986). The power output equivalent to each individual's gaseous exchange threshold (GET) was used for the moderate exercise domain. Using the $\dot{V}O_2$ values reported at GET (first ventilatory threshold) and $\dot{V}O_2$ peak, the power output equivalent to 40% delta (Δ; difference between GET and $\dot{V}O_2$ peak) was calculated (Carter et al., 2002). This was used to reflect the high intensity exercise and ensured that participants were exercising at an equivalent physiological intensity. The GET and 40% Δ exercise intensities were verified by three independent researchers, and were used for the subsequent independent experimental exercise tests.

2.3.3   Exercise Efficiency Tests

Each experimental test was completed following 10-minutes of supine rest and a 5-minute warm-up at 60 W. During the continuous exercise tests subjects exercised at either the power output equivalent to GET (for MICE) or the power output equivalent to 40% Δ (for HICE) for 30 minutes. During the intermittent exercise test (IE), participants exercised at their moderate intensity for 4.5 minutes (IE-M) followed by a 30s sprint at the high exercise intensity (IE-H). This protocol was repeated six times to ensure the completion of 30-minutes of exercise. Participants freely chose their pedal cadence throughout each exercise test.

2.4   Data Analysis

The energy expenditure (EE) from MICE, HICE and IE was quantified using the following equation (Volpe Ayub & Bar-Or, 2003):

$$EE \ (KJ \cdot min^{-1}) = \dot{V}O_2 \ (L \cdot min^{-1}) \times (RER \times 1.232 + 3.815) \times 4.184$$

Gross efficiency (GE) was used to quantify exercise efficiency (Faria et al., 2005; Gaesser et al., 1975; Moseley & Jeukendrup, 2001). GE is the ratio of work done during the specific activity to the total EE:

$$GE \ (\%) = Work \ rate \ [W] \ / \ EE \ [J \ s^{-1}] \times 100\%$$

2.5   Statistical Analyses

A one-way ANOVA was firstly used to compare the mean power output elicited during MICE, HICE and IE. A series of two-factor repeated-measures ANOVAs (Test [MI, HI, IE-M, IE-H] × Time [5, 10, 15, 20, 25 & 30 minutes]) were then used to compare participants' GE between conditions. A similar analysis was used to assess physiological responses. A one way ANOVA compared EE from the MICE, HICE and IE tests. Where assumptions of sphericity were violated, the critical value of F was adjusted by the Greenhouse-Geisser epsilon value following the Mauchly test to reduce the risk of type 1 error. Alpha was set at 0.05 and adjusted accordingly. Tukey's honestly significant difference test detected where statistical differences lay. All data were analysed using SPSS, version 18.

3   Results

3.1   GXT

At the termination of the GXT participants $\dot{V}O_2$ peak, HR, PO and RPE were 38.3 ± 5.5 ml $\cdot$ kg$^{-1}\cdot$min^{-1}, 147 ± 14 b $\cdot$ min^{-1} (86 ± 4 %HRmax), 210 ± 23 W, and 17.6 ± 0.8, respectively. For the experimental tests, HICE elicited a significantly higher mean power output (135 ± 10 W) than MICE (93 ± 12 W) or IE (96 ± 12 W) ($F_{(2,26)} = 1175.75$, $P < .001$).

3.2   Exercise Efficiency Tests

A significant difference in GE was observed between tests ($F_{(1.9.24.6)} = 40.21$, $P < .001$; Table 2). GE was higher during MICE (11.0 ± 2.1 %) than all other exercise tests ($P < .001$), while IE-M (9.6 ± 1.4 %) was greater than HICE (8.8 ± 1.3 %) or IE-H (6.9 ± 1.4 %) (both $P < .01$). A time main effect was observed for GE ($F_{(2.5,32.4)} = 15.71$, $P < .001$), with a significant decrease in exercise efficiency observed between the 5th (10.2 ± 1.3 %) and 10th (9.0 ± 1.2 %) minute of the exercise tests (Table 2).

Test	5	10	15	Time (min) 20	25	30	Mean (SD)	95% CI
MICE	11.9 ± 2.6	10.7 ± 1.7	11.0 ± 2.6	10.8 ± 2.3	10.9 ± 2.3	10.8 ± 2.1	11.0 ± 2.1***	$9.8 - 12.2$
HICE	9.8 ± 1.2	9.0 ± 1.2	8.7 ± 1.8	8.8 ± 1.7	8.2 ± 1.5	8.2 ± 1.5	8.8 ± 1.3	$8.0 - 9.6$
IE-M	11.5 ± 1.9	9.5 ± 1.7	9.3 ± 1.5	9.1 ± 1.5	9.3 ± 1.9	9.1 ± 1.7	9.6 ± 1.4**	$8.8 - 1.5$
IE-H	7.4 ± 1.7	6.8 ± 1.4	6.9 ± 1.4	6.9 ± 1.5	6.9 ± 1.5	6.3 ± 1.4	6.9 ± 1.4	$6.1 - 7.7$
Mean (SD)	10.2 ± 1.3	9.0 ± 1.2*	9.0 ± 1.6	8.9 ± 1.4	8.8 ± 1.6	8.6 ± 1.3		
95% CI	$9.4 - 10.9$	$8.4 - 9.7$	$8.1 - 9.9$	$8.1 - 9.7$	$7.9 - 9.7$	$7.8 - 9.4$		

Test main effect: ***Significantly higher than all other tests ($P < .001$); **Significantly higher than HICE, IE-H (P .01)

Time main effect: *Significantly lower than 5-minutes ($P < .001$)

Table 2: Mean ($\pm$ SD) GE (%) between tests and across time

3.3   Physiological Markers

A test main effect was observed for $\dot{V}O_2$, HR and $\dot{V}_E$ (all $P < .001$; Figure 1). IE-H produced a higher $\dot{V}O_2$ value (74 ± 12 %) than all other exercise tests (50 ± 8 % MICE; 65 ± 5 % HICE; 52 ± 8 % IE-M). For HR, despite similarities between HICE and IE-H (80 ± 8 % & 76 ± 9 %, respectively) both tests elicited a higher HR response than MICE and IE-M (61 ± 8 % & 65 ± 7 %, respectively. A significant time main effect was also observed for $\dot{V}O_2$, HR and $\dot{V}_E$ ($P < .001$). $\dot{V}O_2$ significantly increased at the start (5 to 10 minutes) and end of the tests (20 to 30 minutes; $P < .05$), while HR sequentially increased with each 5 minute increment ($P < .01$). $\dot{V}_E$ increased between 5 and 10 minutes and between 15 and 30 minutes ($P < .05$). With regards to EE, this was significantly greater during HICE (40.1 ± 4.2 KJ$\cdot$min^{-1}) than either MICE (28.6 ± 4.4 KJ $\cdot$ min^{-1}) or IE (32.0 ± 3.5 KJ $\cdot$ min^{-1}) ($F (2,26) = 146.19$, $P < .001$).

4   Discussion

This study assessed the exercise (in)efficiency of ischemic heart disease patients during continuous and intermittent exercise at moderate and high intensities. Unlike previous research (Normandin *et al.*, 2013), ischemic heart disease patients were more efficient during 30-minutes of continuous exercise (MICE) than high-intensity intermittent exercise (IE-H), causing us to reject our study hypothesis. However, high-intensity continuous exercise (HICE) and IE-H elicited a greater energy expenditure (EE) and higher physiological intensity than MICE.

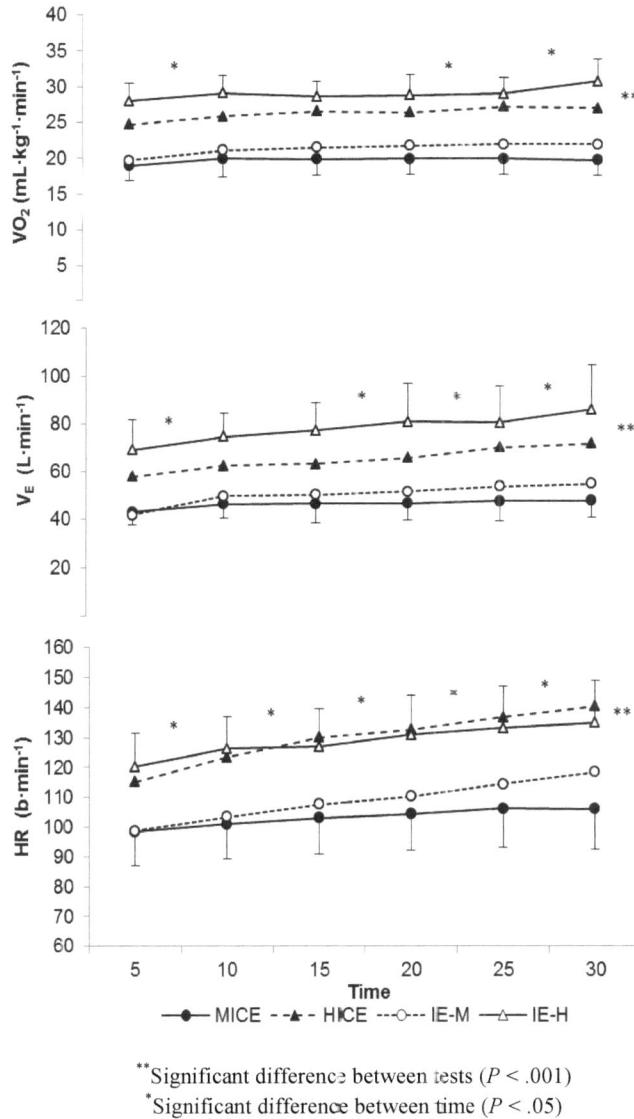

**Significant difference between tests ($P < .001$)
*Significant difference between time ($P < .05$)

Figure 1: Mean ($\pm$ SD) $\dot{V}O_2$, $\dot{V}_E$ and HR from each test.

Participants' gross efficiency during MICE was statistically superior (*i.e.*, 2.2% better) than during continuous exercise of a high intensity (HICE). Similarly, MICE was superior to intermittent exercise of both a moderate- (IE-M) and high intensity (1.4% & 4.1%, respectively). Participants were also more efficient during IE-M than either high-intensity condition (HICE or IE-H; Table 2). An inverse relationship between whole-body exercise economy and exercise intensity has been shown with healthy men and women during isometric plantar flexion (Hunter *et al.*, 2001), treadmill walking (Hunter *et al.*, 2005) and cycling exercise (Lucia *et al.*, 2002). As exercise intensity (and thus force production) increases, skeletal muscle become less economical (Lucia *et al.*, 2002; Hunter *et al.*, 2001; 2005). This is likely due to an increased dependence on inefficient Type II muscle fibres and may be related to differences in muscle fibre shortening velocities (Hopker *et al.*, 2009). Oxygen and energy demand may be greater in Type II than Type I muscle fibres for a given amount of contractile work as Type II muscle fibres consume more ATP (*i.e.*, to drive calcium pumps within the sarcoplasmic reticulum) and hence, this may result in a reduced exercise economy (Coyle *et al.*, 1992; Lucia *et al.*, 2002). However, the findings reported in this study differ from those reported by Normandin and colleagues with heart failure patients (Normandin *et al.*, 2013). In their study, high-intensity interval exercise, which incorporated 2 × 8 minutes of 30 s intervals at 100% peak power output and a 30 s passive recovery interval, proved more efficient (GE = 15%) than a 22-minute continuous cycle at 60 % peak power output (GE = 12.4%). When comparing these results with our study, differences between populations groups (ischemic heart disease cf. heart failure) and exercise protocols (duration, intensity, intervals, etc.) may explain the observed differences in the studies' findings. As fitness levels, physiological responses, pedal cadence, diet, genetics and fibre-type distribution have all been shown to be mediating factors when assessing and interpreting exercise efficiency in healthy populations (Coast *et al.*, 1986; Coyle *et al.*, 1992; Poole & Henson, 1988), further research is necessary to identify the physiological and physical underpinnings for such differences in Exercise efficiency between ischemic heart disease and other cardiac populations.

Ischemic heart disease patients were significantly more efficient in the first five minutes of exercise, regardless of the exercise intensity. A significant decrease in exercise efficiency was typically observed (~1.2%) between the fifth and tenth minute of the exercise tests. In both the continuous (MICE & HICE) and high-intensity intermittent exercise conditions, $\dot{V}O_2$ drift was observed. Elevated $\dot{V}O_2$ responses were noted at the start (5-10 min) and completion (20-30 minutes) of the exercise bout. This gradual increase in $\dot{V}O_2$, which was similarly observed for HR and $\dot{V}_E$, is the primary mediating factor for the change in exercise efficiency over the course of the exercise tests.

This study utilised a high-intensity intermittent protocol which is similar to the type of protocols recently assessed and advocated in the literature (Normandin *et al.*, 2013; Rognmo *et al.*, 2005; Warburton *et al.*, 2005; Wisløff *et al.*, 2007;). Although both high- and moderate intensity exercise may induce a similar cardiac hypertrophy, high-intensity training specifically has been shown to induce important cardiac adaptations such as increased contractility, increased glucose oxidation and improved mitochondrial function (Hafstad *et al.*, 2011). Recent research has advocated the prescription of high-intensity exercise for CAD and heart failure patients (Guiraud *et al.*, 2010; Meyer *et al.*, 2012; Normandin *et al.*, 2013) as it is effective in improving $\dot{V}O_2$ peak, cardiovascular disease risk profile and overall health, which in turn may reduce morbidity and mortality rates (Rognmo *et al.*, 2004). As demonstrated in Figure 1, participants revealed a higher physiological cost during IE-H compared to MICE for $\dot{V}O_2$ (~32%), $\dot{V}_E$ (41%) and HR (20%). Although participants' exercise efficiency was superior during MICE, participants only exercised at 61 ± 8% HRmax which was much lower than that observed during either the HICE or IE-H tests (80 ± 8% & 76 ± 9% HRmax, respectively). Accordingly, higher energy expenditure was observed during the high-intensity exercise bouts. The higher intensity exercise prescribed in this study met recommendations for improving cardio-respiratory fitness (ACSM's guidelines for exercise testing and prescription, 2013).

When trained individuals are matched for fitness, exercise efficiency may prove to be a decisive factor in distinguishing overall athletic performance (Faria et al., 2005). However, in situations whereby maximal functional capacity and elevated energy expenditure may be a more important factor for undertaking activities of daily living, such as with ischemic heart disease patients, exercise (in)efficiency may be of greater importance. For example, Lammert and Hansen (Lammert & Hansen, 1982) demonstrated that long-term benefits of a weight loss programme may be counteracted over-time by improvements in exercise efficiency. However, researchers and practitioners should be cautious when implementing high-intensity exercise as the risk of a cardiac event is greater during high-intensity exercise compared to moderate intensity exercise (Rognmo et al., 2012; Keteyian, 2012). Future research is needed to compare the long-term effect of prescribing moderate intensity exercise, which may elicit an efficient exercise performance, to an exercise intensity that may generate a higher physiological workload and greater energy expenditure in various cardiac populations.

This study has several limitations, including a small number of patients (although in keeping with previous research in this area (Meyer et al., 1990; Normandin et al., 2013)), the high-level of fitness of the study sample, and the inclusion of only one experimental trial for all continuous and intermittent exercise conditions. As such, further research is needed to examine whether similar findings are evident following repeated trials and/or following a specific training programme with cardiac populations of varying fitness. Inter-individual variation in the calculation of the higher exercise intensity may also have been evident. For safety reasons, the test was terminated at a sub-maximal intensity as maximal exercise constitutes a physiologic stress that may pose a great risk for people with previous cardiac diagnoses (Beaver et al., 1986; Heyward 2006). However, at the point of test termination, inter-individual variability may have been present due to prescribed beta blocker use and chronotropic incompetence (Brubaker & Kitzman, 2011). This may have influenced the calculation of the higher exercise intensity domain. As the workload of the intermittent and continuous exercise bouts were not matched by means of power output or energy expenditure, this is an aspect of the research design which should also be considered in the future. Finally, for a more holistic understanding of ischemic heart disease patients' and other cardiac populations' exercise (in)efficiency, it would also be important to implement randomized controlled trials whereby the exercise efficiency pre- and post-rehabilitation (i.e., exercise vs. control [no exercise]) can be examined. By manipulating the exercise programme (intensity, duration, mode, etc.), and by considering a patient's baseline level of fitness, a greater understanding of the importance of exercise intensity and exercise (in)efficiency may be alluded to with this population. For example, as subjects in the present study completed a greater proportion of continuous exercise during their 12-week CR programme, the greater efficiency observed during MICE may have been due to their greater exposure to this type of exercise training.

In conclusion, ischemic heart disease patients were more inefficient during high-intensity exercise (continuous and intermittent) than during continuous moderate intensity exercise. High-intensity exercise may therefore be of a greater benefit for this population group due to eliciting a higher physiological response and energy expenditure. This may be particularly important when considering the potential for improving cardiovascular risk profiles (i.e., blood pressure, blood lipids, and bodyweight) and overall health of ischemic heart disease patients.

References

ACSM's guidelines for exercise testing and prescription (2013). Philadelphia: Lippincott, Williams and Wilkins.

Aggarwal, S., Arena, R., Cuda, L., Hauer, T., Martin, B. J., Austford, L. & Stone, J. A. (2012). The independent effect of traditional cardiac rehabilitation and the LEARN program on weight loss: a comparative analysis. Journal of Cardiopulmonary Rehabilitation & Prevention, 21, 48-52.

Beaver, W., Wasserman, K. & Whipp, B. (1986). A new method for detecting anaerobic threshold by gas exchange. Journal of Applied Physiology, 60, 2020-27.

Brubaker, P. H. & Kitzman, D. W. (2011). Chronotropic incompetence: causes, consequences, and management. Circulation, 123, 1010-20.

Carter, H., Pringle, J. S., Jones, A. M. & Doust, J. H. (2002). Oxygen uptake kinetics during treadmill running across exercise intensity domains. European Journal of Applied Physiology, 86, 347-54.

Coast, J., Cox, R. & Welch, H. (1986). Optimal pedalling rate in prolonged bouts of cycle ergometry. Medicine & Science in Sports & Exercise, 18, 225-30.

Coyle, E. F., Sidossis, L. S., Horowitz, J. F. & Beltz, J. D. (1992). Cycling efficiency is related to the percentage of type I muslce fibers. Medicine & Science in Sports & Exercise, 24, 782-88.

Dimopoulos, S., Anastasiou-Nana, M., Sakellariou, D., Drakos, S., Kapsimalakou, S., Maroulidis, G., Roditis, P., Papazachou, O., Vogiatzis, I., Roussos, C. & Nanas, S. (2006). Effects of exercise rehabilitation program on heart rate recovery in patients with chronic heart failure. European Journal of Cardiovascular Prevention and Rehabilitation, 13, 67-73.

Ehrman, J. K., Gordon, P. M., Visich, P. S. & Keteyian, S. J. (2009). Clinical exercise physiology. Champaign IL: Human Kinetics.

Faria, E. W., Parker, D. L. & Faria, I. E. (2005). The science of cycling: physiology and training - part 1. Sports Medicine, 35, 285-312.

Gaesser, G. A. & Brooks, G. A. (1975). Muscular efficiency during steady-rate exercise: effects of speed and work rate. Journal of Applied Physiology, 38, 1132-39.

Gellish, R. L., Goslin, B. R., Olson, R. E., McDonald, A., Russi, G. D. & Moudgil, V. K. (2007). Longitudinal modeling of the relationship between age and maximal heart rate. Medicine & Science in Sports & Exercise, 39, 822-29

Guiraud, T., Juneau, M., Nigam, A., Gayda, M., Meyer, P., Mekary, S., Paillard, F. & Bosquet, L. (2010). Optimization of high intensity interval exercise in coronary heart disease. European Journal of Applied Physiology, 108, 733-40.

Hafstad, A.D., Boardman, N.T., Lund, J., Hagye, M., Khalid, A. M., Wisløff, U., Larsen, T. S. & Aasum, E. (2011). High intensity interval training alters substrate utilization and reduces oxygen consumption in the heart. Journal of Applied Physiology, 111, 1235-41.

Hagberg, J. M. (1991). Physiologic adaptations to prolonged high-intensity exercise training in patients with coronary artery disease. Medicine & Science in Sports & Exercise, 23, 661-67.

Hambrecht, R., Walther, C., Mobius-Winkler, S., Gielen, S., Linke, A., Condadi, K., Erbs, S., Kluge, R., Kendziorra, K., Sabri, O., Sick, P. & Schuler, G. (2004). Percutaneous coronary angioplasty compared with exercise training in patients with stable coronary artery disease. Circulation, 109, 1371-78.

Hambrecht, R., Wolf, A. & Gielen, G. (2000). Effects of exercise on coronary endothelial function in patients with coronary artery disease. New England Journal of Medicine, 342, 454-60.

Helgerud, J., Hkydal, K., Wang, E., Karlsen, T., Berg, P., Bjerkaas, M., Simonsen, T., Helgesen, C., Hjorth, N., Bach R. & Hoff, J. (2007). Aerobic high-intensity intervals improve VO2max more than moderate training. Medicine & Science in Sports & Exercise, 39, 665-71.

Helgerud, J., Støren, Ø. & Hoff, J. (2010). Are there differences in running economy at different velocities for well-trained distance runners? European Journal of Applied Physiology, 108, 1099-105.

Heyward, V. H. (2006). Advanced fitness assessment and exercise prescription. Champaign IL: Human Kinetics.

Hopker, J., Passfield, L., Coleman, D., Jobson, J., Edwards, L. & Carter, H. (2009). The effects of training on gross efficiency in cycling: a review. International Journal of Sports Medicine, 30, 845-50.

Horowitz, J. F., Sidossis, L. S. & Coyle, E. F. (1994). High efficiency of type I muscle fibers improves performance. International Journal of Sports Medicine, 15, 152-57.

Hunter, G. R., Bamman, M. M., Larson-Meyer, D. E., Joanise, D. R., McCarthy, J. P., Blaudeau, T. E. & Newcomer, B. R. (2005). Inverse relationship between exercise economy and oxidative capacity in muscle. European Journal of Applied Physiology, 94, 558-68.

Hunter, G., Newcomer, B., Larson-Meyer, D., Bamman, M. M. & Weinsier, R. L. (2001). Muscle metabolic economy is inversely related to exercise intensity and type II myofiber distribution. Muscle Nerve, 24, 654-61.

Karlsen, T., Hoff, J., Støylen, A., Skovholdt, M. C., Gulbrandsen Aarhus, K. & Helgerud, J. (2008). Aerobic interval training improves VO2peak in coronary artery disease patients; no additional effect from hyperoxia. Scandinavian Cardiovascular Journal, 42, 303-9.

Keteyian, S. J. (2012). Swing and a miss or inside-the-park home run: which fate awaits high-intensity exercise training? Circulation, 126, 1431-33.

Lammert, O. & Hansen, E. (1982). Effects of excessive caloric intake and caloric restriction on body weight and energy expenditure at rest and light exercise. Acta Physiologica Scandinavica, 114, 135-41.

Lucia, A., Hoyos, J., Perez, M., Santalla, A. & Chicharro, J. L. (2002). Inverse relationship between VO2max and economy/efficiency in world-class cyclists. Medicine & Science in Sports & Exercise, 34, 2079-84.

Meyer, K., Lehmann, M., Sünder, G., Keul, J. & Weidemann, H. (1990). Interval versus continuous exercise training after coronary bypass surgery: a comparison of training-induced acute reactions with respect to the effectiveness of the exercise methods. Clinical Cardiology, 13, 851-61.

Meyer, P., Normandin, E., Gayda, M., Billon, G., Guiraud, T., Bosquet, L., Fortier, A., Juneau, M., White, M. & Nigam, A. (2012). High-intensity interval exercise in chronic heart failure: protocol optimization. Journal of Cardiac Failure, 18, 126-33.

Moseley, L. & Jeukendrup, A. E. (2001). The reliability of cycling efficiency. Medicine & Science in Sports & Exercise, 33, 621-27.

Normandin, E., Nigam, A., Meyer, P., Juneau, M., Guiraud, T., Bosquet, L., Mansour, A. & Gayda, M. (2013). Acute responses to intermittent and continuous exercise in heart failure patients. Canadian Journal of Cardiology, 29, 466-71

Poole, D. & Henson, L. (1988). Effect of acute caloric restriction on work efficiency. American Journal of Clinical Nutrition, 47, 15-8.

Roditis, P., Dimopoulos, S., Sakellariou, D., Sarafoglou, S., Kaldara, E., Venetsanakos, J., Vogiatzis, J., Anastasiou-Nana, M., Roussos, C. & Nanas, S. (2007). The effects of exercise training on the kinetics of oxygen uptake in patients with chronic heart failure. European Journal of Cardiovascular Prevention and Rehabilitation, 14, 304-11.

Rognmo, O., Hetland, E., Helgerud, J., Hoff, J. & Slørdahl, S. A. (2004). High intensity aerobic interval exercise is superior to moderate intensity exercise for increasing aerobic capacity in patients with coronary artery disease. European Journal of Cardiovascular Prevention & Rehabilitation, 11, 216-22.

Rognmo, Ø., Moholdt, T., Bakken, H., Hole, T., Mølstad, P., Myhr, N. E., Grimsmo, J. & Wisløff, U. (2012). Cardiovascular risk of high- versus moderate-intensity aerobic exercise in coronary heart disease patients. Circulation, 126, 1436-40.

Schrauwen, P., Troost, F., Xia, J., Ravussin, E. & Saris, W. H. (1999). Skeletal muscle UCP2 and UCP3 expression in trained and untrained male subjects. International Journal of Obesity Related Metabolic Disorders, 23, 966-72.

Volpe Ayub, B. & Bar-Or, O. (2003). Energy cost of walking in boys who differ in adiposity but are matched for body mass. Medicine & Science in Sports & Exercise, 35, 669-74.

Warburton, D.E.R., McKenzie, D. C., Haykowsky, M. J., Taylor, A., Shoemaker, P., Ignaszewski, A. P. & Chan, S. Y. (2005). Effectiveness of high-intensity interval training for the rehabilitation of patients with coronary artery disease. American Journal of Cardiology, 95, 1080-84.

Wisløff, U., Stoylen, A., Loennechen, J. P., Bruvold, M., Rognmo, O., Haram, P. M., Tjønna, A. e., Helgerud, J., Slødahl, S. A., Lee, S. j., Videm, V., Bye, A., Smith, G. L., Najjar, S. M., Ellingsen, O. & Skjaerpe, T. (2007). Superior cardiovascular effect of aerobic interval training versus moderate continuous training in heart failure patients. Circulation, 115, 3086-94.

Cardiovascular Manifestations in Systemic Lupus Erythematosus: A Clinical Analysis of 1,125 Patients with SLE

Hiroshi Hashimoto

Department of Rheumatology, Juntendo Tokyo Koto Geriatric Medical Center
Juntendo University, Tokyo, Japan

1   Introduction

Systemic lupus erythematosus (SLE), an inflammatory disease of unknown cause, is a representative autoimmune disease that results in the production of autoantibodies, activation of the complement system and immune complex generation (Belmmont *et al.*, 1996; D'Cruz, 1988). In addition, SLE is a collagen-vascular disease along with polyarteritis nodosa, systemic sclerosis and others (Talbott, 1974). SLE has multisystem organ involvement, a predilection for females and a predominant age of onset from the twenties to forties (Wallace, 2007). Multisystem organ involvement includes cardiovascular manifestations, as well as renal, central nervous, pulmonary, and cutaneous manifestations. Cardiac manifestations include pericarditis, myocarditis, endocarditis, myocardial infarction and coronary artery disease. Vascular manifestations include pulmonary hypertension, cerebrovascular disease, intestinal hemorrhage/perforation due to vasculitis and peripheral vasculopathies such as livedo reticularis, subcutaneous nodules, skin ulcers, digital gangrene, thrombophrebitis and Raynaud's phenomenon. Many investigators have studied and reported these cardiovascular manifestations until the present time. However, there are few articles that almost all of the cardiovascular manifestations in SLE have been described and reviewed. In this article, the characteristics of the above-mentioned cardiac and vascular manifestations were analyzed and described using a retrospective review of the medical records of 1125 patients with SLE examined in Juntendo University Hospital between 1955 and 2002.

2   Clinical Presentation of Cardiac and Vascular Manifestations in 1,125 Patients with SLE

One thousand, one hundred and twenty-five SLE patients fulfilling four or more of the revised ACR (American College of Rheumatology) criteria (Hochberg, 1997) were examined and treated at the Department of Internal Medicine and Rheumatology in Juntendo University Hospital between 1955 and 2002. For all patients, the diagnosis and treatment procedures were conducted during a period when the use of steroids and immunosuppressive agents was common. Computerized analysis of the clinical manifestations, laboratory and immunological findings, treatments, complications, causes of death and prognosis was conducted.

Analysis of the distribution of age at diagnosis and the difference in gender revealed that the mean age at diagnosis was 27.1 years and the male to female ratio was 1:9. In adults over the age of 50 and children, the incidence of SLE demonstrated only a slight female predominance; however, for those in their twenties, thirties and forties, close to 90% of patients were women. The frequencies of cardiac and vascular manifestations in SLE are shown in Table 1. Cerebrovascular disease is a nervous disorder resulting from an inadequate cerebral blood flow or emboli, cerebral obstructive disorders, and cranial hemorrhage according to the classification of neuropsychiatric syndrome of SLE which was proposed by the American College of Rheumatology (ACR) in 1999, (ACR Ad Hoc Committee on Neuropsychiatric Lupus Nomenclature, 1999). Although a histological classification of lupus nephritis was proposed by the International Society of Nephrology and Renal Pathology Society (ISN/RPS) in 2004 (Weening *et al.*, 2004), the World Health Organization (WHO) classification based on histopathological findings (Churg *et al.*, 1995) was used in this study. Libman-Sacks type endocarditis was studied using autopsied cases that were experienced until 1980 and histopathological vascular lesions related to prognosis were studied using autopsied cases that were experienced until 1975.

Cardiac manifestations	
Pericarditis	77 (7%)
Myocarditis	25 (2%)
Myocardial infarction and coronary artery disease	5/820 (6%)
Angina pectoris	7/820 (9%)
Endcarditis (Libman-Sacks type due to autopsy)	10/45 (22%)
Neuropsychiatric manifestations	
Cerebrovascular disease	158 (14%)
Pulmonary vascular lesions	
Pulmonary hypertension	17 (2%)
Pulmonary arterial thrombosis and pulmonary emboli	10 (1%)
Renal vascular involvement	
Proteinuria	949 (84%)
Microhematuria	1066 (95%)
Focal segmental glomerulonephritis (WHO: Type III)	35/216 (16%)
Diffuse proliferative glomerulonephritis (WHO: Type IV)	55/216 (25%)
Intestinal vasculitis	
Intestinal haemorrhage and/or perforation due to vasculitis	4 (0.4%)
Cutaneous vasculitis	
Livedo reticularis	58 (5%)
Cutaneous ulcers	165 (15%)
Digital gangrene	30 (3%)
Thrombophrebitis	43 (4%)
Raynaud's phenomenon	539 (48%)
Total 1125 patients	

Table 1: Cardiac and vascular manifestations in SLE.

Glucocorticosteroids (steroids) were a mainstay of treatment for SLE. Although there were several kinds of steroids, prednisolone (PSL) was commonly used to treat SLE. The initial dose of steroids was usually determined according to the severity and activity of the disease. Active and severe diseases required high-dosages of steroids usually of 1mg/kg/day of PSL or more. Sometimes steroid pulse therapy (methylprednisolone 0.5-1g/day, intravenous administration, for 3days) was used followed by high-dosages of steroids. Moderate to mild diseases usually required 0.5-1mg/kg/day and less than 0.5mg/kg/day of PSL, respectively. However, the effectiveness and usefulness of steroids were limited because of severe side effects, unresponsiveness and resistance to steroids. In these situations, immuno-suppressive agents such as cyclophosphamide, azathioprine, mizoribine, tacrolimus and/or plasmaphere-sis or other innovative therapies were usually used in conjunction with steroids.

3   Cardiac Manifestations

3.1   Pericarditis

The most common cardiac abnormality was pericarditis, which has been reported to occur in 8–25% (Bulkley & Roberts, 1975), but this is relatively rare in Japan, with a frequency of 7% (77 out of 1,125 cases) found in the present study (Hashimoto, 2012). Pericarditis was observed in 53% of autopsied cases, showing mostly fibrous findings. Pericarditis is often one of the initial manifestations (Rothfield, 1996). Patients with pericarditis had fever (96%), pleuritis (51%), profuse proteinuria (49%), Raynaud's phenomenon (64%) and positive CRP (84%) more frequently than those without pericarditis. Electrocardiograms (ECG) showed low voltage and pericardial effusion with low complement levels and positive antinuclear antibodies and/or anti-DNA antibodies (Hashimoto, 2012). Most of the cases with pericarditis improved with the administration of prednisolone (PSL) 0.5–1 mg/kg/day showed a favorable outcome, but cases with cardiac tamponade, which was rare in this study, needed high-dosages of PSL of over 1mg/kg/day and/or steroid pulse therapy (Hashimoto, 2012).

3.2   Myocarditis

Myocarditis was rarely observed, occurring in just 2% of cases in this study. In cases with myocarditis, positive CRP, elevated creatine kinase (CK), IgG class anti-dsDNA antibodies, hematuria, in conjunction with tachycardia, cardiac enlargement, and congestive heart failure were often observed (Hashimoto, 2012). Epicarditis and pleuritis were frequently observed simultaneously. Moreover, SLE might be associated with arrhythmia and conductive disturbance (such as sinus-atrial block, atrial-ventricular block and bundle branch block). If tachycardia, cardiac enlargement and congestive heart failure in addition to these findings existed, acute serious myocarditis was suspected. Sometimes myocardial biopsy was performed in order to confirm the diagnosis.

Patients with myocarditis associated with congestive heart failure were treated with high-dosages of steroids (PSL 1–1.5 mg/kg/day, divided into 3~4 doses). All of the patients with myocarditis improved after steroid therapy.

A case report of an SLE patient with myocarditis associated with congestive heart failure is presented as follows. The patient, a 41-year-old male, was diagnosed with SLE and had symptoms including fever, malar rash, arthralgia, anti-nuclear antibodies, and anti-DNA antibodies. He was hospitalized due to shortness of breath at exercise. Although cardiac murmurs were not heard, the first and second heart sounds were slightly reduced, and a third heart sound could be heard. Chest X-ray showed an increase in the cardiothoracic ratio and ECG showed low voltage in the limb lead, poor R wave progression in the chest lead and T-wave inversion in V5 and V6. Cardiac ultrasonography showed the left cardiac ventricle was enlarged; wall motion diffusely reduced and dilative cardiomyopathy-like findings were observed. The ejection fraction (EF) also significantly decreased to 0.32. Although the symptoms related to heart failure improved after treatment with diuretics, digitalis and angiotensin converting enzyme (ACE) inhibitor, the ejection fraction by cardiac ultrasonography decreased from 31% to 21%, indicating that heart function was progressively worsening. No lesions in the coronary arteries were found by a heart catheter examination, hence a myocardial biopsy was conducted. In the histological findings of myocardial biopsy by HE staining, a defect in focal myocardium muscle cells spreading from the sub-endocardium with fibrosis and small round cell infiltration consisting of T cells was observed, as shown in Figure 1.

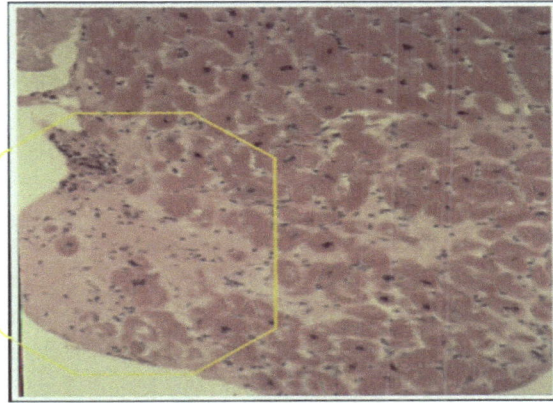

Figure 1: Histological finding of myocarditis by HE staining in SLE patient. Defect of focal myocardium muscle cells spreading from the sub-endocardium with fibrosis and small round cell infiltration was observed.

According to the above findings, the patient was treated with 60mg/day of PSL. The ejection fraction gradually improved to 42%, the cardiothoracic ratio reduced to 45% and ECG findings improved in conjunction with an improvement in serum creatine kinase (CK) and complement levels after treatment. The clinical course of this patient is shown in Figure 2.

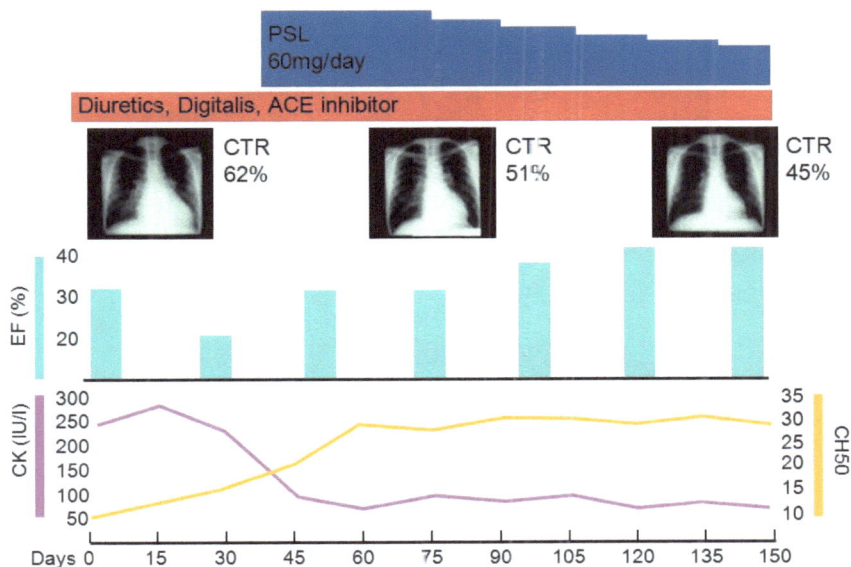

Figure 2: Clinical course of SLE patient (41-year-old male) with myocarditis. PSL; prednisolone, CTR; cardiothoracic ratio, ACE; angiotensin converting enzyme, EF; ejection fraction, CK; creatine kinase. The patient was treated with high-dosages of PSL for myocarditis due to SLE. The EF gradually improved to 42%, CT ratio reduced to 45% and ECK findings improved in conjunction with improvement of serum CK and complement levels after treatment.

According to Rothfield (Rothfield, 1996), myocarditis was diagnosed clinically in only 9% of SLE patients in his series. He also noted that patients with acute myocarditis and congestive heart failure should be treated with a high dosages of PSL (60mg/day in an every-6-hour regimen) and that the objective of the therapy was to relieve the inflammation causing the congestive heart failure.

3.3   Myocardial Infarction and Coronary Artery Disease

In this study, eleven lupus patients with myocardial infarction were analyzed. The average age at diagnosis of SLE was 37 years (range; 26–63 years), and the average age at development of myocardial infarction was 51 years (range; 41–66 years) in these patients. Conservative medical management using anti-hypertensive drugs and statins without high-dosages of steroids was conducted in most cases in this study. Percutaneous transluminal coronary recanalization (PTCA) and coronary artery bypass graft (CABG) were also occasionally conducted.

There were two deaths, including one case from cardiac rupture. Figure 3 shows angiography of coronary artery stenosis in a case of SLE. Figure 4 shows severe coronary atherosclerosis in a 30-year-old man with SLE (autopsied case).

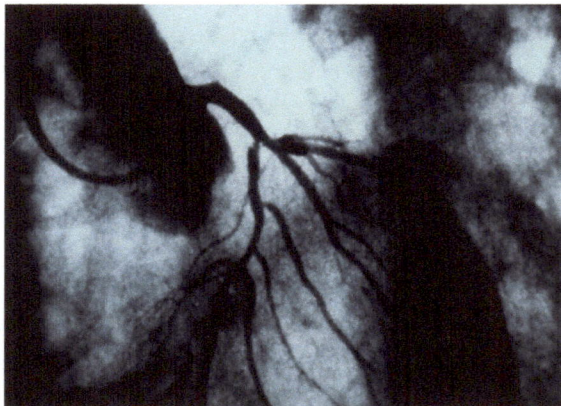

Figure 3: Stenosis of the anterior inter-ventricular branch of the left coronary artery seen by coronary angiography in an SLE patient (38-year-old male). A coronary artery bypass graft was conducted in this patient.

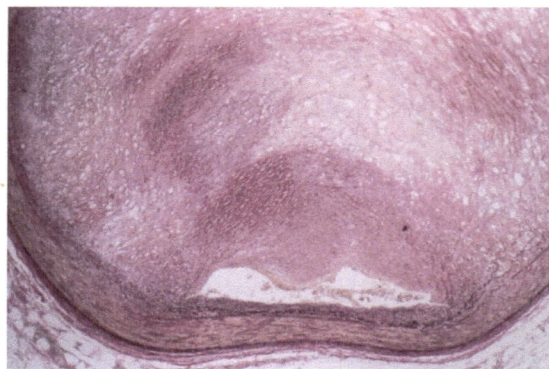

Figure 4: 95% narrowing of the left circum flex coronary artery due to atherosclerosis in an autopsied SLE case (30-year-old male).

Coronary artery disease due to atherosclerotic changes is more common in SLE patients. The frequency of coronary heart disease, including myocardial infarction, in SLE has been reported to be 6–10% (Gladman & Urowitz, 1987; Petri *et al*, 1992; Manzi *et al,* 1997; Bruce *et al*, 2000; Bruce *et al*, 2003). Death from myocardial infarction late in the course of the disease is one of the most frequent causes of death after 10 to 30 years of SLE (Rothfield, 1996). Urowitz et al (Urowitz, 1976) reported that deaths occurring <1year after onset of SLE were directly related to SLE disease activity, whereas mortality in patients with a longer disease duration was primarily attributable to cardiovascular disease, thus showing a bimodal pattern of SLE-associated death. Death from myocardial infarction due to inflammation of the coronary arteries has been reported in SLE patients dying early in the course of their disease, but this is a rare event (Rothfield, 1996).

It has been noted that there are several risk factors for myocardial infarction due to atherosclerosis in SLE including traditional cardiovascular risk factors. These include older age, male gender, smoking, high total cholesterol and LDL levels, high systolic blood pressure, diabetes mellitus, left ventricular hypertrophy, renal involvement, long-term administration of steroids, and anti-phospholipid syndrome (Bruce *et al*, 2003, Faurachou *et al*, 2011, Skaggs, *et al*, 2012, Symmons & Gabriel, 2011).

On the other hand, three case-control studies (Roman *et al.*, 2003; Asanuma *et al.*, 2003; El-Magadmi, *et al.* 2004) confirmed that atherosclerosis developed prematurely, independently of traditional risk factors for cardiovascular disease. SLE itself seems to be a risk factor for the development of atherosclerosis because long-term inflammatory disease activity can result in endothelial and vascular damage (D'Cruz *et al.*, 2007). Antibodies such as anti-phospholipid antibody, anti-oxLDL and anti-ApoA-1 have also been noted as SLE specific cardiovascular risk factors (Salel *et al*, 1977). Although there is also persuasive experimental evidence for a role for anti-phospholipid antibodies, some case-control and epidemiological studies have not reported any relationship (D'Cruz *et al.*, 2007). Therefore, the contribution of anti-phospholipid antibodies to accelerated atherosclerosis in SLE remains unclear.

Svenungsson, *et al.* showed that lupus patients with previous cardiovascular events had a distinct pattern of risk factors. These included increased carotid intima-media thickness, raised concentration of circulating oxidized low density lipoprotein (LDL), triglycerides, and lipoprotein (a), raised α1-antitrypsin and homocysteine concentration, and decreased high density lipoprotein (HDL) cholesterol (Svenungsson *et al.*, 2001).

It has been noted that systemic administration of steroids could be linked to the higher occurrence of vascular diseases such as coronary artery disease, stroke, and peripheral vascular disease, than the expected occurrence in SLE. It was also noted that glucocorticoid (GC)-associated damage accumulated over time constituted most of the damage at 15 years, although disease-activity-related damage occurred early (Gladman, *et al.*, 2003). However, it is unclear whether this reflects pro-atherogenic effects of the underlying disease process or adverse metabolic effects associated with steroid use (Wei *et al.*, 2004). Although no randomized clinical trials of atherosclerosis prevention strategies have been performed specifically in SLE, it has been pointed out that the current guidelines for modifying cardiovascular risk factors in patients with SLE are essentially the same as those aimed at reducing cardiovascular disease in the general population (Skaggs *et al*, 2012).

3.4   Endocarditis

Endocarditis in SLE is reported to consist mostly of verrucous endocarditis, known as Libman-Sackes (L-S) endocarditis (Libman & Sacks, 1924). L-S endocarditis is a pathological diagnosis and is not reflected in the clinical evidence of valvular disease. In this paper, L-S endocarditis was found in 10 out of 45 autopsy cases. L-S lesions were usually microscopic, but macroscopic vegetations were also noted. The vegetations were found on the mitral valve leaflets in 4 cases, on the mitral and tricuspid valve leaflets in 3 cases, on the mitral and aortic valve leaflets in 2cases and on the mitral, tricuspid and aorta valve leaflets in one case. The chordae tendineae and mural endocardium as well as valves were also involved in some cases. The causes of death in these patients who were treated with steroids were mostly uremia. Two patients died of infections without bacterial endocarditis. There was no significant difference in the 3-year-survival rate between the patients with and without L-S endocarditis.

Rothfield reported that L-S endocarditis was found in 1/3 to 2/3 of autopsy cases (Rothfield, 1996). The frequency of L-S endocarditis has been declining, but this decline might be due to the greater use of more vigorous treatments over the past 30 years compared with the period when the lesions were first described (Libman & Sacks, 1924), when no treatment was available (Rothfield, 1996; Gladman & Urowitz, 1987). In general, systolic murmurs due to verrucous endocarditis are not audible. However, as L-S endocarditis may be a secondary infection, SLE patients who are febrile and develop a murmur should be evaluated for bacterial endocarditis. Recently, Doppler echocardiography has shown that there is a high frequency of valvular regurgitation, with the right side more frequently involved than the left. Clinically significant valvular disease was found in about 2% of patients in a large series (Straaton *et al*, 1988). It has also noted that heart valvular disease, a definition based on L-S endocarditis, was the most frequent cardiac manifestation in patients with anti-phospholipid syndrome, with a prevalence of 30% (Zuily *et al*, 2013). The presence of anti-phospholipid antibodies in SLE patients was noted to be associated with a threefold greater risk of heart valve disease, confirming the crucial importance of anti-phospholipid antibodies in the pathogenic process, leading to thrombotic manifestations on valves because of hypercoagulability (Zuily *et al*., 2013).

4   Cerebrovascular Disease

In this study, cerebrovascular diseases were observed in 14% as shown in Table 1. In cerebral infarction, acute local nervous disorders lasted for over 24 hours, and abnormal findings were observed in brain computed tomography (CT) and/or magnetic resonance imaging (MRI). In chronic multifocal disease, a recurrent or progressive decline in neurological function due to cerebrovascular diseases was observed. Hemorrhage findings due to subarachnoid hemorrhage and/or intracranial hemorrhage were observed on either brain CT and/or MRI. In sinus thrombosis, acute local nervous disorders were observed accompanied by intracranial hypertension. Causes of cerebrovascular disease included anti-phospholipid antibodies or anti-phospholipid syndrome. A case report of SLE patient (60-years-old female) with anti-phospholipid syndrome is presented as follows. She was hospitalized in an unconsciousness state due to cerebral infarction and chronic subdural hematoma. She suffered a cerebral infarction again after removal of the subdural hematoma. She subsequently died of disseminated intravascular coagulation due to postoperative complication. The pathological findings at autopsy revealed necrotizing vasculitis with fibrinoid degeneration together with perivascular round-cell infiltration in vessels of the cerebrum (Figure 5).

The frequencies of neuropsychiatric manifestations of SLE, including cerebrovascular disease, in our study in conjunction with the findings of other investigators are shown in Table 2 (Estes & Christian, 1971; West, 2007).

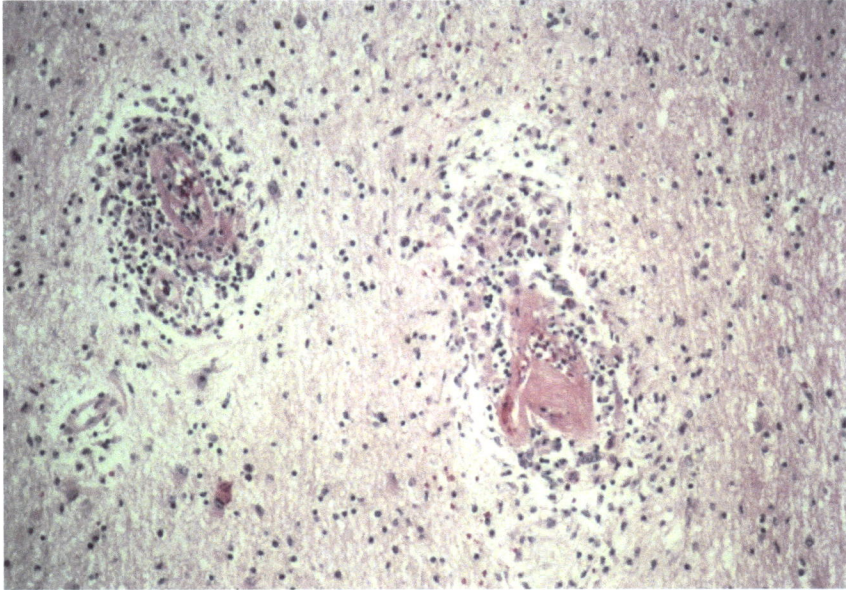

Figure 5: Necrotizing vasculitis with fibrinoid degeneration together with perivascular round-cell infiltration in vessels of cerebrum was observed in a patient with SLE and anti-phospholipid syndrome (60-year-old female, autopsied case).

Investigators		Estes (1971)	Wallace (1990)	Hashimoto (2002)
cases with SLE		150	465	1125
NPSLE		88	232	535
neurological syndrome	seizure and seizure disorder	26%	6%	13%
	cerebrovascular disease	8%	11%	14%
	myelopathy	–	–	4%
	meningitis	–	–	4%
	peripheral neuropathy	7%	5%	7%
	headache	–	–	9%
psychosis		16%	5%	21%

NPSLE: neuropsychiatric syndromes of SLE
SLE: systemic lupus erythematosus

Table 2: Neuropsychiatric manifestations in SLE.

5   Pulmonary Vascular Lesions

5.1   Pulmonary Hypertension (PH)

The frequency of pulmonary hypertension (PH) in SLE was 1.5% in this study. The frequency of PH in SLE was noted to be lower than that in mixed connective-tissue disease (MCTD) (12–15%) and systemic sclerosis (7%) (Burdt, *et al.*, 1999; Wakaki, *et al.*, 1984; Medsger, Jr, 1996). There was a wide range in the estimates of pulmonary hypertension (PH) prevalence in SLE from 0.005% to 14%, because the diagnostic definition and/or procedure for PH varies from reporter to reporter (Johnson & Granton, 2011).

Lupus patients with PH had hypoxia after exercise, an increased P2 sound, enlargement of pulmonary artery segments, enlargement of the right ventricle on chest X-ray, and an increased average pulmonary artery pressure of over 25mmHg on ultrasound echocardiography (UCG). The average pressure of the pulmonary artery in 17 patients with PH in this study was 55.2mmHg. Figure 6 shows chest X-ray (a) and CT features (b) of PH in a case of SLE.

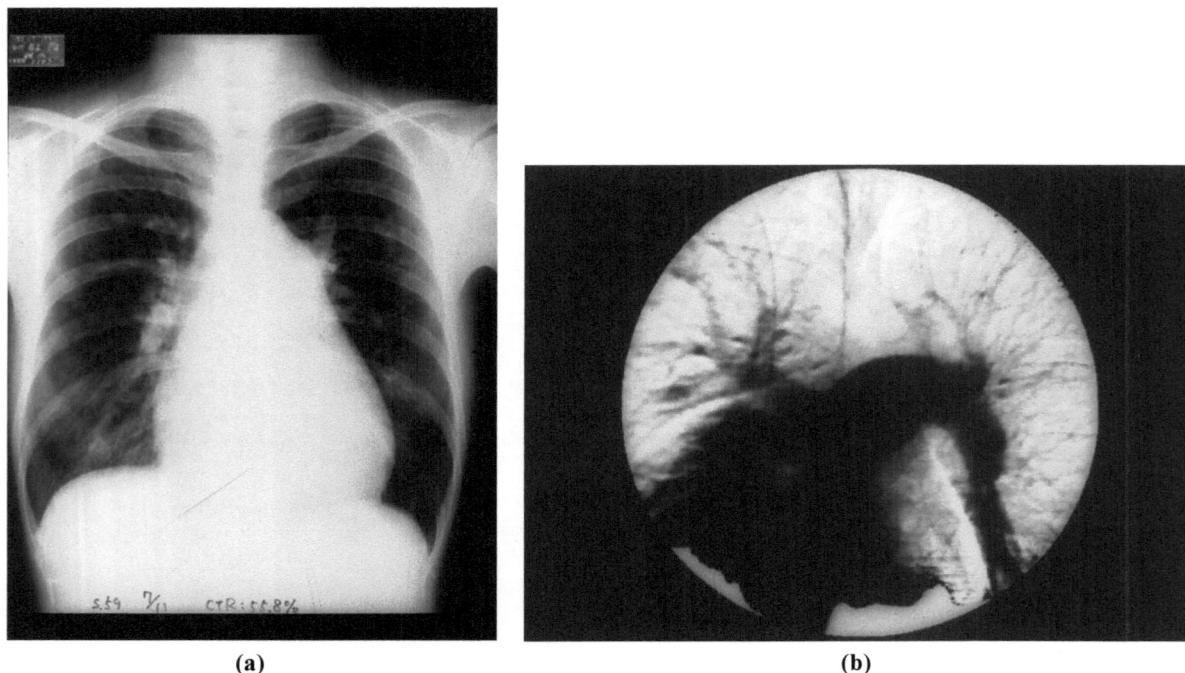

(a)   (b)

Figure 6: (a) Cardiomegaly with the protrusion of the pulmonary artery in a chest X-ray of an SLE patient with PH. **(b)** Dilatation of the main pulmonary artery in the CT feature of an SLE patient with PH.

Although the cause of PH in SLE is unknown, it has been thought that causative factors include spasms and/or thickening of the pulmonary arteries and arterioles, vasculitis, pulmonary arterial thrombosis and multiple pulmonary emboli. Pathological specimens show subintimal connective tissue proliferation in pulmonary arteries and arterioles and medial hypertrophy of the vessels (Johnson & Granton, 2011). Immunoglobulin and C3 deposition have been detected suggesting an autoimmune pathogenesis (Quismorio, et al., 1984). However, there was no evidence of inflammation. It was noted that SLE patients with PH tended to have MCTD-like manifestations, such as Raynaud's phenomenon, arthritis, swollen hands, anti-U1-RNP antibodies, IgG anti-cardiolipin antibodies (Kasukawa, R. et al, 1990, Hashimoto, 2002). Characteristics of clinical findings in SLE patients with PH in conjunction with pulmonary arterial thrombosis and pulmonary emboli (PAT/PE) are shown in Table 3.

		pulmonary hypertension		pulmonary arterial thrombosis and/or pulmonary emboli	
frequency (total 1125 patients)		17 patients	1.50%	10 patients	0.90%
clinical findings	malar rash	13 patients	76.50%	5 patients	50.00%
	arthritis	11 patients	62.50%	6 patients	60.00%
	nephritis	12 patients	70.00%	7 patients	70.00%
	Raynaud's phenomenon	5 patients	29.40%	6 patients	60.00%
	low complementemia	7 patients	38.40%	4 patients	40.00%
	high titer of anti-DNA	10 patients	58.80%	8 patients	80.00%
	positive anti-U!-RNP	7 patients	41.20%	2 patients	20.00%
	lupus anticoagulant	1 patient	5.90%	6 patients	60.00%
treatment	PSL<20mg/day)	4 patients	23.50%	1 patient	10.00%
	PSL 20-40mg/day	6 patients	35.30%	4 patients	40.00%
	PSL >40mg/day	6 patients	35.30%	4 patients	40.00%
	steroid pulse therapy	1 patient	5.90%	1 patient	10.00%
	plasmapheresis	3 patients	18.80%	0	0%
	immunosuppressants	2 patients	12.50%	1 patient	10.00%
	anti-coagulants	17 patients	100.00%	10 patients	100.00%
outcome	improvement	5 patients	29.40%	7 patients	70%
	no change	6 patients	35.30%	0	0%
	death	6 patients	35.30%	3 patients	30.00%
PSL; precnisolone					

Table 3: Clinical findings in SLE patients with pulmonary hypertension and pulmonary arterial thrombosis/emboli

Although recent observational studies suggest that a subset of SLE patients with PH would improve with immunosuppression (Johnson *et al*, 2011), five patients were treated with less than 20mg/day of PSL in this study. In one patient with PH and anti-U1RNP antibodies, steroid pulse therapy following high-dosages of steroids (1 mg/kg/day of PSL) was used in the early stage when PH progressed rapidly. In addition to the above treatment, epoprostenol sodium (prostaglandin I 2), an endothelin receptor antagonist (bosentan hydrate, ambrisentan) and a phosphodiesterase type 5 (PDE-5) inhibitor (sildenafil citrate and tadalafil), which have been used for treatment of primary PH, were also used in lupus patients with PH. Other therapies included oxygen therapy, vasodilating drugs (calcium antagonists, nitrates and prostaglandin E1, and prostaglandin I 2, etc.), anti-clotting/anti-platelet drugs, and diuretic agents.

In term of outcome, the rates of improvement, unchanged and death in SLE patients with PH were almost the same. The patients who showed improvement had mild PH. Six patients died of heart failure and/or sudden death.

According to systemic review of the literature by Johnson SR et al., clinical factors that were associated with survival in SLE patients with PH were as follows; Ppa at diagnosis, thrombosis, thrombocytopenia, concurrent pregnancy, infection, Raynaud's phenomenon, plexiform lesion and pulmonary vasculitis (Chow, *et al.*, 2011). Condliffe et al. reported their 3-year survival rate in SLE patients with PH was 75%, showing a favorable prognosis compared to 47% in patients with systemic sclerosis associated with PH (Condliffe, *et al.* 2009).

5.2   Pulmonary Arterial Thrombosis and Pulmonary Emboli (PAT/PE)

The frequency of PAT/PE in SLE has been reported to be 5.6% in Europe and the United States (Glad-man & Urowitz, 1980) and was 0.9% (ten patients) in this study. PAT/PE are thought to be acute clinical conditions due to vasculitis and abnormalities of coagulability, such as anti-phospholipid syndrome. The lupus anti-coagulant, one of the anti-phospholipid antibodies, was positive in 6 out of 10 cases in this study.

The major treatments of PAT/PE are anticoagulation therapies using agents, such as heparin, war-farin, and antiplatelet agents, in conjunction with steroids and/or immunosuppressive drugs. Recently, new anticoagulants, such as thrombin inhibitor (dabigatran) and Xa inhibitor (rivaroxaban), have been developed. Although the outcome varies depending on the severity of PAT/PE, 7 of 10 patients improved while the remaining 3 patients died in this study.

6   Renal Vascular Involvment

Renal disease in SLE patients is extremely common, showing clinical manifestations of renal involve-ment, namely lupus nephritis (LN), in approximately two-thirds of patients. Clinical manifestations in-clude proteinuria, abnormal urinary sediments such as red blood cells, white blood cells and mixed cellu-lar casts, as well as renal dysfunction. The clinical pictures of LN and the types of the World Health Organization (WHO) classification based on histopathological findings in this study are shown in Table 4.

A. Urinalysis, Reanl function	n=1125 (%)	
No proteinuria	176	(16)
Proteinuria	949	(84)
Intermittent	431	(45)
Persistent	354	(37)
Profuse (>3.5g/day)	164	(17)
Microhematuria	1066	(95)
Urine casts	838	(74)
Elevated BUN	659/1063	(62)
Elevated S-creatinine	429/1047	(41)
B. Histopathological findings (WHO classification)	n= 216 (%)	
I. Minimal change (MC) or Normal	49	(23)
II. Mesagial alteration	34	(16)
III. Focal segmental glomerulonephritis (FGN)	35	(16)
IV. Diffuse proliferative glomerulonephritis (DPGN)	55	(25)
V. Membranous glomerulonephritis (MGN)	39	(18)
VI. Advanced	4	(12)

Table 4: Lupus nephritis in 1125 cases.

The available therapeutic procedures include steroids, immunosuppressive agents, plasmapheresis, anticoagulants and hemodialysis. Steroids were the first choice for treatment of LN. However, dosages of steroids were determined based on urinary findings, renal function and renal histopathological findings used to evaluate the activity and severity of LN. High-dosages of steroids (PSL 1-1.5mg/kg/day) were administered initially as induction therapy for remission in patients with active and /or severe LN, including persistent or profuse proteinuria, renal dysfunction, diffuse proliferative glomerulonephritis (DPGN) of type IV, rapidly progressive glomerulonephritis (RPGN) or membranous GN (MGN) of Type V in conjunction with low serum complement levels and high titers of anti-dsDNA antibodies. Steroid pulse therapy was often administered at first. Figure 7 shows the remission rate after onset according to the WHO classification type and degree of proteinuria. The remission rates of patients with Type IV (DPGN) and profuse peroteiniria or nephrotic syndrome tended to decrease during the course of the disease, while the remission rates of patients with Type II and persistent proteinuria tended to increase. Patients with Type V (MGN) had a low remission rate through out the course of the disease, but no decrease in the remission rate was observed until later time.

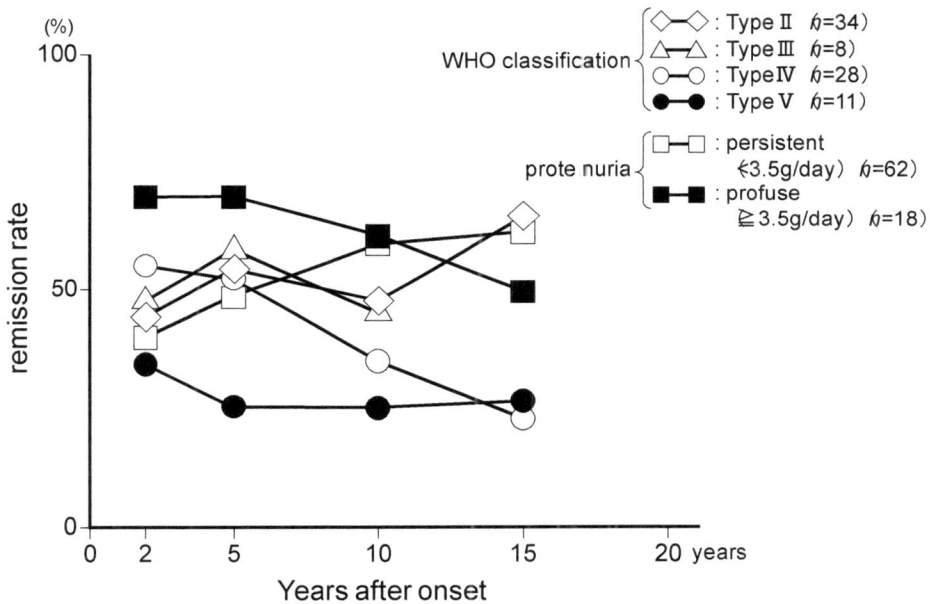

Figure 7: Remission rate of lupus nephritis according the WHO classification type and degree of proteinuria.

Furthermore, of 32 patients who received long-term treatment for over 20 years, the complete remission rate was 27%, the incomplete remission rate was 37.8%, and the worsening rate was 21.6%. Of the treatments used, those that contributed to remission could not be specified. This fact suggests that the underlying disease types had a greater influence on the remission rate than the treatment method.

As LN is thought to be an immune complex disease, deposits of immune complexes in glomeruli can be observed histologically and renal disease activity correlates with a high titer of anti-dsDNA antibodies and low serum complement levels clinically. Renal vascular lesions are most commonly seen in patients with both focal and diffuse proliferative glomerulonephritis (Types III and IV) (Antonovych & Sabnis, 1995). In patients with active lupus nephritis, the most common lesion encountered was lupus vasculopathy involving small arteries and arterioles and consisting of subendothelial hyaline-like materials, seen as fibrinoid changes (Figure 8).

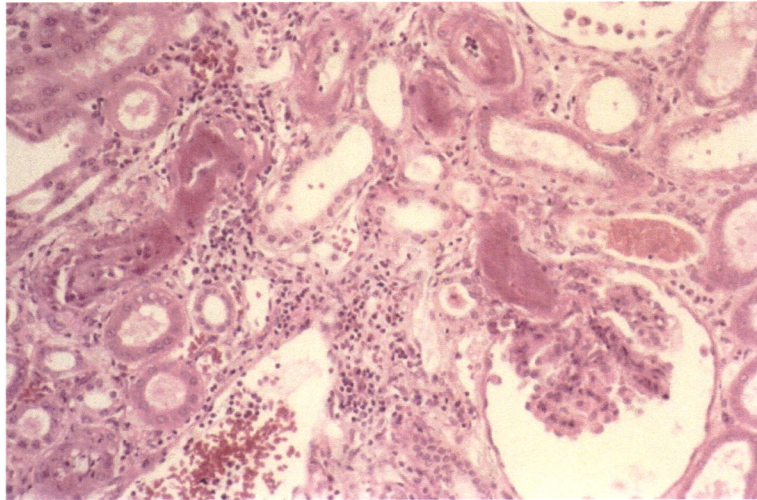

Figure 8: Necrotizing vasculitis with fibrinoid necrosis and thrombosis in the renal efferent arteriole, afferent arteriole and intralobular artery was seen in patient with lupus nephritis (60-years-old female)

A definite diagnosis of lupus vasculopathy can only be confirmed by immunofluorescence microscopy since arteriolar hyaline changes observed by light microscopy and electron-dense proteinaceous material observed by electron microscopy cannot be distinguished from changes in arteriolar sclerosis, with or without hypertension. A hypertensive vascular change is the second most common change, particularly in patients with chronic renal disease and in patients on long-term steroid treatment (Antonovych & Sabnis, 1995).

In rare cases, malignant hypertension, thrombotic thrombocytopenic purpura and microscopic polyangiitis (MPA) can be seen. The association of MPA with an anti-neutrophil cytoplasmic antibody (ANCA) against myeloperoxidase (MPO) has been noted and MPA is well known to present as one form of primary ANCA-associated vasculitis (Merkel, *et al.*, 1997). Clinical manifestations in MPA include RPGN due to necrotizing glomerulonephritis and pulmonary hemorrhage due to pulmonary capillaritis, which are life-threatening visceral involvements (Gillevin, *et al.*, 1999).

7   Intestinal Vasculitis

Acute abdomen caused by intestinal vasculitis was often observed. Occasionally, surgical treatment was needed. In this study, 4 cases had intestinal vasculitis, 3 of whom had intestinal perforation and 3 cases died. Histological features in a patient with intestinal perforation included necrotizing vasculitis with thrombosis (Figure 9). Occasionally, intestinal bleeding and peritoneal bleeding from vasculitis were observed. Colonic pneumatosis cystoides intestinalis occurred in patients with bowel vasculitis. According to the report by Zizic, *et al.* (Zizic, *et al.*, 1982), acute abdomen was observed in 15 of 140 patients with SLE, and 8 of these 15 patients died. In the present study, vasculitis was observed in 9 of 11 cases with acute surgical abdomen, and intestinal perforation was observed in 6 cases. Risk factors for SLE patients who developed severe abdominal involvement included peripheral vasculitis, neuropsychiatric lupus, aseptic osteonecrosis, thrombocytopenia and positive rheumatoid factor (Zizic, *et al.*, 1982).

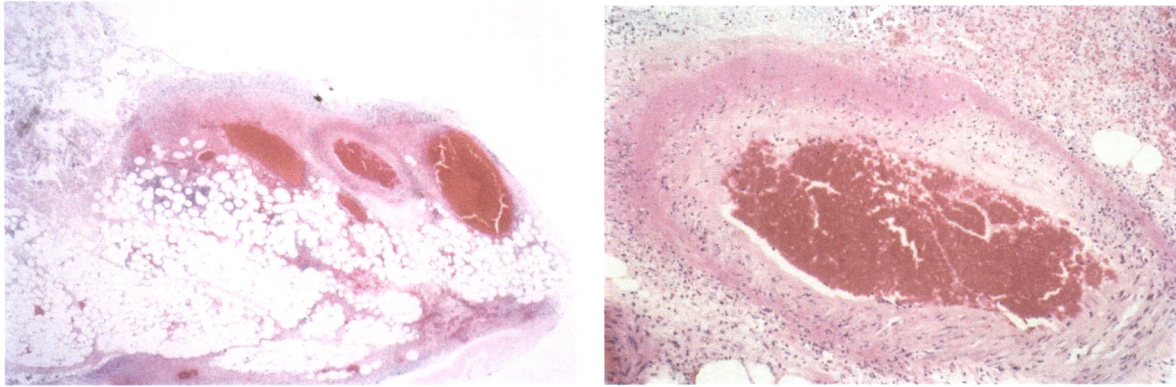

Figure 9: Necrotizing vasculitis with thrombosis observed in an intestinal perforation region (a 49-year-old female patient with anti-phospholipid antibody). Right; features under microscopic magnification.

Although nausea and vomiting, diarrhea, ascites, gastrointestinal bleeding, and fever in conjunction with severe abdominal pains in the intestinal vasculitis were observed, these symptoms might be masked by underlying therapies, such as steroid or immunosuppressive drugs, thus resulting in a delayed diagnosis. The differential diagnosis of intestinal vasculitis was important because it includes other, more common causes of abdominal pain, other lupus-related causes of abdominal pain such as peritonitis and pancreatitis, and other causes of vascular compromise, such as atherosclerosis and anti-phospholipid syndrome. The patients with intestinal vasculitis were commonly treated with high doses of steroids, including intravenous methylprednisolone. If the patients did not rapidly improve, intravenous cyclophosphamide pulse therapy was added. In the usage of the above-mentioned aggressive immunotherapies, antibiotics were mostly administered to prevent infections at the same time.

8   Cutaneous Vasculitis

Cutaneous vasculitis was often observed in SLE and included urticarial vasculitis, leukocytoclastic vasculitis, and polyarteritis nodosa-like vasculitis, livedo reticularis and thrombophlebitis. In addition, cutaneous ulcers (Figure 10), digital gangrene (Figure 11), Raynaud's phenomenon and nail-fold changes were also observed. Urticarial vasculitis often showed low serum complement levels, as well as immune complexes such as cryoglobulin. Cutaneous vasculitis, such as cutaneous ulcers, digital gangrene, splinter hemorrhages, thrombophlebitis and livedo reticularis might be associated with anti-phospholipid antibodies or anti-phospholipid syndrome (McCauliffe & Sontheimer, 1996).

Patients with urticarial vasculitis were treated with non-steroidal anti-inflammatory drugs, steroids and/or immunosuppressive drugs. For patients with severe cutaneous vasculitis, treatment with moderate or high-dosages of steroid and/or immunosuppressive drugs such as cyclophosphamide and azathioprine was needed. In clinical manifestations related to cryoglobulin or anti-phospholipid antibodies, combined therapy of plasmapheresis with steroids or immunosuppressive drugs might be effective (Hashimoto, 2012). For treatment of cutaneous ulcers and digital gangrene/necrosis, prostaglandin agents such as alprostadil (Lipo PGE1) and limaprost alfadex, peripheral vasodilating drugs and antiplatelet drugs such as ticlopidine hydrochloride, clopidogrel sulfate cilostazol, beraprost sodium, sarpogrelate hydrochloride,

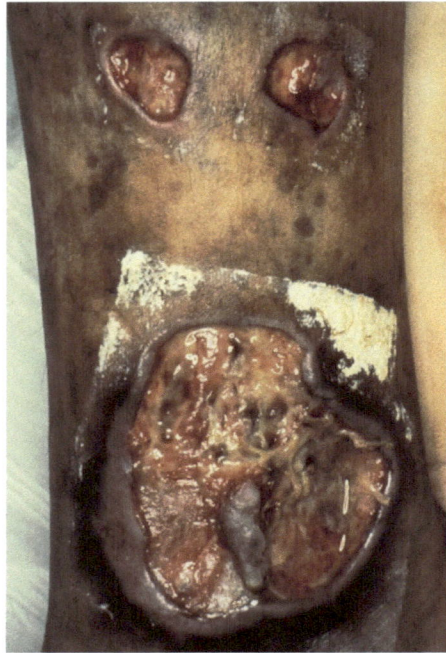

Figure 10: Leg ulcers were observed in an SLE patient (27 year old, male) with lupus nephritis and psychosis.

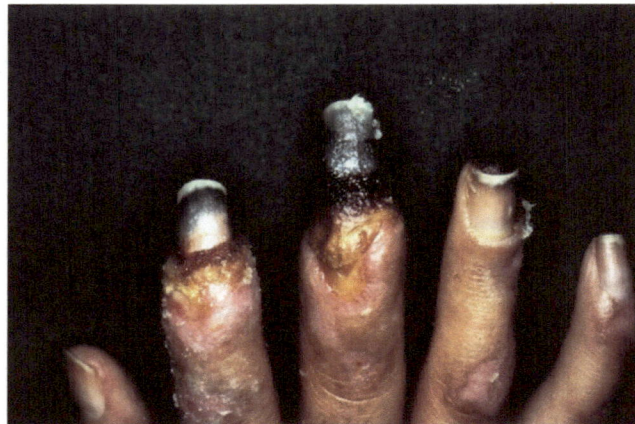

Figure 11: Digital gangrene was observed in an SLE patient (54 year old, female) with Raynaud's phenomenon.

and low-dose aspirin, were used at the same time. Other causes of cutaneous manifestations including infections should be ruled out prior to treatment.

Treatment for Raynaud's phenomenon and peripheral circulatory disturbances included various peripheral vasodilating drugs, such as β-receptor stimulants, nicotinate derivatives and Ca antagonists, and the antiplatelet drugs described above. For refractory cases, a sympathetic ganglion block often was effective. Plasmapheresis might be effective in patients with high viscosity of the plasma (Hashimoto, 2012).

9   Histopathological Vascular Lesions and SLE Prognosis

The relationship between histological vascular lesions and prognosis was studied using 34 autopsied cases (Hashimoto, *et al.*, 1984). These 34 cases were divided into 3 groups according to the size of the involved vessel; (1) medium-sized arteries, (2) small-sized arteries, and (3) without systemic vascular lesions. Vascular lesions were also separated into five groups according to histological findings; (a) fibrinoid degeneration, (b) intimal thickening, (c) thrombosis, (d) sclerosis and (e) without systemic vascular lesions. As a result, cases with involvement of medium-sized arteries causing death were mostly those with central nervous system lupus and had a poor prognosis in comparison to cases with involvement of small-sized arteries and without systemic vascular lesions. According to histological findings, the cause of death in cases with fibrinoid degeneration and thrombosis was mainly renal failure, whereas death from infection was observed in most cases with sclerosis. Cases with thrombosis had the worst prognosis as compared to cases with other histological findings. These histological findings of vascular involvement might be useful for predicting the prognosis of SLE patients.

10   Summary

In this article, the characteristics of cardiovascular manifestations, including cardiac manifestations, cerebrovascular disease, pulmonary vascular involvement, renal vascular involvement, intestinal vasculitis, and cutaneous vasculitis, were analyzed and described using a retrospective review of the medical records of 1125 SLE patients examined in Juntendo University Hospital between 1955 and 2002.

Seventy-seven patients with pericarditis and 25 patients with myocarditis mostly improved after steroid therapy. The average age at development of myocardial infarction (MI) in 11 patients was 51 years. Conservative medical management due to anti-hypertensive drugs and statin without high-dosages of steroids was conducted in most cases with MI. Although several risk factors for MI due to atherosclerosis in SLE have been noted, it has been pointed out that the current guidelines for modifying cardiovascular risk factors in patients with SLE are essentially the same as those aimed at reducing cardiovascular disease in the general population (Skaggs *et al*, 2012). Libman-Sackes (L-S) endocarditis was found in 10 out of 45 autopsied cases. The vegetations of L-S endocarditis were mostly found on the mitral valve leaflets.

Cerebrovascular diseases were observed in 75 patients. A female SLE patient with anti-phospholipid syndrome had necrotizing vasculitis with fibrinoid degeneration together with perivascular round-cell infiltration in vessels of cerebrum. Pulmonary hypertension (PH) was seen in 17 patients (1.5%). The rates of outcomes in terms of improvement, no change and death in patients with PH were almost the same, respectively. Although the patients who improved had mild PH, 6 patients died of heart failure and/or sudden death. Pulmonary arterial thrombosis and/or pulmonary emboli (PAT/PE) were seen in 10 patients and were acute clinical conditions due to vasculitis and abnormal coagulability, including anti-phospholipid syndrome.

Renal vascular lesions in lupus nephritis (LN) were most commonly seen in patients with both focal and diffuse proliferative glomerulonephritis histologically. In the outcome of 32 patients with LN who received long-term treatment for over 20 years, the complete remission rate was 27%, the incomplete remission rate was 37.8%, and the worsening rate was 21.6%. Treatments including steroids, immunosuppressants and plasmapheresis that contributed to remission of LN could not be specified. This fact suggests that the underlying disease types of LN had a greater influence on the remission rate than the treatment method.

Intestinal vasculitis was seen in 4 patients, and 3 of these had intestinal perforation that was the cause of death. Necrotizing vasculitis with thrombosis could be seen histologically in intestinal perforation region in some cases. Cutaneous vasculitis including leukocytoclastic vasculitis, livedo reticularis, thrombophlebitis, cutaneous ulcers, digital gangrene, Raynaud's phenomenon and nail-fold changes, were observed. Combined therapies of plasmapheresis with steroids and/or immunosuppressive drugs were thought to be effective for patients with cutaneous vasculitis, especially when related to cryoglobulinemia or anti-phospholipid antibodies. The histological findings of vascular involvement and the size of the involved vessels might be related to the prognosis of SLE patients.

Acknowledgments

The author acknowledges the helpful contributions of Professors Emeritus Yuichi Shiokawa and Shunichi Hirose, Professors Yoshinari Takasaki, Hiroshi Tsuda and Shigeto Kobayashi, and Dr. Yoshiaki Tokano for their study coordination.

References

ACR Ad Hoc Committee on Neuropsychiatric Lupus Nomenclature. (1999). The American College of Rheumatologynomenclature and case definitions for neuropsychiatric lupus syndrome. Arthritis Rheumatism, 42, 599–608.

Antonovych, T.T., & Sabnis, S.G. (1995). Renal manifestations of systemic lupus erythematosus. In Pathology of Systemic Lupus Erythematosus., (Ed, Antonovych, T.T.) Armed Forces Institute of Pathology American Registry of Pathology, Washington, D.C., (pp. 11–44).

Asanuma, Y., Oeser, A., Shintani, A.K., Turner, E., Olsen, N., Fazio, S., Linton, M.F., Raggi, P & Stein, C.M. (2003). Premature coronary artery atherosclerosis in systemic lupus erythematosus. New England Journal of Medicine, 349, 2407–2415.

Belmont, H.M., Abramson, S.B. & Lie, J.T. (1996). Pathology and pathogenesis of vascular injury in systemic lupus erythematosus. Arthritis Rheumatism, 39, 9–22.

Bruce, I.N., Gladman, D.D. & Urowitz, M.B. (2000). Premature atherosclerosis in SLE. Rheumatic Disease Clinical North America, 26, 257–278.

Bruce, I.N., Urowitz, M.B., Gladman, D.D., Ibanez, D. & Steiner, G. (2003). Risk factors for coronary heart disease in women with systemic lupus erythematosus. The Toronto risk factor study. Arthritis & Rheumatism, 48, 3159–3167.

Bulkley, B.H. & Roberts, W.C. (1975). The heart in systemic lupus erythematosus and the changes induced in it by corticosteroid therapy. A study of 36 necropsy patients. American Journal of Medicine, 58, 243–264.

Burdt, M.A., Hoffman, R.W., Deutsher, S.L., Wang, G.S., Johnson, J.C. & Sharp, G.C.(1999). Long-term outcome in mixed connective tissue disease; longitudinal clinical and serological findings, Arthritis & Rheumatism, 42, 899–909.

Chow, S.L., Chandran, V., Fazelzad, R. & Johnson, S.R. (2011). Prognostic factors for survival in systemic lupus erythematosus associated pulmonary hypertension, Lupus, 21, 353–364.

Churg, J., Bernstein, J., & Glassock, R.J. (1995). Lupus nephritis. In Renal Disease: Classification and Atlas of Glomerular Diseases. 2nd. Ed. New York: Igaku-Shoin (pp151).

Condliffe, R., Kiely, D.G., Peacock, A.J., Corris, P.A., Gibbs, J.S., Vrapi, F.D., Das, C., Elliot, C.A., Johnson, M., DeSoyza, J., Torpy, C., Goldsmith, K., Hodgkins, D., Hughes, R.J., Pepke-Zaba, J. & Coglan, I.G. (2009). Connective tissue disease-associated pulmonary arterial hypertension in the modern treatment era, American Journal Respiratory Critical Care Medicine, 179, 151–157.

D'Cruz, D. (1988). Vasculitis in systemic lupus erythematosus. Lupus, 7, 270–274.

D'Cruz, D.P., Khamashta, M.A. & Hughes, G.R.V. (2007). Systemic lupus erythematosus, Lancet, 369, 587–596.

El-Magadmi, M., Bodill, H., Ahmad, Y., Durrington, P.N., Mackness, M., Walker, M., Bernstein, R.M. & Bruce I.N. (2004), Systemic lupus erythematosus: an independent risk factor for endothelial dysfunction in women, Circulation, 110, 399–404.

Estes, D. & Christian, C.L. (1971). The natural history of systemic lupus erythematosus prospective analysis, Medicine, 50, 85–95.

Faurschou, M., Mellemkjaer, L., Starklint, H., Kamper, A.L., Tarp, U., Voss, A. & Jacobsen, S. (2011). High risk of ischemic heart disease in patients with lupus nephritis. Journal of Rheumatology, 38, 2400–2405.

Gillevin, L., Durand-Gasselin, R., Cevallos, R.(1999). Microscopic polyangiitis: clinical and laboratory findings in eighty-five patients, Arthritis Rheumatism, 42, 421–430.

Gladman, D.D. & Urowitz, M.B. (1980). Venous syndrome and pulmonary embolism in systemic lupus erythematosus, Annals Rheumatic Disease, 39, 340–343.

Gladman. D.D. & Urowitz. M.B. (1987). Morbidity in systemic lupus erythematosus. Journal of Rheumatology, 14 (supplement), 223–226.

Gladman, D.D., Urowitz, M.B., Rahman, P., Ibanez, D. & Tam, L.S. (2003). Accrual of organ damage over time in patients with systemic lupus erythematosus. Journal of Rheumatology, 30, 1955–1959.

Hashimoto, H. (2012). Systemic Lupus Erythematosus – Clinical Manual, 2nd ed., Nihon-ijishinposha, Tokyo, (pp. 238–246). (Japanese).

Hashimoto, H. (2012). Glucocorticoid therapy in systemic lupus erythematosus – clinical analysis of 1125 patients with systemic lupus erytehmatosus. In Glucocorticoids. (Ed. Xiaoxiao, Q.), Intec, Croatia, (pp. 481–500).

Hashimoto, H., Maekawa, S., Nasu, H., Okada, T., Shikawa, Y. & Fukuda, Y. (1984). Systemic vascular lesions and prognosis in systemic lupus erythematosus. Scandinavian Journal of Rheumatology, 13, 45–55.

Hochberg, M.C. (1997). Updating the American College of Rheumatology revised criteria for the classification of systemic lupus erythematosus [letter]. Arthritis & Rheumatism, 40, 1725.

Johnson, S.R. & Granton, J.T. (2011). Pulmonary hypertension in systemic lupus erythematosus, European Respiratory Review, 20, 277–286.

Kasukawa, R., Nishimaki. T., Takagi, T., Miyawaki, S., Yokohari, R. & Tsunematsu, T. (1990). Pulmonary hypertension in connective tissue disease. Clinical Rheumatology, 9, 55–62.

Libman, E. & Sacks, B. (1924). A hitherto undescribed form of valvular and mural endocarditis. Archive Internal Medicine. 33, 701–738.

Manzi, S., Meilahn, E.N., Rairie, J.E, Conte, C.G., Medsger, T.A.Jr. & Jansen-McWilliams, L. (1997). Age-specific incidence rates of myocardial infarction and angina in women with systemic lupus erythematosus: comparison with the Framingham study. American Journal of Epidemiology, 145, 408–415.

McCauliffe, D. P. & Sontheimer, R.D. (1996). Cutaneous lupus erythematosus.. In The Clinical management of Systemic Lupus Erythematosus, 2nd ed., (Ed. Shur, P.H.). Lippincott-Raven, Philadelphia (pp. 67–82).

Medsger, Jr., T. (1996). Pulmonary manifestations. In The Clinical management of Systemic Lupus Erythematosus, 2nd ed., (Ed. Shur, P.H.). Lippincott-Raven, Philadelphia (pp.87).

Merkel, P.A., Polisson, R.P., Chang,Y., Skaters, S. & Niles, J.L. (1997). Prevalence of anti-neutrophil cytoplasmic antibodies in a large inception cohort of patients with connective tissue disease. Annals of Internal medicine, 126, 866–873.

Petri, M., Perez-Gutthan, S., Spence, D. & Hochberg, M.C. (1992). Risk factors for coronary artery disease in patients with systemic lupus erythematosus. American Journal of Medicine, 93, 513–519.

Quismorio, F.P.J., Sharna, O., Koss, M., Boylen, T., Edmiston, A.W., Thornton, P.J. & Tatter, D. (1984). Immunopathologic and clinical studies in pulmonary hypertension associated with systemic lupus erythematosus, Seminer Arthritis Rheumatism, 13, 349–359.

Roman, M.J., Shanker, B.A., Davis, A., Michael, D., Lockshin, M.D., Sammaritano, L. & Simantov, R. (2003). Prevalence and correlates of accelerated atherosclerosis in systemic lupus erythematosus. New England Journal of Medicine, 349, 2399–2406.

Rothfield, N.F. (1996). Cardiac aspect. In The Clinical management of Systemic Lupus Erythematosus, 2nd ed., (Ed. Shur, P.H.). Lippincott-Raven, Philadelphia (pp.83–86).

Salel, A.F., Fong, A. & Zelis, R. (1977). Accuracy of coronary profile: correlation of risk factors with arteriographically documented severity of atherosclerosis, New England Journal of Medicine, 296, 1447–1450.

Skaggs, B.J., Hahn, B.H. & MacMahon, M. (2012). Accelerated atherosclerosis in patients with SLE – mechanisms and management. National Review Rheumatology, 8, 214–223.

Straaton, K.V., Chatham, W.W., Reveille, J.D., Koopman, W.J. & Smith, S.H., (1988). Clinically significant valvular heart disease in systemic lupus erythematosus, American Journal Medicine, 85, 648.

Svenungsson, E., Jensen-Urstad, K., Heimburger, M., Silveira, A., Hamsten, A.,Faire, U., Witztum, J. & Frostegard, J. (2001), Risk factors for cardiovascular disease in systemic lupus erythematosus, Circulation, 104, 1887–1893.

Symmons, D.R. & Gabriel, S.E. (2011). Epidemiology of CVD in rheumatic disease, with a focus on RA and SLE. National Review Rheumatology, 7, 399–408.

Talbott, J.H. (1974). Collagen-Vascular Disease, Gruce & Stratton, INC., New York.

Urowitz,MB, Bookman, A.A., Koehler, B.E., Gordon, D.A., Smythe, H.A. & Ogryzio, M.A. (1976). The bimodal mortality pattern of systemic lupus erythematosus. American Journal Medicine 60: 221–225, 1976.

Wakaki, K., Koizumi, F. & Fukase, M. (1984). Vascular lesions in systemic lupus erythematosus (SLE) with pulmonary hypertension. Acta Pathological Japonica, 34, 593–604.

Wallace, D.J. (2007). The clinical presentation of systemic lupus erythematosus. In Dubois' Lupus Erythematosus, seventh edition. (Edts. Wallace, D.J. & Hahn, B.H.), Lippincott Williams & Wilkins, Philadelphia, (pp. 638–646).

Weening, J.J., D'Agali, V.D., Schwartz, M.M., Seshan, S.V., Alpers, C.E., Apel, G.B., Balow, J.E., Brulin, J.A., Cook, T., Ferrario, F., Fogo, A.B., Ginzler, E.M., Hebert, L., Hill, G., Hill, P., Jennette, J.C., Kong, N.C., Lesavre, P., Lockshin, M., Looi, L., Makino, H., Moura, L.A. & Nagata, M. (2004). The classification of glomerulonephritis in systemic lupus erythematosus. Kidney International, 65, 521–530.

Wel, L., MacDonald, T. & Walker, B. (2004). Taking glucocorticoids by prescription is associated with subsequent cardiovascular disease. Annals Internal Medicine 141, 764–770.

West, S.G. (2007). The nervous system, In Dubois' Lupus Erythematosus, seven edition, (Ed. Wallace, D.J., Hahn, B.H.) Lippincott Williams & Wilkins, Philadelphia, (pp. 707–746).

Zizic, T.M., Classen, J.N. & Stevens, M.B. (1982). Acute abdominal complications of systemic lupus erythematosus and polyarteritis nodosa. American Journal of Medicine 73, 525–531.

Zuily, S., Huttin, O., Mchamed, S., Marie, P.Y., Selton-Suty, C. & Wahl, D. (2013). Valvular heart diseases in antiphospholipid syndrome, Current Rheumatology Reports, 15, 320–328.

The Roles of Novel Vasoactive Agents in Atherosclerotic Cardiovascular Diseases: Good or Bad Guys?

Takuya Watanabe, Hanae Konii, Kengo Sato, Fumiko Itoh
Laboratory of Cardiovascular Medicine
Tokyo University of Pharmacy and Life Sciences
Tokyo, Japan

1   Introduction

Coronary artery disease (CAD) is the most common manifestation of atherosclerosis, which leads to acute coronary syndrome, and it continues to be the most common cause of mortality and morbidity worldwide (Weber & Noels, 2011). Over the past 50 years, it has become clear that the cascade of thrombotic events following atherosclerotic plaque rupture causes occlusion of the coronary artery, interrupting the supply of blood and oxygen to the myocardium, thus resulting in severe ischemia and infarction. Myocardial infarction is followed by heart failure, myocardial rupture, or arrhythmia. Early treatment of myocardial ischemia to prevent infarction using fibrinolysis, coronary artery bypass grafting, and percutaneous coronary intervention has improved the prognosis (Weber & Noels, 2011). Timely diagnosis is important for such treatments to be of maximal benefit. Biomarkers may help to improve diagnostic accuracy during the earlier stages of diseases when preventive measures and more effective treatments can be implemented with lower risks. Further, biomarkers providing prognostic information assist clinicians in deciding how aggressively they need to be treated.

However, only a limited number of markers have demonstrated significant diagnostic and/or therapeutic impact. Deeper insights into the pathophysiology of atherosclerosis have led to the discovery of additional novel biomarkers (Watanabe et al., 2012c). High levels of oxidized low-density lipoprotein (oxLDL), inflammatory cytokines, such as high-sensitivity C-reactive protein (hs-CRP), interleukin-6 (IL-6), and cardiotrophin-1, and potent vasoconstrictors, such as serotonin and urotensin II, can be used as biomarkers for CAD (Holvoet et al., 2001; Noto et al., 2007; Talwar et al., 2000; Watanabe et al., 2009, 2012a). In contrast, reduced circulating levels of antiatherogenic vasoactive agents can also be regarded as indicators for CAD (Watanabe et al., 2012c). New bioactive peptides that have attracted attention have been implicated as potential biomarkers (Watanabe et al., 2013). These include the adipocytokine adiponectin (Barseghian et al., 2011), the glial growth factor heregulin-β_1 (neuregulin-1 type I) (Watanabe et al., 2012b), the incretin hormones glucagon-like peptide-1 (GLP-1) and glucose-dependent insulinotropic polypeptide (GIP) (Ussher & Druker, 2012), and cardio-depressant peptides recently identified by the *in silico* approach, salusin-α and salusin-β (Shichiri et al., 2003).

Risk factors for CAD are well known to include lifestyle-related diseases, such as hypertension, diabetes, dyslipidemia, obesity, smoking, stress, and chronic inflammatory diseases (periodontitis and rheumatoid arthritis), as well as genetic factors. Although these risk factors are treated individually in clinical practice, the occurrence of CAD has not yet been markedly reduced. Therefore, new therapeutic approaches are required for cardiovascular diseases. In the field of cardiovascular medicine, atrial natriuretic peptide and adrenomedullin have been applied to heart failure treatment (Yoshimura et al., 2001; Rademaker et al., 2003). Novel peptides recently discovered by bioinformatics analyses directly affecting vascular cells have attracted attention and have been suggested as potential therapeutic targets for atherosclerotic CAD (Watanabe et al., 2013). Therefore, we sorted a variety of peptides according to their good or bad properties for atherosclerosis by cellular, animal, and clinical experiments.

Atherosclerosis is a chronic inflammatory response to the injury in the arterial wall (Weber & Noels, 2011). As shown in Figure 1, endothelial inflammation is characterized by increased endothelial production of inflammatory cytokines, such as IL-1β and IL-6, monocyte chemoattractant protein-1 (MCP-1), and adhesion molecules, such as vascular cell adhesion molecule-1 (VCAM-1) and intercellular adhesion molecule-1 (ICAM-1). Monocytes adhere to endothelial cells (ECs) and then infiltrate into the neointimal lesion, followed by oxLDL-induced transformation of macrophages into foam cells (Allahverdian et al., 2012). Subsequently, the migration and proliferation of vascular smooth muscle cells (VSMCs) accelerate the development of atherosclerotic plaques (Figure 1). Acute vascular events are provoked by rupture of atherosclerotic plaques and subsequent thrombotic occlusion of the arterial lumen, which interrupts blood flow and causes ischemia in downstream peripheral tissue (Weber & Noels, 2011).

This article focuses on the stimulatory effects on atherosclerosis exerted by serotonin, angiotensin II, urotensin II, cardiotrophin-1, and salusin-β, and the contrasting suppressive effects of adiponectin, GLP-1, GIP, heregulin-β$_1$, and salusin-α. Here, we highlight the emerging roles of recently identified bioactive peptides in addition to classical vasoactive agents that act directly on the arterial wall, which consists of VSMCs, ECs, and monocyte-derived macrophages, as biomarkers and therapeutic targets for CAD.

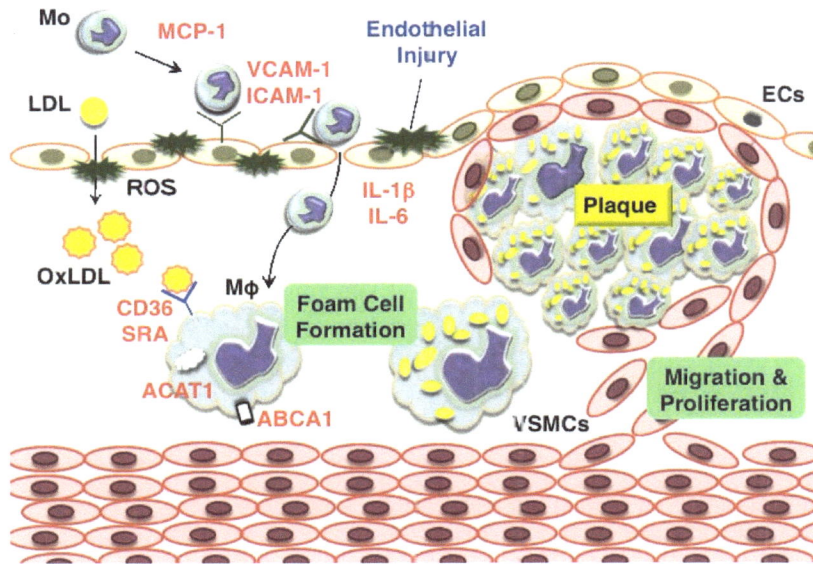

Figure 1: Mechanisms of atherosclerosis. Cellular and molecular phenomena in response to vasoactive agents are described in red in Figure.

2   Roles of Vasoactive Agents in the Cardiovascular System

Serotonin (5-hydroxytryptamine) is secreted from activated platelets and induces both platelet aggregation and VSMC contraction (Watanabe & Koba, 2012). These phenomena are mediated through 5-HT$_{2A}$ receptors, which are present in monocytes/macrophages and ECs, as well as VSMCs and platelets (Watanabe & Koba 2012). Human angiotensin II is a hypertensive polypeptide of 8 amino acids, and is produced by angiotensin-converting enzyme from angiotensin I, which is converted from angiotensinogen by renin in the cardiovascular-renal system. Angiotensin II exerts hypertension-induced cardiovascular remodeling effects, such as hypertrophy of VSMCs and cardiomyocytes through AT$_1$ receptors. Human urotensin II, the most potent vasoconstrictor peptide, consists of 11 amino acids and is produced from preprourotensin by urotensin-converting enzyme (Watanabe et al., 2009). The receptor of urotensin II, the so-called UT receptor, is present in monocytes/macrophages, VSMCs, ECs, and cardiomyocytes (Watanabe et al., 2009). Human cardiotrophin-1, an IL-6 superfamily peptide of 201 amino acids that is dominantly produced from cardiomyocytes and ECs, stimulates hypertension-induced cardiac hypertrophy (López-Andrés *et al.*, 2010). The cardiotrophin-1 receptors, the complex of leukemia inhibitory factor receptor and glycoprotein-13, are present in monocytes/macrophages, VSMCs, ECs, and cardiac fibroblasts (López-Andrés *et al.*, 2010). Human salusin-β is a peptide of 20 amino acids and has potent hypotensive and bradycardic effects (Watanabe *et al.*, 2011). Salusin-β and salusin-α are theoretically produced simultaneously from the same precursor, preprosalusin, following alternative splicing of the torsin-related peptide TOR2a (Shichiri *et al.*, 2003). Salusin-β is expressed in macrophages, VSMCs, and ECs, but receptors for salusin-β have not yet been identified (Watanabe *et al.*, 2011).

Human adiponectin, heregulin-β$_1$, GIP, GLP-1, and salusin-α are peptides of 247, 71, 42, 30, and 28 amino acids, respectively (Barseghian *et al.*, 2011; Watanabe *et al.*, 2011, 2012b; Ussher & Druker, 2012). Adiponectin, GIP, and GLP-1 are predominantly produced in adipose tissue, the K-cells of the upper gut, and the L-cells of the lower gut, respectively, and to a lesser extent by the cardiovascular system (Barseghian *et al.*, 2011; Ussher & Druker, 2012). Salusin-α and heregulin-β$_1$ are both expressed in monocytes/macrophages, VSMCs, and ECs (Watanabe *et al.*, 2011, 2012b). Receptors of adiponectin (AdipoR1 and AdipoR2) and heregulin-β$_1$ (ErbB3 and ErbB4) are abundantly expressed in human monocytes/macrophages, ECs, VSMCs, and cardiomyocytes (Barseghian *et al.*, 2011; Watanabe *et al.*, 2012b). Both GLP-1 receptor (GLP-1R) and GIP receptor (GIPR) are also expressed in these vascular cells and cardiomyocytes as well as pancreatic islet β-cells (Ussher & Druker, 2012; Nagashima *et al.*, 2011). However, salusin-α receptors have not yet been identified (Watanabe *et al.*, 2011). Adiponectin, heregulin-β$_1$, and GLP-1 exert antiinflammatory and antioxidant effects, and promote endothelial nitric oxide production (Barseghian *et al.*, 2011; Watanabe *et al.*, 2012b; Ussher & Druker, 2012). Adiponectin, GLP-1, and heregulin-β$_1$ exhibit cardioprotective effects against ischemic injury (Shibata *et al.*, 2007; Nikolaidis *et al.*, 2005; Hedhli *et al.*, 2011). GLP-1 and GIP stimulate insulin secretion from pancreatic islet β-cells and GLP-1 lowers blood pressure (Ussher & Druker, 2012). Adiponectin and GLP-1 are also known to ameliorate insulin resistance, lipid metabolism, and obesity, whereas GIP induces obesity (Barseghian *et al.*, 2011; Ussher & Druker, 2012). Salusin-α mildly lowers blood pressure and suppresses cardiomyocyte apoptosis, but has no effect on endothelial nitric oxide production (Shichiri *et al.*, 2003; Watanabe *et al.*, 2011).

3   Modulatory Effects of Vasoactive Agents on Atherosclerosis

These vasoactive agents exert opposite effects on foam cell formation, as indicated by cholesterol ester accumulation induced by oxLDL or acetylated LDL in primary cultured human monocyte-derived macrophages (Table 1). Foam cell formation is enhanced by serotonin, angiotensin II, urotensin II, cardiotrophin-1, and salusin-β, but is suppressed by adiponectin, GLP-1, GIP, heregulin-β$_1$, and salusin-α in human monocyte-derived macrophages (Aviram *et al.*, 1992; Kanome *et al.*, 2008; Watanabe *et al.*, 2005, 2008; Konii *et al.*, 2013; Furukawa *et al.*, 2004; Xu *et al.*, 2009; Tashiro *et al.*, 2014). The intracellular free cholesterol level is increased by the endocytic uptake of oxLDL and acetylated LDL *via* CD36 and scavenger receptor class A (SRA), respectively, and is decreased by efflux of free cholesterol mediated mainly by ATP-binding cassette transporter A1 (ABCA1) (Watanabe *et al.*, 2008; Xu *et al.*, 2009). As excessive free cholesterol accumulation is toxic to cells, free cholesterol must be either removed through efflux to extracellular acceptors, such as apolipoprotein (apo) A1 and high-density lipoprotein, or esterified to cholesterol ester by the microsomal enzyme acyl-CoA:cholesterol acyltransferase-1 (ACAT1)

(Watanabe *et al.*, 2008; Xu *et al.*, 2009). As shown in Table 1, ACAT1 expression is stimulated by serotonin, angiotensin II, urotensin II, cardiotrophin-1, and salusin-β, but suppressed by adiponectin, GLP-1, GIP, heregulin-β$_1$, and salusin-α in human monocyte-derived macrophages (Suguro *et al.*, 2006; Kanome *et al.*, 2008; Watanabe *et al.*, 2005, 2008; Konii *et al.*, 2013; Furukawa *et al.*, 2004; Xu *et al.*, 2009; Tashiro *et al.*, 2014). Expression of CD36 and/or SRA is upregulated by cardiotrophin-1 (Konii *et al.*, 2013), and downregulated by serotonin, adiponectin, GLP-1, GIP, and heregulin-β$_1$ (Aviram *et al.*, 1989; Ouchi *et al.*, 2001; Xu *et al.*, 2009; Tashiro *et al.*, 2014), but not altered by angiotensin II, urotensin II, or salusins in human monocyte-derived macrophages (Kanome *et al.*, 2008; Watanabe *et al.*, 2005, 2008). Table 1 shows that ABCA1 is upregulated by adiponectin, GLP-1, GIP, and heregulin-β$_1$ in human monocyte-derived macrophages (Tsubakio-Yamamoto *et al.*, 2008; Xu *et al.*, 2009; Tashiro *et al.*, 2014).

	Foam Cell Formation	ACAT1	CD36/SRA	ABCA1
Serotonin	↑	↑	↓	NE
Angiotensin II	↑	↑	→	→
Urotensin II	↑	↑	→	→
Cardiotrophin-1	↑	↑	↑	→
Salusin-β	↑	↑	→	→
Adiponectin	↓	↓	↓	↑
GLP-1	↓	↓	↓	↑
GIP	↓	↓	↓	↑
Heregulin-β$_1$	↓	↓	↓	↑
Salusin-α	↓	↓	→	→

Table 1: Effects of vasoactive agents on foam cell formation and related gene expression in macrophages. NE: not examined. Arrows indicate stimulatory, suppressive, or negative effects.

Further, we and other groups have documented proatherogenic effects of serotonin, angiotensin II, urotensin II, cardiotrophin-1, and salusin-β, and anti-atherosclerotic effects of adiponectin, GLP-1, GIP, heregulin-β$_1$, and salusin-α in established animal models of atherosclerosis, apoE-knockout mice. Angiotensin II, urotensin II, cardiotrophin-1, and salusin-β accelerate the development of atherosclerotic lesions and macrophage infiltration in aortic walls (Nobuhiko *et al.*, 2004; Shiraishi *et al.*, 2008; Konii *et al.*, 2013; Nagashima *et al.*, 2010). In contrast, adiponectin, GLP-1, GIP, salusin-α, and heregulin-β$_1$ significantly attenuate aortic atherosclerotic lesions accompanied by a significant decrease in macrophage infiltration (Okamaoto *et al.*, 2002; Nagashima *et al.*, 2010, 2011; Xu *et al.*, 2009). Significant changes in oxLDL-induced foam cell formation and ACAT1 expression have been documented *ex vivo* in exudate peritoneal macrophages from apoE-knockout mice infused with these peptides. In our studies, oxLDL-induced foam cell formation and ACAT1 expression were enhanced by urotensin II, cardiotrophin-1, and salusin-β (Shiraishi *et al.*, 2008; Konii *et al.*, 2013; Nagashima *et al.*, 2010), but suppressed by GLP-1, GIP, salusin-α, and heregulin-β$_1$ (Nagashima *et al.*, 2010, 2011; Xu *et al.*, 2009). CD36 expression was upregulated by angiotensin II and cardiotrophin-1 (Keidar *et al.*, 2001; Konii *et al.*, 2013), but downregulated by GLP-1 and GIP (Nagashima *et al.*, 2011). Macrophage foam cell formation was found to be reduced in aortic atherosclerotic lesions from adiponectin-transgenic LDL receptor-knockout mice fed a high-fat diet (Luo *et al.*, 2010). Serotonin receptor 5-HT$_{2A}$-selective antagonists markedly suppress the development of atherosclerotic lesions in rabbits on a high-cholesterol diet (Hayashi *et al.*, 2003), suggesting that endogenous serotonin may play a crucial role in atherosclerosis, as described below.

4   Other Effects of Vasoactive Agents on Vascular Cells

As shown in Table 2, ICAM-1 and/or VCAM-1 expression in ECs are stimulated by angiotensin II, urotensin II, cardiotrophin-1, and salusin-β, but suppressed by adiponectin, GLP-1, GIP, and heregulin-β$_1$, and unaffected by serotonin and salusin-α (Pastore *et al.*, 1999; Cirillo *et al,* 2008; Ichiki *et al.*, 2008; Koya *et al.*, 2012; Nagashima *et al.*, 2011; Xu *et al.*, 2005; Li F *et al.*, 1997). MCP-1 expression is stimulated by serotonin, angiotensin II, urotensin II, cardiotrophin-1, and salusin-β, but reduced by GLP-1, GIP, and heregulin-β$_1$ (Mikulski *et al.*, 2010; Chen *et al.*, 1998; Watson *et al.*, 2013; Ichiki *et al.*, 2008; Koya *et al*; 2012; Nagashima *et al.*, 2011; Xu *et al.*, 2005). Contradictory effects of adiponectin on MCP-1 expression have been reported previously (Watanabe *et al.*, 2013). IL-1β/IL-6 production is stimulated by serotonin, angiotensin II, urotensin II, cardiotrophin-1, salusin-β, and GIP, decreased by adiponectin, GLP-1, and heregulin-β$_1$, and unaffected by salusin-α (Ito *et al.*, 2000; Funakoshi *et al.*, 1999; Johns *et al.*, 2004; Fritzenwanger *et al.*, 2006; Koya *et al.*, 2012; Timper *et al.*, 2013; Neumeier *et al.*, 2006; Iwai *et al.*, 2006; Xu *et al*, 2005).

Table 2 also shows the effects of these agents on VSMC proliferation. Serotonin, angiotensin II, urotensin II, cardiotrophin-1, and salusin-β stimulate VSMC proliferation (Watanabe *et al.*, 2001a, 2001b; Konii *et al.*, 2013; Shichiri *et al.*, 2003). Heregulin-β$_1$ and salusin-α show relatively weak inductive effects on VSMC proliferation (Watanabe *et al.*, 2011, 2012b). In contrast, adiponectin, GLP-1, and GIP suppress proliferation of VSMCs (Wang *et al.*, 2005; Nagashima *et al.*, 2011).

	ICAM-1/VCAM-1 Expression	MCP-1 Expression	IL-1β/IL-6 Expression	VSMC Proliferation
Serotonin	→	↑	↑	↑
Angiotensin II	↑	↑	↑	↑
Urotensin II	↑	↑	↑	↑
Cardiotrophin-1	↑	↑	↑	↑
Salusin-β	↑	↑	↑	↑
Adiponectin	↓	↓ or ↑	↓	↓
GLP-1	↓	↓	↓	↓
GIP	↓	↓	↑	↓
Heregulin-β$_1$	↓	↓	↓	↗
Salusin-α	→	→	→	↗

Table 2: Effects of vasoactive agents on vascular cells

5   Presence of Vasoactive Agents in Human Coronary Artery Lesions and Circulating Blood

High serotonin levels are found in the diseased coronary arteries of patients with CAD (van den Berg *et al.*, 1989). In human coronary arterial lesions, IL-6, angiotensin II, urotensin II, and salusin-β are expressed at high levels (Schieffer *et al.*, 2000; Hassan *et al.*, 2005; Watanabe *et al.*, 2008), whereas salusin-α and heregulin-β$_1$ are expressed at trace levels (Watanabe *et al.*, 2008; Xu *et al*, 2009). In patients with CAD, the expression of adiponectin in epicardial adipose tissues is significantly lower than in non-CAD controls, leading to inflammation and atherosclerosis in coronary arteries (Zhou *et al.*, 2011).

These findings suggest that these peptides could act as accelerators or suppressors in the development of human coronary atherosclerotic lesions and serve as biomarkers for CAD.

Circulating markers are more convenient for diagnosis of CAD. As specific antibodies against these peptides have been developed, their concentrations in blood samples could be quantified using radioimmunoassay and enzyme-linked immunosorbent assay (ELISA). Serum adiponectin levels and plasma levels of hs-CRP, IL-6, heregulin-β_1, GLP-1, and GIP were measured by ELISA, and serum salusin-α levels were measured by radioimmunoassay. It has been difficult to measure salusin-β levels, because of its unique physiochemical features characteristic that salusin-β tightly adheres to polypropylene, polystyrene, and glass commonly used in laboratory handling of blood samples (Shichiri, 2007). We have proposed technical procedures to avoid the adhesive features of this peptide (Sato *et al.*, 2009), and recently succeeded in determining plasma salusin-β levels using a highly sensitive sandwich ELISA (Fujimoto *et al.*, 2013).

To assess essential levels of peptide hormones, the confounding factors that influence peptide production must be taken into consideration. In general, these include food intake, smoking, gender, and the presence of obesity, diabetes, hypertension, or heart failure. Salusin-α, salusin-β, and heregulin-β_1 levels have been demonstrated to be unaffected by a number of physiological stimuli (Watanabe *et al.*, 2012c; Fujimoto *et al.*, 2013). Since adiponectin is known to show sexual dimorphism with higher levels in women than men, serum adiponectin levels have been mostly determined in male subjects. Because GLP-1 and GIP are transiently increased after food intake, plasma incretin levels have been measured in the fasting state and/or after 75-g oral glucose tolerance test. Similar to adiponectin measurements, we determined circulating levels of salusin-α, salusin-β, heregulin-β_1 in the fasting state (Watanabe *et al.*, 2008; Fujimoto *et al.*, 2013; Xu *et al.*, 2009).

6   Relationships Between Circulating Vasoactive Agent Levels and CAD

As shown in Table 3, circulating levels of oxLDL, IL-6, serotonin, angiotensin II, urotensin II, cardiotrophin-1, and salusin-β are significantly higher in patients with CAD than in subjects without CAD (Holvoet *et al.*, 2001; Noto *et al.*, 2007; Vikenes *et al.*, 1999; Li SM *et al.*, 1997; Chai *et al.*, 2010; Talwar *et al.*, 2000; Watanabe *et al.*, 2008). Plasma urotensin II levels are increased in accordance with the severity of CAD. In contrast, circulating levels of adiponectin, GLP-1, heregulin-β_1, and salusin-α are significantly lower in patients with CAD than in those without CAD (El-Menyar *et al.*, 2009; Matsubara *et al.*, 2012; Xu *et al.*, 2009; Watanabe *et al.*, 2008). Serum adiponectin and salusin-α levels and plasma heregulin-β_1 levels are reduced in accordance with the severity of CAD (von Eynatten *et al.*, 2008; Watanabe *et al.*, 2008; Xu *et al.*, 2009). However, serum GIP levels are not significantly correlated with high risk of CAD (Yamaoka-Tojo *et al.* 2010).

Receiver operating characteristic curve analyses have shown that IL-6 (AUC: 0.936), oxLDL (0.935), and salusin-α (0.916) are more powerful biomarkers for CAD, with better sensitivity and specificity, than salusin-β (0.781), adiponectin (0.718), and heregulin-β_1 (0.706) (Noto *et al.*, 2007; Watanabe *et al.*, 2012c).

	Non-CAD Subjects	CAD Patients	P-value
OxLDL (mg/dl)	1.30±0.88	3.11±1.19*	<0.001
IL-6 (pg/ml)	1.7 (0.6–6.8)	15 (3.6–66)	<0.0001
Serotonin (µM)	0.84±0.06	1.05±0.05*	<0.01
Angiotensin II (pg/ml)	39.7±22.8	68.3±31.7	<0.01
Urotensin II (pg/ml)	20.9±7.0	71.9±11.6	<0.01
Cardiotrophin-1 (pM)	27 (6.9–54.1)	114.8 (41.5–527.4)	<0.0001
Salusin-β (nM)	4.09±0.09	5.26±0.20	<0.0001
Adiponectin (µg/ml)	3.1±0.3	1.9±0.2	<0.005
GLP-1 (pM)	4.00 (3.10–5.90)	3.10 (2.40–3.62)	<0.001
Heregulin-β₁ (ng/ml)	7.69±1.51	1.68±0.26	<0.0005
Salusin-α (pM)	18.4±1.0	4.9±0.6	<0.0001

Table 3: Circulating levels of vasoactive agents in CAD patients and non-CAD subjects. CAD was defined as one or more lesions with ≥75% (* ≥50%) diameter stenosis by coronary arteriography.

7   Effects of Antagonists or Agonists for Vasoactive Agent Receptors on Atherosclerosis

The modulatory effects of the above-mentioned agents on atherosclerosis have been clarified. With regard to proatherogenic agents, receptor antagonists for serotonin, angiotensin II, and urotensin II can be applied for treatment of atherosclerosis based on the following experimental and clinical evidence. As salusin-β receptors have not yet been identified, anti-salusin-β neutralizing antibody, as a surrogate for its receptor antagonist, shows therapeutic efficiency in experimental atherosclerosis (Nagashima *et al.*, 2010). Sarpogrelate, a 5-HT$_{2A}$ receptor-selective antagonist, prevents the development of atherosclerotic lesions in rabbits fed a high-cholesterol diet (Hayashi *et al.*, 2003). This reagent suppresses macrophage ACAT1 expression (Suguro *et al.*, 2006), vascular oxidative stress (Sun *et al.*, 2001), and VSMC proliferation (Watanabe *et al.*, 2001a), upregulates endothelial nitric oxide synthase (Hayashi *et al.*, 2003), and reduces the expression of matrix metalloproteinase-1 (Hayashi *et al.*, 2003), contributing to stabilization of vulnerable plaque. Several studies have reported potential clinical benefits that sarpogrelate increases collateral perfusion and decreases myocardial ischemia, and prevents restenosis after coronary angioplasty in patients with CAD (Satomura *et al.*, 2002; Fujita *et al.*, 2003). In patients with peripheral artery disease, sarpogrelate also improves limb ischemic symptoms by increasing plasma adiponectin levels and decreasing platelet aggregation and the release of platelet-derived growth factor, soluble P-selectin, and transforming growth factor-β₁ from platelets, as well as IL-18 (Nakamura *et al.*, 2001; Yamakawa *et al.*, 2003, 2004). Candesartan, one of a number of AT₁ receptor blockers (ARBs) widely used in the treatment of hypertension, significantly retards the development of atherosclerotic lesions in apoE-knockout mice (Hayashi *et al.*, 2012), possibly by suppressing macrophage foam cell formation and VSMC proliferation (Kanome *et al.*, 2008; Watanabe *et al.*, 2001a). This drug reduces carotid atherosclerosis by enhancing nitric oxide and decreasing oxidative stress in patients with hypertension (Ono *et al.*, 2008). Combination therapy of candesartan with statin inhibits the progression of atherosclerosis more potently than statin alone in patients with CAD (Suzuki *et al.*, 2011). Other ARBs also have the similar antiatherosclerotic effects other than blood-pressure-lowing effects (Honjo *et al.*, 2011). We have shown that 4-aminoquinoline, a UT receptor antagonist, attenuates the development of macrophage-driven atherosclerotic lesions in apoE-knockout mice (Shiraishi *et al.*, 2008). Recent clinical studies have shown that palosuran, a UT receptor antagonist, did not affect insulin secretion in patients with type 2 diabetes and albuminuria in hypertensive patients with type 2 diabetic nephropathy (Vogt *et al.*, 2010; Sidharta *et al.*, 2009). Other UT receptor antagonists should be investigated for antiatherogenic effects in patients with atherosclerotic cardiovascular diseases. All receptor antagonists described above have been shown to have pleiotropic effects, such as antiinflammatory and antioxidant effects, as well as antiatherosclerotic effects. Our recent study showed that chronic infusion of anti-cardiotrophin-1 neutralizing antibody into apoE-knockout mice prevents the development of atherosclerotic lesions by suppressing monocyte infiltration into aortic walls (Konii *et al.*, 2013).

With regard to antiatherogenic peptides, such as adiponectin, GLP-1, GIP, heregulin-β_1, and salusin-α, these receptor agonists and analogs (mimetics) have become useful as therapeutic agents for atherosclerosis (Watanabe *et al.*, 2013). In particular, incretin-based therapies are attractive for treatment of diabetes in clinical practice. Both GLP-1 and GIP are rapidly degraded by dipeptidyl peptidase-4 (DPP-4) in the blood or various tissues (Ussher & Druker, 2012). Incretin-based therapies involve long-acting GLP-1 analogs and DPP-4 inhibitors that increase endogenous GLP-1 and GIP levels (Ussher & Druker, 2012). Recently, we and other groups have demonstrated that these incretin-based treatments prevent the development of atherosclerotic lesions in apoE-knockout mice (Nagashima *et al.*, 2011; Terasaki *et al.*, 2012; Vittone *et al.*, 2012; Ta *et al.*, 2011; Arakawa *et al.*, 2010; Gaspari *et al.*, 2011), and restenosis after vascular injury in murines (Goto *et al.*, 2011; Lim *et al.*, 2012). Several recent studies have shown that administration of GLP-1 or heregulin-β_1 improves cardiac dysfunction in patients with heart failure (Read *et al.*, 2012; Mendes-Ferreira *et al.*, 2013). A recent study indicated that exenatide, a GLP-1 analog, increases myocardial blood flow in type 2 diabetic patients without CAD (Gejl *et al.*, 2012). Major clinical trials have shown the cardioprotective effects of exenatide in patients with acute coronary syndrome, successfully treated with percutaneous coronary intervention (Scholte *et al.*, 2011). Intracoronary administration of adiponectin leads to a reduction in myocardial infarct size and improvement of cardiac function after ischemia/reperfusion injury in pigs (Kondo *et al.*, 2010). However, the cardioprotective effects of adiponectin and salusin-α have not yet been reported in humans. In the near future, agonists for adiponectin, salusin-α, and heregulin-β_1 receptors or their analogs may become candidates for treatment of atherosclerosis and related diseases (Watanabe *et al.*, 2011, 2012b, 2013).

8   Conclusions

Serotonin, angiotensin II, urotensin II, cardiotrophin-1, and salusin-β exert proatherogenic effects, whereas adiponectin, GLP-1, GIP, heregulin-β_1, and salusin-α have antiatherogenic effects. These agents may become useful therapeutic targets for atherosclerotic cardiovascular diseases as evidenced by recent studies using the antagonists for AT1, 5-HT2A, UT, cardiotrophin-1 receptor, and salusin-β receptor and/or agonists for AdipoR1, AdipoR2, GLP-1R, GIPR, ErbB3, ErbB4, and salusin-α receptor. In addition, high levels of these proatherogenic agents and/or extremely low levels of these antiatherogenic agents are candidate biomarkers for predicting CAD. Combined use of various biomarkers rather than single use may be useful for the early detection of atherosclerotic cardiovascular diseases.

References

Arakawa, M., Mita, T., Azuma, K., Ebato, C., Goto, H., Nomiyama, T., Fujitani, Y., Hirose, T., Kawamori, R., & Watada, H. (2010). Inhibition of monocyte adhesion to endothelial cells and attenuation of atherosclerotic lesion by a glucagon-like peptide-1 receptor agonist, exendin-4. Diabetes, 59, 1030–1037.

Aviram, M. (1989). Platelet secretory products enhance LDL receptor activity and inhibit scavenger receptor activity in human monocyte derived macrophages. Metabolism, 38, 425–430.

Aviram, M., Fuhrman, B., Maor, I., & Brook, G.J. (1992). Serotonin increases macrophage uptake of oxidized low density lipoprotein. Eur J Clin Chem Clin Biochem, 30, 55–61.

Barseghian, A., Gawande, D., & Bajaj, M. (2011). Adiponectin and vulnerable atherosclerotic plaques. J Am Coll Cardiol, 57, 761–770.

Chai, S.B., Li, X.M., Pang, Y.Z., Qi, Y.F., & Tang, C.S. (2010). Increased plasma levels of endothelin-1 and urotensin-II in patients with coronary heart disease. Heart Vessels, 25, 138–143.

Chen, X.L., Tummala, P.E., Olbrych, M.T., Alexander, R.W., & Medford, R.M. (1998). Angiotensin II induces monocyte chemoattractant protein-1 gene expression in rat vascular smooth muscle cells. Circ Res, 83, 952–959.

Cirillo, P., de Rosa, S., Pacileo, M., Gargiulo, A., Angri, V., Fiorentino, I., Prevete, N., Petrillo, G., de Palma, R., Leonardi, A., de Paulis, A., & Chiariello, M. (2008). Human urotensin II induces tissue factor and cellular adhesion molecules expression in human coronary endothelial cells: an emerging role for urotensin II in cardiovascular disease. J Thromb Haemost, 6, 726–736.

El-Menyar, A., Rizk, N., Al Nabti, A.D., Hassira, S.A., Singh, R., Abdel Rahman, M.O., & Suwaidi, J.A. (2009). Total and high molecular weight adiponectin in patients with coronary artery disease. J Cardiovasc Med, 10, 310–315.

Fritzenwanger, M., Meusel, K., Foerster, M., Kuethe, F., Krack, A., & Figulla, H.R. (2006). Cardiotrophin-1 induces interleukin-6 synthesis in human umbilical vein endothelial cells. Cytokine, 36, 101–106.

Fujimoto, K., Hayashi, A., Kamata, Y., Ogawa, A., Watanabe, T., Ichikawa, R., Iso, Y., Koba, S., Kobayashi, Y., Koyama, T., & Shichiri, M. (2013). Circulating levels of human salusin-β, a potent hemodynamic and atherogenesis regulator. PLoS One, 8, e76714.

Fujita, M., Mizuno, K., Ho, M., Tsukahara, R., Miyamoto, A., Miki, O., Ishii, K., & Miwa, K. (2003). Sarpogrelate treatment reduces restenosis after coronary stenting. Am Heart J, 145, E16.

Funakoshi, Y., Ichiki, T., Ito, K., & Takeshita, A. (1999). Induction of interleukin-6 expression by angiotensin II in rat vascular smooth muscle cells. Hypertension, 34, 118–125.

Furukawa, K., Hori, M., Ouchi, N., Kihara, S., Funahashi, T., Matsuzawa, Y., Miyazaki, A., Nakayama, H., & Horiuchi, S. (2004). Adiponectin down-regulates acyl-coenzyme A:cholesterol acyltransferase-1 in cultured human monocyte-derived macrophages. Biochem Biophys Res Commun, 317, 831–836.

Gaspari, T., Liu, H., Welungoda, I., Hu, Y., Widdop, R.E., Knudsen, L.B., Simpson, R.W., & Dear, A.E. (2011). A GLP-1 receptor agonist liraglutide inhibits endothelial cell dysfunction and vascular adhesion molecule expression in an ApoE$^{-/-}$ mouse model. Diab Vasc Dis Res, 8, 117–124.

Gejl, M., Søndergaard, H.M., Stecher, C., Bibby, B.M., Møller, N., Bøtker, H.E., Hansen, S.B., Gjedde, A., Rungby, J., & Brock, B. (2012). Exenatide alters myocardial glucose transport and uptake depending on insulin resistance and increases myocardial blood flow in patients with type 2 diabetes. J Clin Endocrinol Metab, 97, E1165–E1169.

Goto, H., Nomiyama, T., Mita, T., Yasunari, E., Azuma, K., Komiya, K., Arakawa, M., Jin, W.L., Kanazawa, A., Kawamori, R., Fujitani, Y., Hirose, T., & Watada, H. (2011). Exendin-4, a glucagon-like peptide-1 receptor agonist, reduces intimal thickening after vascular injury. Biochem Biophys Res Commun, 405, 79–84.

Hassan, G.S., Douglas, S.A., Ohlstein, E.H., & Giaid, A. (2005). Expression of urotensin-II in human coronary atherosclerosis. Peptides, 26, 2464–2472.

Hayashi, K., Sasamura, H., Azegami, T., & Itoh, H. (2012). Regression of atherosclerosis in apolipoprotein E-deficient mice is feasible using high-dose angiotensin receptor blocker, Candesartan. J Atheroscler Thromb, 19, 736–746.

Hayashi, T., Sumi, D., Matsui-Hirai, H., Fukatsu, A., Arockia, J., Rani P.J.A., Kano, H., Tsunekawa, T., & Iguchi, A. (2003). Sarpogrelate HCl, a selective 5-HT$_{2A}$ antagonist, retards the progression of atherosclerosis through a novel mechanism. Atherosclerosis, 168, 23–31.

Hedhli, N., Huang, Q., Kalinowski, A., Palmeri, M., Hu, X., Russell, R.R., & Russell, K.S. (2011). Endothelium-derived neuregulin protects the heart against ischemic injury. Circulation, 123, 2254–2262.

Holvoet, P., Mertens, A., Verhamme, P., Bogaerts, K., Beyens, G., Verhaeghe, R., Collen, D., Muls, E., & de Werf, F.V. (2001). Circulating oxidized LDL is a useful marker for identifying patients with coronary artery disease. Arterioscler Thromb Vasc Biol, 21, 844–848.

Honjo, T., Yamaoka-Tojo, M., & Inoue, N. (2011). Pleiotropic effects of ARB in vascular metabolism–focusing on atherosclerosis-based cardiovascular disease. Curr Vasc Pharmacol, 9, 145–152.

Ichiki, T., Jougasaki, M., Setoguchi, M., Imamura, J., Nakashima, H., Matsuoka, T., Sonoda, M., Nakamura, K., Minagoe, S., & Tei, C. (2008). Cardiotrophin-1 stimulates intercellular adhesion molecule-1 and monocyte chemoattractant protein-1 in human aortic endothelial cells. Am J Physiol Heart Circ Physiol, 294, H750–H763.

Ito, T., Ikeda, U., Shimpo, M., Yamamoto, K., & Shimada, K. (2000). Serotonin increases interleukin-6 synthesis in human vascular smooth muscle cells. Circulation, 102, 2522–2527.

Iwai, T., Ito, S., Tanimitsu, K., Udagawa, S., & Oka, J. (2006). Glucagon-like peptide-1 inhibits LPS-induced IL-1β production in cultured rat astrocytes. Neurosci Res, 55, 352–360.

Johns, D.G., Ao, Z., Naselsky, D., Herold, C.L., Maniscalco, K., Sarov-Blat, L., Steplewski, K., Aiyar, N., & Douglas, S.A. (2004). Urotensin-II-mediated cardiomyocyte hypertrophy: effect of receptor antagonism and role of inflammatory mediators. Naunyn Schmiedebergs Arch Pharmacol, 370, 238–250.

Kanome, T., Watanabe, T., Nishio, K., Takahashi, K., Hongo, S., & Miyazaki, A. (2008). Angiotensin II upregulates acyl-CoA:cholesterol acyltransferase-1 via the angiotensin II type 1 receptor in human monocyte-macrophages. Hypertens Res, 31, 1801–1810.

Keidar, S., Heinrich, R., Kaplan, M., Hayek, T., & Aviram, M. (2001). Angiotensin II administration to atherosclerotic mice increases macrophage uptake of oxidized LDL: a possible role for interleukin-6. Arterioscler Thromb Vasc Biol, 21, 1464–1469.

Kondo, K., Shibata, R., Unno, K., Shimano, M., Ishii, M., Kito, T., Shintani, S., Walsh, K., Ouchi, N., & Murohara, T. (2010). Impact of a single intracoronary administration of adiponectin on myocardial ischemia/reperfusion injury in a pig model. Circ Cardiovasc Interv, 3, 166–173.

Konii, H., Sato, K., Kikuchi, S., Okiyama, H., Watanabe, R., Hasegawa, A., Yamamoto, K., Itoh, F., Hirano, T., & Watanabe, T. (2013). Stimulatory effects of cardiotrophin 1 on atherosclerosis. Hypertension, 62, 942-950.

Koya, T., Miyazaki, T., Watanabe, T., Shichiri, M., Atsumi, T., Kim-Kaneyama, J.R., & Miyazaki, A. (2012). Salusin-β accelerates inflammatory responses in vascular endothelial cells via NF-κB signaling in LDL receptor-deficient mice in vivo and HUVECs in vitro. Am J Physiol Heart Circ Physiol, 303, H96–H105.

Li, F., Joshua, I.G., Lian, R., & Justus, D.E. (1997). Differing regulation of major histocompatibility class II and adhesion molecules on human umbilical vein endothelial cells by serotonin. Int Arch Allergy Immunol, 112, 145–151.

Li, S.M., Liu, B., & Chen, H.F. (1997). Effect of puerarin on plasma endothelin, renin activity and angiotensin II in patients with acute myocardial infarction. Zhongguo Zhong Xi Yi Jie He Za Zhi, 17, 339–341.

Lim, S., Choi, S.H., Shin, H., Cho, B.J., Park, H.S., Ahn, B.Y., Kang, S.M., Yoon, J.W., Jang, H.C., Kim, Y.B., & Park, K.S. (2012). Effect of a dipeptidyl peptidase-IV inhibitor, des-fluoro-sitagliptin, on neointimal formation after balloon injury in rats. PLoS One, 7, e35007.

López-Andrés, N., Fortuno, M.A., Diez, J., Zannad, F., Lacolley, P., & Rossignol, P. (2010). Vascular effects of cardiotrophin-1: a role in hypertension? J Hypertens, 28, 1261–1272.

Luo, N., Liu, J., Chung, B.H., Yang, Q., Klein, R.L., Garvey, W.T., & Fu, Y. (2010). Macrophage adiponectin expression improves insulin sensitivity and protects against inflammation and atherosclerosis. Diabetes, 59, 791–799.

Matsubara, J., Sugiyama, S., Sugamura, K., Nakamura, T., Fujiwara, Y., Akiyama, E., Kurokawa, H., Nozaki, T., Ohba, K., Konishi, M., Maeda, H., Izumiya, Y., Kaikita, K., Sumida, H., Jinnouchi, H., Matsui, K., Kim-Mitsuyama, S., Takeya, M., & Ogawa, H. (2012). A dipeptidyl peptidase-4 inhibitor, des-fluoro-sitagliptin, improves endothelial function and reduces atherosclerotic lesion formation in apolipoprotein E-deficient mice. J Am Coll Cardiol, 59, 265–276.

Mendes-Ferreira, P., De Keulenaer, G.W., Leite-Moreira, A.F., & Brás-Silva, C. (2013). Therapeutic potential of neuregulin-1 in cardiovascular desease. Drug Discov Today, 18, 836–842.

Mikulski, Z., Zaslona, Z., Cakarova, L., Hartmann, P., Wilhelm, J., Tecott, L.H., Lohmeyer, J., & Kummer, W. (2010). Serotonin activates murine alveolar macrophages through 5-HT$_{2C}$ receptors. Am J Physiol Lung Cell Mol Physiol, 299, L272–L280.

Nagashima, M., Watanabe, T., Shiraishi, Y., Morita, R., Terasaki, M., Arita, S., Hongo, S., Sato, K., Shichiri, M., Miyazaki, A., & Hirano, T. (2010). Chronic infusion of salusin-α and -β exerts opposite effects on atherosclerotic lesion development in apolipoprotein E-deficient mice. Atherosclerosis, 212, 70–77.

Nagashima, M., Watanabe, T., Terasaki, M., Tomoyasu, M., Nohtomi, K., Kim-Kaneyama, J., Miyazaki, A., & Hirano T. (2011). Native incretins prevent the development of atherosclerotic lesions in apolipoprotein E knockout mice. Diabetologia, 54, 2649–2659.

Nakamura, K., Kariyazono, H., Masuda, H., Sakata, R., & Yamada, K. (2001). Effects of sarpogrelate hydrochloride on adenosine diphosphate- or collagen-induced platelet responses in arteriosclerosis obliterans. Blood Coagul Fibrinolysis, 12, 391–397.

Neumeier, M., Weigert, J., Schäffler, A., Wehrwein, G., Müller-Ladner, U., Schölmerich, J., Wrede, C., & Buechler, C. (2006). Different effects of adiponectin isoforms in human monocytic cells. J Leukoc Biol, 79, 803–808.

Nikolaidis, L.A., Doverspike, A., Hentosz, T., Zourelias, L., Shen, Y.T., Elahi, D., Shannon, R.P. (2005). Glucagon-like peptide-1 limits myocardial stunning following brief coronary occlusion and reperfusion in conscious canines. J Pharmacol Exp Ther, 312, 303–308.

Nobuhiko, A., Suganuma, E., Babaev, V.R., Fogo, A., Swift, L.L., Linton, M.F., Fazio, S., Ichikawa, I., & Kon, V. (2004). Angiotensin II amplifies macrophage-driven atherosclerosis. Arterioscler Thromb Vasc Biol, 24, 2143–2148.

Noto, D., Cottone, S., Baldassare, C.A., Vadala, A., Barbagallo, C.M., Rizzo, M., Pernice, V., Mina, M., Fayer, F., Cerasola, G., Notarbartolo, A., & Rocco A.M. (2007). Interleukin 6 plasma levels predict with high sensitivity and specificity coronary stenosis detected by coronary angiography. Thromb Haemost, 98, 1362–1367.

Okamoto, Y., Kihara, S., Ouchi, N., Nishida, M., Arita, Y., Kumada, M., Ohashi, K., Sakai, N., Shimomura, I., Kobayashi, H., Terasaka, N., Inaba, T., Funahashi, T., & Matsuzawa, Y. (2002). Adiponectin reduces atherosclerosis in apolipoprotein E-deficient mice. Circulation, 106, 2767–2770.

Ono, H., Minatoguchi, S., Watanabe, K., Yamada, Y., Mizukusa, T., Kawasaki, H., Takahashi, H., Uno, T., Tsukamoto, T., Hiei, K., & Fujiwara, H. (2008). Candesartan decreases carotid intima-media thickness by enhancing nitric oxide and decreasing oxidative stress in patients with hypertension. Hypertens Res, 31, 271–279.

Ouchi, N., Kihara, S., Arita, Y., Maeda, K., Kuriyama, H., Okamoto, Y., Hotta, K., Nishida, M., Takahashi, M., Nakamura, T., Yamashita, S., Funahashi, T., & Matsuzawa, Y. (1999). Novel modulator for endothelial adhesion molecules: adipocyte-derived plasma protein adiponectin. Circulation, 100, 2473–2476.

Ouchi, N., Kihara, S., Arita, Y., Nishida, M., Matsuyama, A., Okamoto, Y., Ishigami, M., Kuriyama, H., Kishida, K., Nishizawa, H., Hotta, K., Muraguchi, M., Ohmoto, Y., Yamashita, S., Funahashi, T., & Matsuzawa, Y. (2001). Adipocyte-derived plasma protein, adiponectin, suppresses lipid accumulation and class A scavenger receptor expression in human monocyte-derived macrophages. Circulation, 103, 1057–1063.

Pastore, L., Tessitore, A., Martinotti, S., Toniato, E., Alesse, E., Bravi, M.C., Ferri, C., Desideri, G., Gulino, A., & Santucci, A. (1999). Angiotensin II stimulates intercellular adhesion molecule-1 (ICAM-1) expression by human vascular endothelial cells and increases soluble ICAM-1 release in vivo. Circulation, 100, 1646–1652.

Rademaker, M.T., Cameron, V.A., Charles, C.J., Lainchbury, J.G., Nicholls, M.G., & Richards, A.M. (2003). Adrenomedullin and heart failure. Regul Pept, 112, 51–60.

Read, P.A., Khan, F.Z., & Dutka, D.P. (2012). Cardioprotection against ischemia induced by dobutamine stress using glucagon-like peptide-1 in patients with coronary artery disease. Heart, 98, 408–413.

Sato, K., Sato, T., Susumu, T., Koyama, T., & Shichiri, M. (2009). Presence of immunoreactive salusin-β in human plasma and urine. Regul Pept, 158, 63–67.

Satomura, K., Takase, B., Hamabe, A., Ashida, K., Hosaka, H., Ohsuzu, F. & Kurita, A. (2002). Sarpogrelate, a specific 5-HT₂-receptor antagonist, improves the coronary microcirculation in coronary artery disease. Clin Cardiol, 25, 28–32.

Schieffer, B., Schieffer, E., Hilfiker-Kleiner, D., Hilfiker, A., Kovanen, P.T., Kaartinen, M., Nussberger, J., Harringer, W., & Drexler, H. (2000). Expression of angiotensin II and interleukin 6 in human coronary atherosclerotic plaques: potential implications for inflammation and plaque instability. Circulation, 101, 1372–1378.

Scholte, M., Timmers, L., Bernink, F.J., Denham, R.N., Beek, A.M., Kamp, O., Diamant, M., Horrevoets, A.J., Niessen, H.W., Chen, W.J., van Rossum, A.C., van Royen, N., Doevendans, P.A., & Appelman, Y. (2011). Effect of additional treatment with EXenatide in patients with an Acute Myocardial Infarction (EXAMI): study protocol for a randomized controlled trial. Trials, 12, 240.

Shibata, R., Izumiya, Y., Sato, K., Papanicolaou, K., Kihara, S., Colucci, W.S., Sam, F., Ouchi, N., & Walsh, K. (2007). Adiponectin protects against the development of systolic dysfunction following myocardial infarction. J Mol Cell Cardiol, 42, 1065–1074.

Shichiri, M., Ishimaru, S., Ota, T., Nishikawa, T., Isogai, T., & Hirata, Y. (2003). Salusins: newly identified bioactive peptides with hemodynamic and mitogenic activities. Nat Med, 9, 1166–1172.

Shichiri, M. (2007). Reply to 'Salusins; newly identified bioactive peptides with hemodynamic and mitogenic activities.' Nat Med, 13, 661–662.

Shiraishi, Y., Watanabe, T., Suguro, T., Nagashima, M., Kato, R., Hongo S., Itabe, H., Miyazaki, A., Hirano, T., & Adachi, M. (2008). Chronic urotensin II infusion enhances macrophage foam cell formation and atherosclerosis in apolipoprotein E-knockout mice. J Hypertens, 26, 1955–1965.

Sidharta, P.N., Rave, K., Heinemann, L., Chiossi, E., Krähenbühl, S., & Dingemanse, J. (2009). Effect of the urotensin-II receptor antagonist palosuran on secretion of and sensitivity to insulin in patients with type 2 diabetes mellitus. Br J Clin Pharmacol, 68, 502–510.

Suguro, T., Watanabe, T., Kanome, T., Kodate, S., Hirano, T. Miyazaki, A., & Adachi, M. (2006). Serotonin acts as an upregulator of acyl-coenzyme A:cholesterol acyltransferase-1 in human monocyte-macrophages. Atherosclerosis, 186, 275–281.

Sun, Y.M., Su, Y., Jin, H.B., Li, J., & Bi, S. (2001). Sarpogrelate protects against high glucose-induced endothelial dysfunction and oxidative stress. Int J Cardiol, 147, 383–387.

Suzuki, T., Nozawa, T., Fujii, N., Sobajima, M., Ohori, T., Shida, T., Matsuki, A., Kameyama, T., & Inoue, H. (2011). Combination therapy of candesartan with statin inhibits progression of atherosclerosis more than statin alone in patients with coronary artery disease. Coron Artery Dis, 22, 352–358.

Ta, N.N., Schuyler, C.A., Li, Y., Lopes-Virella, M.F., & Huang, Y. (2011). DPP-4 (CD26) inhibitor alogliptin inhibits atherosclerosis in diabetic apolipoprotein E-deficient mice. J Cardiovasc Pharmacol, 58, 157–166.

Talwar, S., Squire, I.B., Downie, P.F., Davies, J.E., & Ng, L.L. (2000). Plasma N terminal pro-brain natriuretic peptide and cardiotrophin 1 are raised in unstable angina. Heart, 84, 421–424.

Tashiro, Y., Sato., K., Watanabe, T., Nohttomi, K., Terasaki, M., Nagashima, M., & Hirano, T. (2014). A glucagon-like peptide-1 analog liraglutide suppresses macrophage foam cell formation and atherosclerosis. Peptides, 54, 19-26.

Terasaki, M., Nagashima, M., Watanabe, T., Miyazaki, A., & Hirano, T. (2012). Preventive effects of dipeptidyl peptidase-4 inhibitor on the development of atherosclerotic lesions in apolipoprotein E-null mice. Metabolism, 61, 974–977.

Timper, K., Grisouard, J., Sauter, N.S., Herzog-Radimerski, T., Dembinski, K., Peterli, R., Frey, D.M., Zulewski, H., Keller, U., Müller, B., & Christ-Crain, M. (2013). Glucose-dependent insulinotropic polypeptide induces cytokine expression, lipolysis, and insulin resistance in human adipocytes. Am J Physiol Endocrinol Metab, 304, E1–E13.

Tsubakio-Yamamoto, K., Matsuura, F., Koseki, M., Oku, H., Sandoval, J.C., Inagaki, M., Nakatani, K., Nakaoka, H., Kawase, R., Yuasa-Kawase, M., Masuda, D., Ohama, T., Maeda, N., Nakagawa-Toyama, Y., Ishigami, M., Nishida, M., Kihara, S., Shimomura, I., & Yamashita, S. (2008). Adiponectin prevents atherosclerosis by increasing cholesterol efflux from macrophages. Biochem Biophys Res Commun, 375, 390–394.

Ussher, J.R. & Drucker, D.J. (2012). Cardiovascular biology of the incretin system. Endocr Rev, 33, 187–215.

van den Berg, E.K., Schmitz, J.M., Benedict, C.R., Malloy, C.R., Willerson, J.T., & Dehmer, G.J. (1989). Transcardiac serotonin concentration is increased in selected patients with limiting angina and complex coronary lesion morphology. Circulation, 79, 116–124.

Vikenes, K., Farstad, M., & Nordrehaug, J.E. (1999). Serotonin is associated with coronary artery disease and cardiac events. Circulation, 100, 483–489.

Vittone, F., Liberman, A., Vasic, D., Ostertag, R., Esser, M., Walcher, D., Ludwig, A., Marx, N., & Burgmaier, M. (2012). Sitagliptin reduces plaque macrophage content and stabilizes arteriosclerotic lesions in Apoe$^{-/-}$ mice. Diabetologia, 55, 2267–2275.

Vogt, L., Chiurchiu, C., Chadha-Boreham, H., Danaietash, P., Dingemanse, J., Hadjadj, S., Krum, H., Navis, G., Neuhart, E., Parvanova, A.I., Ruggenenti, P., Woittiez, A.J., Zimlichman, R., Remuzzi, G., de Zeeuw, D., & PROLONG (PROteinuria Lowering with urOteNsin receptor antaGonists) Study Group. (2010). Effect of the urotensin receptor antagonist palosuran in hypertensive patients with type 2 diabetic nephropathy. Hypertension, 55, 1206–1209.

von Eynatten, M., Humpert, P.M., Bluemm, A., Lepper, P.M., Hamann, A., Allolio, B., Nawroth, P.P., Bierhaus, A., & Dugi, K.A. (2008). High-molecular weight adiponectin is independently associated with the extent of coronary artery disease in men. Atherosclerosis, 99, 123–128.

Wang, Y., Lam, K.S., Xu, J.Y., Lu, G., Xu, L.Y., Cooper, G.J., & Xu, A. (2005). Adiponectin inhibits cell proliferation by interacting with several growth factors in an oligomerization-dependent manner. J Biol Chem, 280, 18341–18347.

Watanabe, T., Pakala, R., Katagiri, T., & Benedict, C.R. (2001a). Serotonin potentiates angiotensin II-induced vascular smooth muscle cell proliferation. Atherosclerosis, 159, 269–279.

Watanabe, T., Pakala, R., Katagiri, T., & Benedict, C.R. (2001b). Synergistic effect of urotensin II with mildly oxidized LDL on DNA synthesis in vascular smooth muscle cells. Circulation, 104, 16–18.

Watanabe, T., Suguro, T., Kanome, T., Sakamoto, Y., Kodate, S., Hagiwara, T., Hongo, S., Hirano, T., Adachi, M., & Miyazaki, A. (2005). Human urotensin II accelerates foam cell formation in human monocyte-derived macrophages. Hypertension, 46, 738–744.

Watanabe, T., Nishio, K., Kanome, T., Matsuyama, T., Koba, S., Sakai, T., Sato, K., Hongo, S., Nose, K., Ota, H., Kobayashi, Y., Katagiri, T., Shichiri, M., & Miyazaki, A. (2008). Impact of salusin-α and -β on human macrophage foam cell formation and coronary atherosclerosis. Circulation, 117, 638–648.

Watanabe, T., Arita, S., Shiraishi, Y., Suguro, T., Sakai, T., Hongo, S., & Miyazaki, A. (2009). Human urotensin II promotes hypertension and atherosclerotic cardiovascular diseases. Curr Med Chem, 16, 550–563.

Watanabe, T., Sato, K., Itoh, F., Iso, Y., Nagashima, M., Hirano, T., & Shichiri, M. (2011). The roles of salusins in atherosclerosis and related cardiovascular diseases. J Am Soc Hypertens, 5, 359–365.

Watanabe, T. & Koba, S. (2012a). Roles of serotonin in atherothrombosis and related diseases. In: Traditional and Novel Risk Factors in Atherothrombosis; Efrain Gaxiola, Ed.; InTech: Rijeka, Croatia, pp. 57–70.

Watanabe, T., Sato, K., Itoh, F., & Iso, Y. (2012b). Pathogenic involvement of heregulin-β$_1$ in anti-atherogenesis. Regul Pept, 175, 11–14.

Watanabe, T., Sato, K., Itoh, F., Wakabayashi, K., Shichiri, M., & Hirano, T. (2012c). Endogenous bioactive peptides as potential biomarkers for atherosclerotic coronary heart disease. Sensors (Basel), 12, 4974–4985.

Watanabe, T., Sato, K., Itoh, F., Noguchi, Y., Fujimoto, K., Koyama, T., & Shichiri, M. (2013). Emerging roles for vasoactive peptides in diagnostic and therapeutic strategies against atherosclerotic cardiovascular diseases. Curr Protein Pept Sci, 14, 472–480.

Watson, A.M., Olukman, M., Koulis, C., Tu, Y., Samijono, D. Yuen, D. Lee, C., Behm, D.J., Cooper, M.E., Jandeleit-Dahm, K.A., Calkin, A.C., & Allen, T.J. (2013). Urotensin II receptor antagonism confers vasoprotective effects in diabetes associated atherosclerosis: studies in humans and in a mouse model of diabetes. Diabetologia, 56, 1155–1165.

Weber, C. & Noels, H. (2011). Atherosclerosis: current pathogenesis and therapeutic options. Nat Med, 17, 1410–1422.

Xu, G., Watanabe, T., Iso, Y., Koba, S., Sakai, T., Nagashima, M., Arita S., Hongo, S., Ota, H., Kobayashi, Y., Miyazaki, A., & Hirano, T. (2009). Preventive effects of heregulin-β_1 on macrophage foam cell formation and atherosclerosis. Circ Res, 105, 500–510.

Xu, Z., Ford, G.D., Croslan, D.R., Jiang, J., Gates, A., Allen, R., & Ford, B.D. (2005). Neuroprotection by neuregulin-1 following focal stroke is associated with the attenuation of ischemia-induced pro-inflammatory and stress gene expression. Neurobiol Dis, 19, 461–470.

Yamakawa, J., Takahashi, T., Itoh, T., Kusaka, K., Kawaura, K., Wang, X.Q., & Kanda, T. (2003). A novel serotonin blocker, sarpogrelate, increases circulating adiponectin levels in diabetic patients with arteriosclerosis obliterans. Diabetes Care, 26, 2477–2478.

Yamakawa, J., Takahashi, T., Saegusa, S., Moriya, J., Itoh, T., Kusaka, K., Kawaura, K., Wang, X.Q., & Kanda, T. (2004). Effect of the serotonin blocker sarpogrelate on circulating interleukin-18 levels in patients with diabetes and arteriosclerosis obliterans. J Int Med Res, 32, 166–169.

Yamaoka-Tojo, M., Tojo, T., Takahira, N., Matsunaga, A., Aoyama, N., Masuda, T., & Izumi, T. (2010). Elevated circulating levels of an incretin hormone, glucagon-like peptide-1, are associated with metabolic components in high-risk patients with cardiovascular disease. Cardiovasc Diabetol, 9, 17.

Yoshimura, M., Yasue, H., & Ogawa, H. (2001). Pathophysiological significance and clinical application of ANP and BNP in patients with heart failure. Can J Physiol Pharmacol, 79, 730–735.

Zhou, Y., Wei, Y., Wang, L., Wang, X., Du, X., Sun, Z., Dong, N., & Chen, X. (2011). Decreased adiponectin and increased inflammation expression in epicardial adipose tissue in coronary artery disease. Cardiovasc Diabetol, 10, 2.

Mutations of Mitochondrial Genome and Atherosclerosis: Possible Mechanistic Relationship

Igor A. Sobenin
Laboratory of Medical Genetics, A.L. Myasnikov Institute of Clinical Cardiology
Russian Cardiology Research and Production Complex, Russia

Yuri V. Bobryshev
Faculty of Medicine, School of Medical Sciences
University of New South Wales, Australia

Elena B. Romanenko
A.N. Belozersky Research Institute of Physico-Chemical Biology
M.V. Lomonosov Moscow State University, Russia

Alexander N. Orekhov
Institute for Atherosclerosis Research
Skolkovo Innovative Center, Russia

1   Introduction

In humans, several diseases such as coronary stenosis, some forms of diabetes, myocardial infarction, cardiomyopathy, neurodegenerative diseases, and other pathologies have been associated with mutations in the mitochondrial genome (Taylor & Turnbull, 2005; Raule *et al.*, 2007; Sevini *et al.*, 2007; Reeve *et al.*, 2008; Fayssoil, 2009; Wallace, 2010; Weakley *et al.*, 2010; Yarham *et al.*, 2010; Craigen, 2012; Gratchev *et al.*, 2012; Griffiths, 2012; Limongelli *et al.*, 2012; Mohammed *et al.*, 2012; Park & Larsson, 2011; Rötig, 2011; Schapira, 2012; Schon *et al.*, 2012). Atherosclerosis, the most common pathology in modern society, underlies the development of most cardiovascular diseases, which are the leading cause of death in the 21st century. Atherosclerosis is a multifactorial disease, in the development and progression of which an interaction of phenotypic, environmental, socioeconomic and genetic factors plays a significant role. Numerous polymorphisms of the nuclear genome considered as genetic risk factors for atherosclerotic diseases, can help explaining for only a few percentages of the variability of clinical manifestations of atherosclerosis, such as coronary heart disease (CHD) (John *et al.*, 2009). At the same time, mutations of the mitochondrial genome have remained out of focus for a long time. However, these mutations may play a pathogenic role in the formation of atherosclerotic lesions of human arteries causing various defects in the protein chains of some energy-generating enzymes and transfer RNA (tRNA), synthesized directly in the mitochondria (Weakley *et al.*, 2010). This leads to a decrease in the concentration of these enzymes and their tRNA or total dysfunction, which contributes to the development of oxidative stress, deterioration of ATP production and, presumably, to accelerated development of atherosclerosis (Griffiths, 2012). Thus, mutations occurring within the mitochondrial genome may be a probable cause of atherosclerosis development in humans. Studying associations between mitochondrial mutations and focal development of atherosclerotic lesions in human arteries is of high theoretical and practical impact. Nowadays there is a growing body of evidence in support of a non-redundant role of mitochondrial factors in the pathogenesis of atherosclerosis.

2   Structural Changes of Mitochondria in Atherosclerosis

The utltramicroscopic structure of intimal cells in atherosclerotic lesions has been in focus for of a number of electron-microscopic studies for decades (Geer *et al.*, 1961; Balis *et al*, 1964; Simionescu & Sima, 2012); however, the information on the structural changes of mitochondria in atherosclerosis is insufficient. It has been shown recently that mitochondria in blood leukocytes from atherosclerotic patients are structurally more heterogeneous than mitochondria in leukocytes in the blood of healthy individuals (Sobenin *et al.*, 2012a). Our recent electron-microscopic study of human atherosclerotic lesions, obtained during urgent autopsies carried out within 1.5-3 hours after sudden death, revealed the existence of profound structural alterations of mitochondria in cells (Sobenin *et al.*, 2012b, Sobenin *et al.*, 2013c) (Figure 1). Whereas in some mitochondria cristae were well-defined (Figure 1A), other mitochondria displayed different degrees of the structural alterations of cristae, which were manifested as in a reduction of the number of cristae as in changes in the crista shapes (Figure 1A). In mitochondria with disrupted crista architectonics, the formation of membrane-surrounded structures, which perhaps represent degenerating cristae, was also observed, and the zones of mitochondrial matrix with the membrane-surrounded structures are usually characterized by oedema (Figure 1B, C). Some mitochondria demonstrated focal damages of the integrity of their surrounding membranes. Even though some mitochondria were observed in direct contact with lysosomes that results in the formation of autophagosomal bodies, the vast majority of altered mitochondria do not prompt the process of authophagocytos (Sobenin *et al.*, 2013c). In some mitochondria, cristae were completely destroyed (Figure 1D).

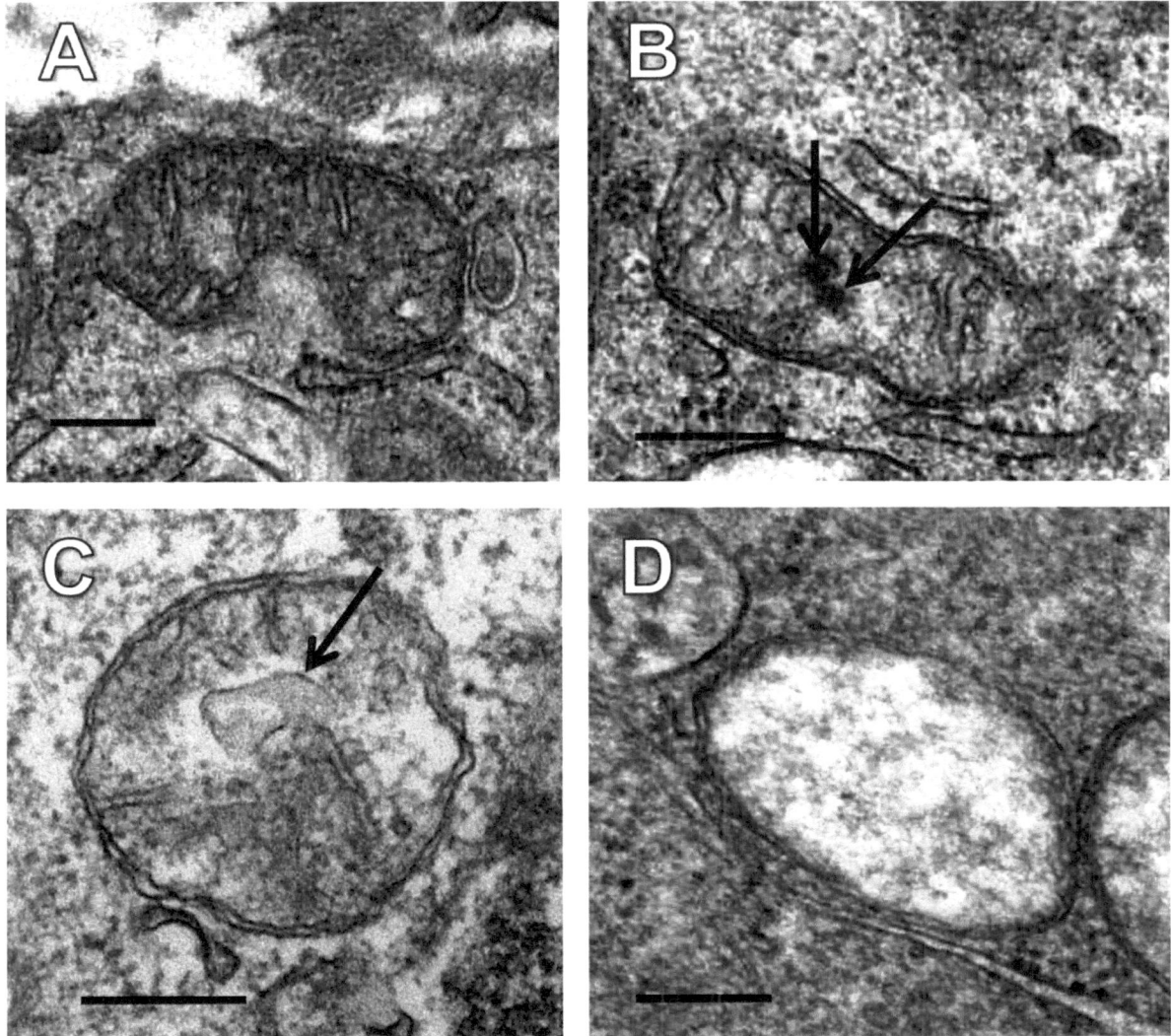

Figure 1: Different ultrastructural characteristics of mitochondria in cells in human atherosclerotic lesions. (**A**): "Intact" mitochondria with well-defined cristae and well-preserved surrounding membranes. (**B, C**): Alterations of cristae and the formation of vacuole-like structures (shown by arrows) in zones of edematous matrix of mitochondria. (**D**): Complete disappearance of cristae from swollen mitochondrion. Electron microscopy; Scales = 200 nm (**A-D**).

In some mitochondria present in intimal cells in atherosclerotic lesions, the destruction of cristae was accompanied by formation of electron-dense bodies located in matrix of swollen mitochondria (Sobenin *et al.*, 2012b) (Figure 2 A-D).

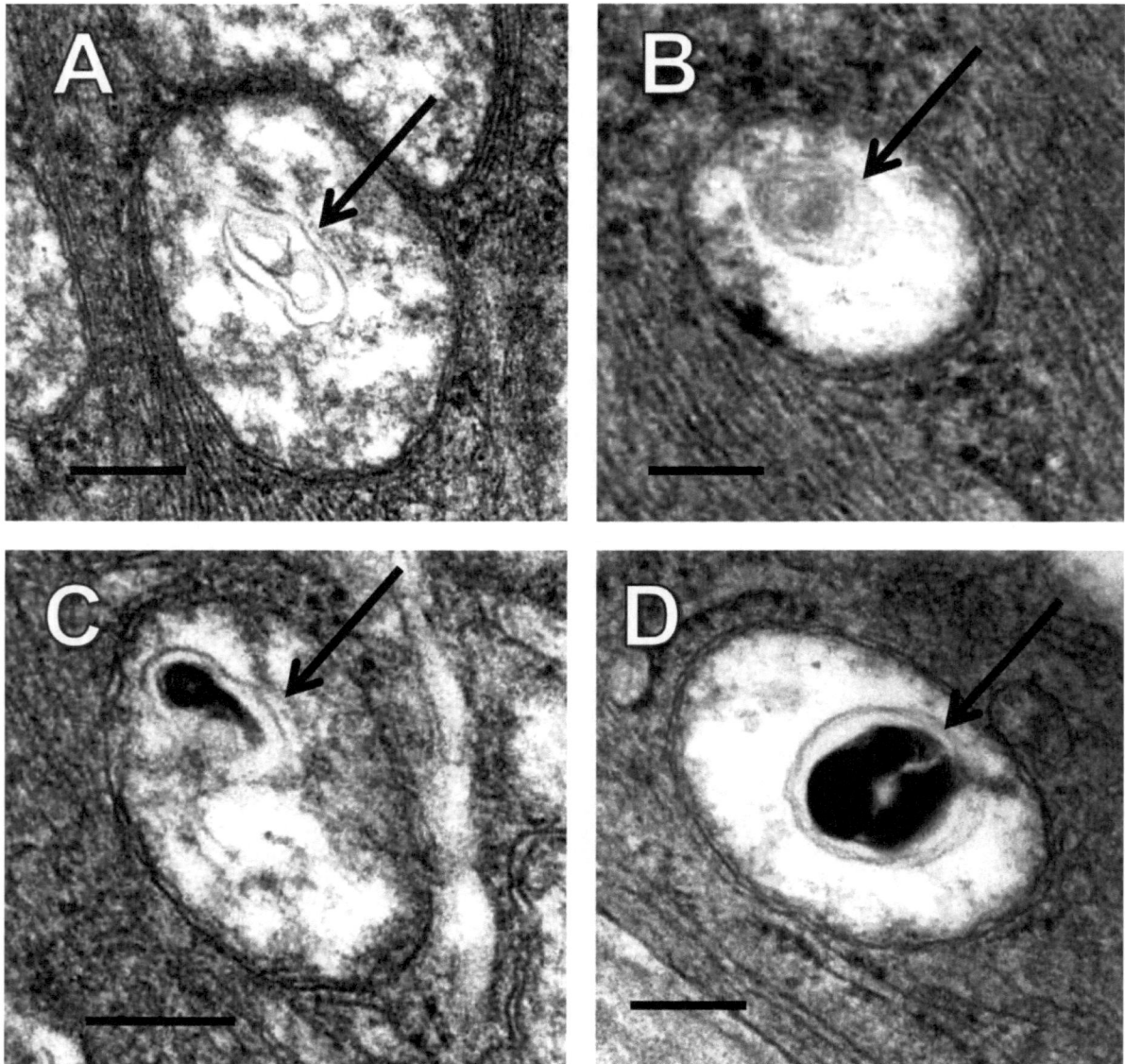

Figure 2: Destructive alterations of mitochondria in intimal cells in human atherosclerotic lesions (**A-C**). Formation of round-shaped membrane-surrounded structures (**A, B**; shown by arrows) and formation of electron-dense bodies on the base of round-shaped membrane-surrounded structures within mitochondrial matrix (**C, D**; shown by arrows). In (**C**), note destruction of the integrity of the surrounding membrane. Electron microscopy; Scales = 200 nm (**A-D**).

As intact mitochondria and mitochondria with structural alterations are both present in the same tissue specimens, the observed changes of mitochondria cannot be considered as a result of autolytic degeneration which potentially could occur in autopsy material. More possibly, they reflect the existence of *in situ* morphological heterogeneity of mitochondria. The observation that the surrounding membranes in some mitochondria were damaged (Figure 2D) may indicate that some components of mitochondrial matrix could enter to the cytoplasm. It is well established that a large number of cells in atherosclerotic lesions undergo cell death (Björkerud & Björkerud, 1996; Bobryshev *et al.*, 1997), with many of them undergoing necrotic mode of death which is accompanied by the release of cytoplasmic content in the extracellular space (Bobryshev *et al.*, 1997; Martinet *et al.*, 2011). Even though a possibility of the presence of antibodies against mitochondrial components in atherosclerosis have not yet been investigated, it is known that antibodies to other structural components of atherosclerotic lesions and circulating immune complexes can also be identified in atherosclerotic lesions (Burut *et al.*, 2011). Mitochondria also play a role in immunity (Cloonan & Choi, 2012) but the contribution of mitochondria in immune reactions in atherosclerosis is not recognized so far. So, electron-microscopic analysis of atherosclerotic lesions demonstrates a high variability in the ultrastructural appearance of mitochondria in human aortic atherosclerotic lesions compared with the appearance of mitochondria in the unaffected parts of the aortic intima. The observed structural variations in the appearance of mitochondria may be a phenotypic and morphologic reflection or go in parallel with mutations in the human mitochondrial DNA (mtDNA), which, in turn, could be a determinant of atherosclerosis.

3   The Background: ROS-Induced Oxidation and Damage of mtDNA

The mitochondria are among the chief producers of oxygen free radicals within the cell. The electron transport chain constantly produces superoxide radical anions, which, in the case of mitochondrial dysfunction, cause the escape of electrons that readily form hydroxyl radicals and hydrogen peroxide from superoxide. These extremely reactive oxygen species (ROS) are risk factors for atherosclerosis associated with lipid and protein oxidation in the vascular wall. ROS formation triggers a cascade of events, such as modification of low density lipoprotein, inflammation, cellular apoptosis and endothelium injury. In atherosclerotic lesions, advanced ROS production positively correlates with multiple mitochondrial abnormalities including impaired mitochondrial dynamics, mitochondrial dysfunction, altered oxidative phosphorylation capacity, induction of the mitochondrial-dependent apoptosis, and other pathologic changes (Davidson & Duchen, 2007). During oxidative phosphorylation, 5% of the oxygen used in respiration is converted to superoxide anions or other ROS (Aitken *et al.*, 1992). The close proximity of mtDNA to the harmful ROS makes mtDNA vulnerable to oxidative attack.

It is estimated mtDNA has a mutation rate 10-20 times higher than nuclear DNA (Yakes & Van Houten, 1997). Two factors contribute to the vulnerability of mtDNA as compared to nuclear DNA. First, coupled with the close proximity to ROS, mtDNA is also lacking the protective strategies associated with nuclear DNA such as protective histones, chromatin structure, and introns (Wallace, 1992), and second, the proof reading apparatus for mtDNA is much less efficient than that of nuclear DNA (Croteau & Bohr, 1997). Though mtDNA is packaged by proteins and harbors some DNA repair capacity, these protective functions are less robust than those functions operating on nuclear DNA and therefore are thought to contribute to the enhanced susceptibility of mtDNA to oxidative damage. Mutations in mtDNA can have a significant detrimental effect due to decreased noncoding regions.

Increased oxidative stress induced by ROS was shown to directly damage mtDNA (Wu *et al.*, 2004). One of the products of DNA oxidation resulted from the attack of DNA nucleosides by hydroxyl radicals, 8-hydroxy-2'-deoxyguanosine (8-OHdG), is generated from oxidized mtDNA at rates 3-23 fold higher than from nuclear DNA (Hamilton *et al.*, 2001).

Severe oxidative stress leads also to reduction in copy number of mtDNA in peripheral blood mononuclear cells (PMBCs) (Liu *et al.*, 2003; Chen *et al.*, 2008; Wang *et al.*, 2011). A lower copy number of mtDNA is associated with the increased levels of 8-OHdG thereby reflecting the relationship with advanced rate of DNA damage, and correlates with the severity of independent risk factors of atherosclerosis such as hyperlipidemia (Liu *et al.*, 2005). In macrophages, reduced ability of mitochondria to utilize oxidized lipids can accelerate transformation of macrophages to foam cells and therefore participate in atherogenesis.

4   Heteroplasmy of mtDNA and Mutational Threshold

Mitochondrial mutations can be both somatic and inherited through the maternal line. They are characterized by the phenomenon of heteroplasmy, which is defined as the presence of a mixture of more than one type of an organellar genome within a cell or individual. Mitochondrial DNA is present in hundreds to thousands of copies per cell and has a very high mutation rate. New mtDNA mutations arise in cells, coexist with wild-type mtDNA, and segregate randomly during cell division. The penetrance and expression of mitochondrial mutations vary greatly between relatives and depend mainly on a genotype and the level of heteroplasmy (a proportion of mutant molecules of mtDNA). The mixtures of wild-type and mutant mtDNA coexisting in the same mitochondria are referred to as heteroplasmic mutations. Therefore, both a qualitative and a quantitative evaluation of a mutant allele of mitochondrial genome are necessary for studying the association of mitochondrial mutations with human diseases.

A mitochondrial disorder can result from the substitution, deletion, and duplication of mtDNA bases and depletion of mtDNA copies. To add to the complexity of mitochondrial disorders, they can arise from one mtDNA mutation or from a number of independent mutations that in turn can lead to more than one disease type. The number of mutations can increase in a particular tissue, while not being reflected in other parts of the body. Mitochondrial mutations can also be homoplasmic in nature when cellular mitochondria contain all of the same mutant mtDNA.

Repeated cell division leads to the separation of heteroplasmic and homoplasmic cell lines in a phenomenon of random segregation. Mutant mtDNA increases with aging, thus decreasing cellular energy capacity. This decrease in turn affects the threshold of a minimal cell function (Diehl & Hoek, 1999). Although cells may harbor mutant mtDNA, the expression of disease is dependent on the level of heteroplasmy. Modeling approaches suggest that an upper threshold level might exist for mutations beyond which the mitochondrial population collapses with a concomitant decrease in ATP (Kowald & Kirkwood, 1993). This decrease in ATP results in the phenotypic expression of disease (Schapira, 2012). It is estimated that in many patients with clinical manifestations of mitochondrial disorders the proportion of mutant DNA exceeds 50% (Smith & Lightowlers, 2011).

Regardless of the type of mutation or the amount of heteroplasmy in affected mitochondria, unrepaired damage leads to a decrease in ATP, which in turn causes the phenotypic manifestation of disease. The manifestation of disease not only depends on the ATP level but also on the tissue affected. For example, the tissue threshold for muscle or neuronal tissue is thought to be as high as or higher than 90% for damaged mtDNA (Moraes *et al.*, 1993). This means the proportions of damaged mtDNA in the total cellular pool must exceed 90% before onset of biochemical abnormalities. For biochemical malfunctions to occur, threshold values for complex I dysfunction have been calculated to be 70-80% for muscle, liver, and kidney, 64% for the heart, and 50% for the brain. For complex III dysfunction, threshold values were found to be high and showed little tissue variation. For complex IV dysfunction, threshold values for the heart and skeletal muscle were calculated to be 67% while kidney and brain were 86%. An 80% decrease in activity of complex IV will lead to a small decrease in liver function, while the heart will experience a 40% decrease in function (Rossignol *et al.*, 1999). Thus, the threshold of malfunction in a given tissue is dependent on the energy demand and the sensitivity of the tissue to mitochondrial dysfunction.

5   Quantitative Assessment of Heteroplasmy

The above considerations raise important methodological problem, since quantitative evaluation of a mutant allele of mitochondrial genome may be a keystone for diagnostics of individual genetic predisposition to the disease, including atherosclerosis. Routine methods of direct sequencing, like Sanger sequencing are generally inappropriate due to erroneous results in the case of polynucleotide sequences, very often observed in mtDNA, although such method has been used for the measurement of heteroplasmy level (Irvin *et al.*, 2009). As a rule, sequence analysis of heteroplasmy around 50% provides clear results in terms of the presence of heteroplasmy, but not in a quantitative manner. Lower level heteroplasmy is often undetectable by direct sequencing. As an example, Meierhofer et al. have used denaturing high performance liquid chromatography to rapidly screen the entire mtDNA for mutations; this approach yielded straightforward interpretation of results with a detection limit down to 1% mtDNA heteroplasmy. However, direct sequencing analysis has become informative only after collection and re-amplification of low degree heteroduplex peak-fractions (Meierhofer *et al.*, 2005).

The high frequency of sporadic mtDNA mutations and their close proximity to each other in mtDNA sequence greatly restricts the possibilities and capacities of well-recognized qPCR methodology; however, the use of locked nucleic acids (LNA), chemically modified ribonucleotides containing additional covalent bond between the oxygen in position 2 'and the carbon at position 4' in the molecule of D-ribose can help solve the problem (Koshkin *et al.*, 1998). This additional bond captures a well-defined conformation of TaqMan probe. The inclusion of several (2-6) LNA molecules in the hybridization probe can significantly improve its characteristics while reducing the overall length to 14-16 nucleotides. This approach was successfully used for the simultaneous measurement of high-level heteroplasmy of two mitochondrial mutations, A3243AG and T8993T G which made possible to identify extremely low levels of heteroplasmy (about 0.01%) (Strand *et al.*, 2008).

There are several methodological approaches, which allow estimating the proportion of mutant allele in heteroplasmic mtDNA sample. Among them, the following can be mentioned: high performance liquid chromatography (HPLC) (Meierhofer *et al.*, 2005), SnapShot analysis (Cassandrini *et al.*, 2006), temporal temperature gradient gel electrophoresis (Wong *et al.*, 2004), high resolution melt profiling (HRM) (Dobrowolski *et al.*, 2009), invader assay (Mashima *et al.*, 2004), amplification refractory mutation system (Bai and Wong, 2004), endonuclease methodology using Surveyor nuclease (Bannwarth *et al.*, 2005), pyrosequencing (Sazonova *et al.*, 2009), and next generation sequencing (NGS) (Zaragoza *et al.*, 2010). Every strategy possesses its own advantages and disadvantages. For example, the approaches employing HRM, HPLC and endonuclease method are exactly suitable for identification of heteroplasmy itself, but they have insufficient resolution for the quantitative measurement of the proportion of mutant allele in the case of mtDNA heteroplasmy. On the opposite, the strategies employing pyrosequencing or NGS provide high accuracy for the quantitative determination of heteroplasmy levels, but they are very expensive, thus effective only for the analysis of a limited number of samples.

However, pyrosequencing is supposed to be a method of choice, in spite of its limitations, as it provides the best value for money, and has been reported in recent basic and clinical studies as a methodology for quantitative measurements of mtDNA heteroplasmy (Sazonova *et al.*, 2009; Sobenin *et al.*, 2012a; Sobenin *et al.*, 2012b; Sobenin *et al.*, 2013). It is a novel sequencing method of relatively short DNA fragments based on real-time (quantitative) pyrophosphate release (Alderborn *et al.*, 2000). A DNA fragment consisting of a sequencing primer hybridized to a single stranded DNA fragment is incubated with the enzymes (DNA polymerase, ATP sulfurylase, firefly luciferase and a nucleotide degrading enzyme). The deoxynucleotides dATP, dCTP, dGTP and dTTP are added sequentially in an iterative manner. In case of complementarity to the base of the DNA template, each time the DNA polymerase incorporates a nucleotide to the new DNA strand, pyrophosphate is released in equal molarity to that of the incorporated deoxynucleotide. Then pyrophosphate is used as a substrate for the enzyme ATP sulfurylase converting pyrophosphate into ATP. Subsequently, the concentration of ATP is detected by the enzyme luciferase as a visible and measurable real-time light signal. Between each addition of deoxynucleotides, unincorporated nucleotides and ATP are degraded by the nucleotide-degrading enzyme. Properties of this enzyme include a slower degradation of nucleotides than the nucleotide incorporation by the DNA polymerase and a slower degradation of ATP than ATP synthesis by the sulfurylase. Sequences of 20-100 bases, such as those in which SNPs are found, can be accurately determined by pyrosequencing. Pyrosequencing can be successfully used for SNPs and insertion/deletions detection, genotype identification and characterization, and in general for applications focusing on the variation of short DNA fragments (Alderborn *et al.*, 2000; Chen *et al.*, 2003; Sinclair *et al.*, 2003). It can be used for accurate quantification of ratios of variant bases in a DNA sample, but is inappropriate for full-length sequencing even of the mitochondrial genome, in spite of its relatively small size.

Within this methodology, PCR amplification of mtDNA fragments containing polymorphic site is performed before pyrosequencing. To quantitatively evaluate the proportion of defective allele, the peak heights in the pyrogram of one-chained PCR-fragments of a mitochondrial genome are analyzed. The levels of heteroplasmy are calculated, taking into account the expected sequence and the dimension of peaks for the homozygotes possessing either 100% of the normal or 100% of the mutant allele (Sazonova *et al.*, 2009). As the validity of heteroplasmy measurements seems to be crucial, and pyrosequencing method is not so common and self-explanatory, an experimental proof with the introduction of different proportion of a mutated allele was obtained (Sobenin *et al.*, 2013b). In brief, the mixtures of mtDNA samples with the ratio of normal and mutant allele 1:0 (homoplasmy), 4:1 (20% heteroplasmy), 2:3 (40% heteroplasmy), 1:2 (67% heteroplasmy), and 0:1 (homopasmy). The results of measurements were very close to the expected values, and accounted for 0%, 18%, 42%, 66%, and 100%, respectively. It was estimated that for determining the level of heteroplasmy higher than 10%, the coefficient of variation does not exceed 10%, and the results of quantitative heteroplasmy measurements are accurate and reproducible. However, for low heteroplasmy levels (less than 5%), this method is effective for the assessment of the presence of heteroplasmy, but does not provide precise measurements. On the other hand, low heteroplasmy levels will hardly result in clinical consequences. Based on this assumption, the heteroplasmy levels below 5% may be considered negligible.

6   Heteroplasmic mtDNA Mutations and Atherosclerosis

During ageing, mtDNA accumulates more and more somatic mutations because of the aggregation of DNA damage due to the limited efficiency of DNA repair machinery. In experiments in mice deficient for mitochondrial DNA polymerase (mtDNA-mutator mice), it has been demonstrated that premature aging is unlikely to result from advanced oxidative stress but from increase in mtDNA mutations, which primarily altered protein-coding genes of the respiratory chain enzymes and thereby causing reduced steady-state levels of complex I, III, and IV (Trufinovic et al., 2005). Therefore, insufficient mitochondrial biogenesis (i.e. respiratory function decline) may be the primary inducer of premature aging in mtDNA mutator mice (Edgar & Trifunovic, 2009). Due to the large number of mitochondrial genome copies within each cell, it is the ratio of mutated to wild-type mtDNA that is a significant determinant of phenotype (Krishnan et al., 2008). Indeed, accumulation of heteroplasmic point mutations in mtDNA may be primarily responsible for mitochondrial respiratory function decline. Several studies demonstrated the monoclonality of amplification of vascular smooth muscle cells in atherosclerotic lesions (Chung et al, 1998; Schwartz & Murry, 1998). Thus, the monoclonal origin of atherosclerotic plaques may represent a likely mechanism of expansion of cells containing mtDNA with a high content of mutated mtDNA within an atherosclerotic plaque.

To date, only few studies have evaluated whether heteroplasmic mutations of mtDNA are associated with atherosclerosis. In two studies, the mtDNA mutation del4977 (a deletion of a nearly 5-kb mtDNA region containing 5 genes for tRNA and 7 genes for respiratory chain enzymes) was assessed, but no significant difference in heteroplasmy levels was found between healthy subjects and patients with coronary atherosclerosis (Bogliolo et al., 1999; Botto et al., 2005). On the other hand, the frequency of this mutation was 5-fold higher in atherosclerotic patients then in apparently healthy individuals (Botto et al., 2005). The heteroplasmy levels of mutation A3243G located in the mitochondrial tRNALeu 1 (UUA/G) gene in diabetic patients with atherosclerosis was 4-fold higher as compared to age-matched non-diabetic subjects (Nomiyama et al., 2004).

Mutation T16189C occurring in the hypervariable D-loop of the control region of mtDNA has attracted research interest because of its suspected association with various multifactorial diseases. In the study performed in 482 in patients with coronary artery disease (CAD), 505 type 2 diabetic patients, and 1481 healthy individuals it has been demonstrated that the prevalence of T16189C was significantly higher in patients with CAD, as well as in diabetics (Mueller et al., 2011).

Recently, the results of a comprehensive analysis of somatic mtDNA mutations in atherosclerotic tussues have been reported. Ten of 40 analyzed mutations were characterized by the levels of heteroplasmy significantly differing in atherosclerotic lesions compared to those in normal aortas (Sazonova et al., 2009; Sobenin et al., 2012a). Mutations of mtDNA associated with lipofibrosis plaques have been found in mitochondrial genes that encode rRNA12S, tRNA-Leu (UUR recognition codon), tRNA-Leu (CUN recognition codon), subunits of 1, 2, 5, and 6 NADH-dehydrogenase, and cytochromeB. From 29% up to 86% aortic samples had demonstrated a significant difference in the level of heteroplasmy for the above mutations between atherosclerotic plaques and unaffected tissue (Sobenin et al., 2012a). Further, the homogenates of affected and normal intimae of 10 aortas were compared to reveal the average level of heteroplasmy for these 10 mutations. For five mutations (A1555G, C3256T, T3336C, G13513A, and G15059A), the mean level of heteroplasmy was different in atherosclerotic intimal homogenates in comparison with the unaffected tissue; the integral mutation burden of mtDNA in intimal tissue independently explained not less than 14% variability of atherosclerosis (Sobenin et al., 2013a). These results allow to suggest that mutations in the human mitochondrial genome play a role in the development of atherosclerosis.

The cross-sectional clinical study was undertaken to examine the association between the level of heteroplasmy for the mutation C3256T in human white blood cells and the extent of carotid atherosclerosis, as well as the presence of coronary heart disease (CHD), the major clinical manifestation of atherosclerosis (Sobenin et al., 2012b). Totally, 191 participants (84 men, 107 women) aged 65.0 years were recruited in the study; 45 (24%) of them had CHD. High-resolution B-mode ultrasonography of carotids followed by quantitative measurement of carotid intima-media thickness (cIMT) was used to estimate the extent of atherosclerosis. Pyrosequencing was used to estimate the level of C3256T heteroplasmy. The highly significant relationship between C3256T heteroplasmy level and predisposition to atherosclerosis was revealed. In individuals with low predisposition to atherosclerosis, as judged by cIMT measurement, the mean level of C3256T heteroplasmy accounted for 17%, as compared to 24% in moderately predisposed subjects, and further to 25% and 28% in significantly and highly predisposed subjects, respectively. Therefore, the level of C3256T heteroplasmy of mitochondrial genome in human white blood cells was suggested to be a novel genetic risk factor for atherosclerosis, which can be used as an informative marker of genetic susceptibility to atherosclerosis, coronary heart disease and myocardial infarction.

Further, the association of mitochondrial genetic variation with the severity of carotid atherosclerosis, as assessed by carotid intima-media thickness and the presence of coronary heart disease, was analyzed (Sobenin et al., 2013b). Significant correlations have been found between carotid intima-media thickness (cIMT) and the levels of heteroplasmy for C3256T, T3336C, G12315A, G13513A, and G15059A mutations of mtDNA. However, the levels of heteroplasmy for A1555G, C5178A, G14459A, and G14846A mtDNA mutations did not correlate with cIMT, although these mutation have been reported earlier to be associated with atherosclerotic plaques in human aortic intima. The levels of heteroplasmy for mutations C3256T, T3336C, G12315A, G13513A, G14459A, G14846A, and G15059A correlated significantly with the size of atherosclerotic plaques visualized in any segment of carotid arteries. Of the conventional coronary risk factors, age had the strongest association with the studied mtDNA heteroplasmies. Age correlated with the level of heteroplasmy for C3256T, C5178A, G12315A, G13513A, G14459A, and G15059A mutations of mitochondrial genome of circulating leukocytes. A significant correlation was found between systolic blood pressure and the G15059A heteroplasmy level, and between triglycerides and T3336C and G12315A heteroplasmies. At the same time, none of the studied heteroplasmies correlated with either diastolic blood pressure, serum total cholesterol or LDL cholesterol.

For better explanation of the relationship between mtDNA mutations and atherosclerosis, a regression analysis has been performed, in which the positive or negative correlation was factored for deriving the statistical association. Each mutation was tested separately for mediation/moderation. Initially, paired regression model was estimated (e.g., cIMT vs. mutation, or the presence/absence of atherosclerotic plaque vs. mutation), and then the multiple regression model was built, which also included conventional risk factors, to avoid false correlations. For this analysis, cIMT and the levels of heteroplasmy were taken as quantitative values. Two models were tested to assess whether the inclusion of mutations adds a significant contribution to the increase of explanatory power of the model for cIMT variability. The first model included only conventional risk factors (age, gender, diabetes, hypertension, triglycerides, LDL cholesterol, HDL cholesterol), and the second model also included the levels of heteroplasmy for mtDNA mutations. The residues in the second model were significantly lower than those in in the model employing only conventional risk factors. The model, which included both conventional risk factors and mutations provided significantly better explanatory level than the first one (adjusted R^2, 33.5% vs. 24.5%). The similar approach was used to assess whether the inclusion of mutations adds a significant contribution to the increase of explanatory power for diagnostics of the presence of atherosclerotic plaque in carotids. Mutations provided statistically significant information for diagnostics (p <0.001). Therefore, in-depth statistical analysis have supported the assumption on significant association for atherosclerosis and CHD with heteroplasmy level of mtDNA mutations (Sobenin et al., 2013b).

Taken together, these findings indicate that mutations of mitochondrial genome play a substantial role in the development of atherosclerosis. However, mechanistic explanations of this role are not available yet. As an example, C3256T mutation is located in coding sequence of the MT-TL1 gene (codon recognizing UUR) which encodes tRNA leucine, and is expressed at the cellular level as a reduced amount of cellular organelles and impaired protein synthesis (Moraes et al., 1993; Rossmanith & Karwan, 1998; Levinger et al., 2004). Mutations G13513A, G14459A, G14846A, and G15059A occur in coding regions of genes responsible for the synthesis of respiratory chain enzymes (MT-ND5 and MT-ND6 genes encoding the subunits 5 and 6 of NADH dehydrogenase, respectively, and MT-CYB gene encoding cytochrome B). An impairment of NADH dehydrogenase activity can be expected to attenuate NADH oxidation and CoQ (ubiquinone) reduction and thus promote oxidative stress. Mutation G13513A (MT-ND5 gene) is believed to be associated with hereditary encephalomyopathy, cardiomyopathy, and the WPW syndrome (Sudo et al., 2004; Shanske et al., 2006; Lim et al., 2009; Valente et al., 2009). Mutation G14459A (MT-ND6 gene) results in alanine to valine substitution in a conserved region of ND6 protein at position 72, and is associated with hereditary ocular neuropathy, atrophy of visual nerve, Leber's hereditary visual neuropathy, dysfunction of basal ganglia, musculospastic syndrome and encephalopathy (Man et al., 2003; Funalot et al., 2002; Kirby et al., 2003; Tarnopolsky et al., 2004). Mutations G14846A and G15059A may lead to the damage of cytochrome B: the first one results in glycine to serine substitution in position 34, thus affecting intermediate transfer of electrons in mitochondrial respiratory chains; the second one results in glycine to stop codon substitution at position 190, thus stopping translation and leading to the loss of 244 amino acids at C-terminal of protein. Both mutations are capable of reducing enzymatic function of cytochrome B, and associated with mitochondrial myopathies (Andreu et al., 1999; Filosto et al., 2003). It is obvious that the current knowledge of the mechanisms whereby mitochondrial mutations can induce and accelerate atherogenesis at the cellular and molecular level is absolutely insufficient; further in-depths basic study are necessary.

The most recent studies provide a link between mtDNA mutation load in circulating blood cells and predisposition to atherosclerosis and its clinical manifestations. Leukocytes play a special role in atherogenesis (Galkina & Ley, 2007). The migration of variety of leukocyte subtypes in the subendothelial layer in arteries and their participation in the processes of inflammation and atherosclerotic plaque formation is well documented (Galkina & Ley, 2009). It is possible to expect that a high level of mtDNA mutation load in circulating cells might provide a high likelihood that the defective leukocytes with impaired mitochondrial function would enter into the arterial intimal layer. If leukocyte function is inhibited due to the presence of mutations in coding regions of mtDNA, this may lead to local oxidative stress and other pathologic events, which could promote atherosclerosis formation. Thus, one can assume that mtDNA heteroplasmy, being a biomarker of defective mitochondrial function in leukocytes, can also be regarded as a biomarker for atherosclerosis and consequent clinical manifestations such as CHD.

7   Closing Remarks

Atherogenesis is a complex multi-step pathogenic process. Alterations in many biological pathways related to vascular function substantially contribute to the pathogenesis of atheroslerosis at different stages of lesion formation. Among those, oxidative stress is probably the most significant factor occurring in atherosclerotic disease. Advanced oxidative stress is someway linked to mitochondrial dysfunction causing increased damage and mutagenesis of mtDNA. Impaired mitochondrial function and alterations in mtDNA could in turn enhance ROS production and oxidative stress.

At present, it is clear that mitochondrial factor may play a pivotal role in susceptibility, induction and progression of arterial atherosclerosis and its clinical manifestations. However, the impact of certain mtDNA mutations to atherogenesis is widely unknown. More studies focused on the assessment of new heteroplasmic mtDNA mutations affecting mitochondrial function in relation to atherosclerosis are definitely required. The deep knowledge about the pathophysiological relevance of each coronary artery disease-associated mtDNA mutation to atherosclerosis is of great importance.

In the field of clinical and epidemiological studies of atherosclerotic disease, the good portion of efforts is aimed to the development of novel tools for more precise risk prediction to allow preventive treatment targeted at high-risk individuals. These tools usually include direct visualization of preclinical atherosclerotic disease as well as an evaluation of a variety of risk factors, including markers of the activity of atherosclerotic disease, thrombogenic risk, and genetic polymorphisms. Within this aspect, the search of novel risk factors and markers of atherosclerosis is highly encouraged. Novel methodologies like Next Generation Sequencing may provide more and more genetic biomarkers of predisposition to atherosclerosis and other chronic diseases. As an example, full-length mtDNA sequencing using Roche's 454 Sequencing technique in 30 randomly selected persons allowed to detect some about 160 novel mutations of mtDNA; among them, 24 mutations were detected in 10-60% cases, in which the heteroplasmy level varied from 7% to 64% (Sobenin, personal communication). By now, the list of mtDNA mutations associated with atherosclerosis is formed due more to random findings than to systematic screening.

The further important areas of research should include the studies evaluating the mechanistic role of mtDNA mutations in cellular and molecular mechanisms of atherogenesis. This understanding is of direct clinical relevance because increased mtDNA damage can be an important pathogenic factor, an additional prognostic predictor, and a potential target of therapeutic strategies in atherosclerosis.

Acknowledgement

This work was supported in part by the Ministry of Education and Science of the Russian Federation, contract No.11.512.11.0027.

References

Aitken, R.J., Buckingham, D.W., & West, K.M. (1992). Reactive oxygen species and human spermatozoa: analysis of the cellular mechanisms involved in luminol- and lucigenin-dependent chemiluminescence. Journal of Cell Physiology, 151, 466–477.

Alderborn, A., Kristofferson, A., & Hammerling, U. (2000). Determination of single-nucleotide polymorphisms by real-time pyrophosphate DNA sequencing. Genome Research, 10, 1249–1258.

Andreu, A.L., Bruno, C., Dunne, T.C., Tanji, K., Shanske, S., Sue, C.M., Krishna, S., Hadjigeorgiou, G.M., Shtilbans, A., Bonilla, E., & DiMauro, S. (1999). A nonsense mutation (G15059A) in the cytochrome b gene in a patient with exercise intolerance and myoglobinuria. Annals of Neurology, 45, 127–130.

Bai, R.K., & Wong, L.J.C. (2004). Detection and quantification of heteroplasmic mutant mitochondrial DNA by real-time amplification refractory mutation system quantitative PCR analysis: a single-step approach. Clinical Chemistry, 50, 996–1001.

Balis, J.U., Haust, M.D., & Morea, R.H. (1964). Electron-microscopic studies in human atherosclerosis cellular elements in aortic fatty streaks. Experimental and Molecular Pathology, 3, 511–525.

Bannwarth, S., Procaccio, V., & Paquis-Flucklinger, V. (2005). Surveyor Nuclease: a new strategy for a rapid identification of heteroplasmic mitochondrial DNA mutations in patients with respiratory chain defects. Human Mutations, 25, 575–582.

Björkerud, S., & Björkerud, B. (1996). Apoptosis is abundant in human atherosclerotic lesions, especially in inflammatory cells (macrophages and T cells), and may contribute to the accumulation of gruel and plaque instability. American Journal of Pathology, 149, 367–380.

Bobryshev, Y.V., Babaev, V.R., Lord, R.S., & Watanabe, T. (1997). Cell death in atheromatous plaque of the carotid artery occurs through necrosis rather than apoptosis. In Vivo, 11, 441–452.

Bogliolo, M., Izzotti, A., De Flora, S., Carli, C., Abbondandolo, A., & Degan, P. (1999). Detection of the '4977 bp' mitochondrial DNA deletion in human atherosclerotic lesions. Mutagenesis, 14. 77–82.

Botto, N., Berti, S., Manfredi, S., Al-Jabri, A., Federici, C., Clerico, A., Ciofini, E., Biagini, A., & Andreassi, M.G. (2005). Detection of mtDNA with 4977 bp deletion in blood cells and atherosclerotic lesions of patients with coronary artery disease. Mutation Research, 570, 81–88.

Burut, D.F., Karim, Y., & Ferns, G.A. (2010). The role of immune complexes in atherogenesis. Angiology, 61, 679–689.

Cassandrini, D., Calevo, M.G., Tessa, A., Manfredi, G., Fattori, F., Meschini, M.C., Carrozzo, R., Tonoli, E., Pedemonte, M., & Minetti, C. (2006). A new method for analysis of mitochondrial DNA point mutations and assess levels of heteroplasmy. Biochemical and Biophysical Research Communications, 342, 387–393.

Chen, D.C., Saarela, J., Nuotio, I., Jokiaho, A., Peltonen, L., & Palotie, A. (2003). Comparison of GenFlex Tag array and pyrosequencing in SNP genotyping. Journal of Molecular Diagnostics, 5, 243–249.

Chen, J.B., Lin, T.K., Liou, C.W., Liao, S.C., Lee, L.C., Wang, P.W., & Tiao, M.M. (2008). Correlation of oxidative stress biomarkers and peritoneal urea clearance with mitochondrial DNA copy number in continuous ambulatory peritoneal dialysis patients. American Journal of Nephrology, 28, 853–859.

Chung, I.M., Schwartz, S.M., & Murry, C.E. (1998). Clonal architecture of normal and atherosclerotic aorta: implications for atherogenesis and vascular development. American Journal of Pathology, 152, 913–923.

Cloonan, S.M., & Choi, A.M. (2012). Mitochondria: commanders of innate immunity and disease? Current Opinion in Immunology, 24, 32–40.

Craigen, W.J. (2012). Mitochondrial DNA mutations: an overview of clinical and molecular aspects. Methods in Molecular Biology, 837, 3–15.

Croteau, D.L., & Bohr, V.A. (1997). Repair of oxidative damage to nuclear and mitochondrial DNA in mammalian cells. Journal of Biological Chemistry, 272, 25409–25412.

Davidson, S.M., & Duchen, M.R. (2007). Endothelial mitochondria: contributing to vascular function and disease. Circulation Research, 100, 1128–1141.

Diehl, A.M., & Hoek, J.B. (1999). Mitochondrial uncoupling: role of uncoupling protein anion carriers and relationship to thermogenesis and weight control "the benefits of losing control." Journal of Bioenergetics and Biomembranes, 31, 493–506.

Dobrowolski, S.F., Hendrickx, A.T., van den Bosch, B.J., Smeets, H.J., Gray, J., Miller, T., & Sears, M. (2009). Identifying sequence variants in the human mitochondrial genome using high-resolution melt (HRM) profiling. Human Mutations, 30, 891–898.

Edgar, D., & Trifunovic, A. (2009). The mtDNA mutator mouse: Dissecting mitochondrial involvement in aging. Aging (Albany NY), 1, 1028–1032.

Fayssoil, A. (2009). Heart diseases in mitochondrial encephalomyopathy, lactic acidosis, and stroke syndrome. Congestive Heart Failure, 15, 284–287.

Filosto, M., Mancuso, M., Vives-Bauza, C., Vila, M.R., Shanske, S., Hirano, M., Andreu, A.L., & DiMauro, S. (2003). Lack of paternal inheritance of muscle mitochondrial DNA in sporadic mitochondrial myopathies. Annals of Neurology, 54, 524–526.

Funalot, B., Reynier, P., Vighetto, A,. Ranoux, D., Bonnefont, J.P., Godinot, C., Malthiery, Y., & Mas, J.L. (2002). Leigh-like encephalopathy complicating Leber's hereditary optic neuropathy. Annals of Neurology, 52, 374–377.

Galkina, E., & Ley, K. (2007). Leukocyte influx in atherosclerosis. Current Drug Targets, 8, 1239–1248.

Galkina, E., & Ley, K. (2009). Immune and inflammatory mechanisms of atherosclerosis. Annual Reviews in Immunology, 27, 165–197.

Geer, J.C., McGill, H.C., & Strong, J.P. (1961). The fine structure of human atherosclerotic lesions. American Journal of Pathology, 38, 263–287.

Gratchev, A., Sobenin, I., Orekhov, A., & Kzhyshkowska, J. (2012). Monocytes as a diagnostic marker of cardiovascular diseases. Immunobiology, 217, 476–482.

Griffiths, E.J. (2012). Mitochondria and heart disease. Advances in Experimental Medicine and Biology, 942, 249–267.

Hamilton, M.L., Guo, Z., Fuller, C.D., Van Remmen, H., Ward, W.F., Austad, S.N., Troyer, D.A., Thompson, I., & Richardson, A. (2001). A reliable assessment of 8-oxo-2-deoxyguanosine levels in nuclear and mitochondrial DNA using the sodium iodide method to isolate DNA. Nucleic Acids Research, 29, 2117–2126.

Irwin, J.A., Saunier, J.L., Niederstätter, H., Strouss, K.M., Sturk, K.A., Diegoli, T.M., Brandstätter, A., Parson, W., & Parsons, T.J. (2009). Investigation of heteroplasmy in the human mitochondrial DNA control region: a synthesis of observations from more than 5000 global population samples. Journal of Molecular Evolution, 68, 516–527.

John, P.A., & Ioannidis, M.D. (2009). Prediction of cardiovascular disease outcomes and established cardiovascular risk factors by genome-wide association markers. Circulation Cardiovascular Genetics, 2, 7–15.

Kirby, D.M., Boneh, A., Chow, C.W., Ohtake, A., Ryan, M.T., Thyagarajan, D., & Thorburn, D.R. (2003). Low mutant load of mitochondrial DNA G13513A mutation can cause Leigh's disease. Annals of Neurology, 54, 473–478.

Koshkin, K.A., Singh, S.K., Nielsen, P., Rajwanshi, V.K., Kumar, R., Meldgaard, M., Olsen, C.E., & Wengel, J. (1998). LNA (Locked Nucleic Acids): Synthesis of the adenine, cytosine, guanine, 5-methylcytosine, thymine and uracil bicyclonucleoside monomers, oligomerisation, and unprecedented nucleic acid recognition. Tetrahedron, 54, 3607–3630.

Kowald, A., & Kirkwood, T.B. (1993). Mitochondrial mutations, cellular instability and ageing: modeling the population dynamics of mitochondria. Mutation Research, 295, 93–103.

Krishnan, K.J., Reeve, A.K., Samuels, D.C., Chinnery, P.F., Blackwood, J.K., Taylor, R.W., Wanrooij, S., Spelbrink, J.N., Lightowlers, R.N., & Turnbull, D.M. (2008). What causes mitochondrial DNA deletions in human cells? Nature Genetics, 40, 275–279.

Levinger, L., Morl, M., & Florentz, C. (2004). Mitochondrial tRNA 3' end metabolism and human disease. Nuclear Acids Research, 32, 5430–5441.

Lim, B.C., Park, J.D., Hwang, H., Kim, K.J., Hwang, Y.S., Chae, J.H., Cheon, J.E., Kim, I.O., Lee, R., & Moon, H.K. (2009). Mutations in ND subunits of complex I are an important genetic cause of childhood mitochondrial encephalopathies. Journal of Child Neurology, 24, 828–832.

Limongelli, G., Masarone, D., D'Alessandro, R., & Elliott, P.M. (2012). Mitochondrial diseases and the heart: an overview of molecular basis, diagnosis, treatment and clinical course. Future Cardiology, 8, 71–88.

Liu, C.S., Kuo, C.L., Cheng, W.L., Huang, C.S., Lee, C.F., & Wei, Y.H. (2005). Alteration of the copy number of mitochondrial DNA in leukocytes of patients with hyperlipidemia. Annals of New York Academy of Sciences, 1042, 70–75.

Liu, C.S., Tsai, C.S., Kuo, C.L., Chen, H.W., Lii, C.K., Ma, Y.S., & Wei, Y.H. (2003). Oxidative stress-related alteration of the copy number of mitochondrial DNA in human leukocytes. Free Radical Research, 37, 1307–1317.

Man, P.Y., Griffiths, P.G., Brown, D.T., Howell, N., Turnbull, D.M., & Chinnery, P.F. (2003). The epidemiology of Leber hereditary optic neuropathy in the North East of England American Journal of Human Genetics, 72, 333–339.

Martinet, W., Schrijvers, D.M., & De Meyer, G.R. (2011). Necrotic cell death in atherosclerosis. Basic Research in Cardiology. 106, 749–760.

Meierhofer D., Mayr, J.A., Ebner, S., Sperl, W., & Kofler, B. (2005). Rapid screening of the entire mitochondrial DNA for low-level heteroplasmic mutations. Mitochondrion, 5, 282–296.

Mohammed, S., Bahitham, W., Chan, A., Chiu, B., Bamforth, F., & Sergi, C. (2012). Mitochondrial DNA related cardiomyopathies. Frontiers in Bioscience (Elite Ed), 4, 1706–1716.

Moraes, C.T., Ciacci, F., Bonilla, E., Jansen, C., Hirano, M., Rao, N., Lovelace, R.E., Rowland, L.P., Schon, E.A., & DiMauro, S. (1993). Two novel pathogenic mitochondrial DNA mutations affecting organelle number and protein synthesis. Is the tRNALeu(UUR) gene an etiologic hot spot? Journal of Clinical Investigations, 92, 2906–2915.

Mueller, E.E., Eder, W., Ebner, S., Schwaiger, E., Santic, D., Kreindl, T., Stanger, O., Paulweber, B., Iglseder, B., Oberkofler, H., Maier, R., Mayr, J.A., Krempler, F., Weitgasser, R., Patsch, W., Sperl, W., & Kofler, B. (2011). The mitochondrial T16189C polymorphism is associated with coronary artery disease in Middle European populations. PLoS One, 6, e16455.

Nomiyama, T., Tanaka, Y., Piao, L., Hattori, N., Uchino, H., Watada, H. Kawamori, R., & Ohtam S. (2004). Accumulation of somatic mutation in mitochondrial DNA and atherosclerosis in diabetic patients. Annals of New York Academy of Sciences, 1011, 193–204.

Park, C.B., & Larsson, N.G. (2011). Mitochondrial DNA mutations in disease and aging. Journal of Cell Biology, 193, 809–818.

Raule, N., Sevini, F., Santoro, A., Altilia, S., & Franceschi, C. (2007). Association studies on human mitochondrial DNA: methodological aspects and results in the most common age-related diseases. Mitochondrion, 7, 29–38.

Reeve, A.K., Krishnan, K.J., & Turnbull, D. (2008). Mitochondrial DNA mutations in disease, aging, and neurodegeneration. Annals of New York Academy of Sciences, 1147, 21–29.

Rossignol, R., Malgat, M., Mazat, J.P., & Letellier, T. (1999). Threshold effect and tissue specificity. Implication for mitochondrial cytopathies. Journal of Biological Chemistry, 274, 33426–33432.

Rossmanith, W., & Karwan, R.M. (1998). Impairment of tRNA processing by point mutations in mitochondrial tRNA(Leu) (UUR) associated with mitochondrial diseases. FEBS Letters, 433, 269–274.

Rötig, A. (2011). Human diseases with impaired mitochondrial protein synthesis. Biochimica et Biophysica Acta, 1807, 1198–1205.

Sazonova, M., Budnikov, E., Khasanova, Z., Sobenin, I., Postnov, A., Orekhov, A. (2009). Studies of the human aortic intima by a direct quantitative assay of mutant alleles in the mitochondrial genome. Atherosclerosis, 204, 184–190.

Schapira, A.H. (2012). Mitochondrial diseases. Lancet, 379, 1825–1834.

Schon, E.A., DiMauro, S., & Hirano, M. (2012). Human mitochondrial DNA: roles of inherited and somatic mutations. Nature Reviews Genetics, 13, 878–890.

Schwartz, S.M., & Murry, C.E. (1998). Proliferation and the monoclonal origins of atherosclerotic lesions. Annual Review of Medicine, 49, 437–460.

Sevini, F., Santoro, A., Raule, N., Lescai, F., & Franceschi, C. (2007). Role of mitochondrial DNA in longevity, aging and age-related diseases in humans: a reappraisal. Italian Journal of Biochemistry, 56, 243–253.

Shanske, S., Coku, J., Lu, J., Ganesh, J., Krishna, S., Tanji, K., Bonilla, E., Naini, A.B., Hirano, M., & DiMauro, S. (2008). The G13513A mutation in the ND5 gene of mitochondrial DNA as a common cause of MELAS or Leigh syndrome: evidence from 12 cases. Archives of Neurology, 65, 368–372.

Simionescu, M., & Sima, A.V. (2012). Morphology of Atherosclerotic Lesions. In: Wick G, Grundtman C, Eds. Inflammation and Atherosclerosis. Wien, New York: Springer (pp. 19–37).

Sinclair, A., Arnold, C., & Woodford, N. (2003). Rapid detection and estimation by pyrosequencing of 23S rRNA genes with a single nucleotide polymorphism conferring linezolid resistance in Enterococci. Antimicrobial Agents and Chemotherapy, 47, 3620–3622.

Smith, P.M., & Lightowlers, R.N. (2011). Altering the balance between healthy and mutated mitochondrial DNA. Journal of Inherited Metabolic Diseases, 34, 309–313.

Sobenin, I.A., Sazonova, M.A., Postnov, A.Y., Bobryshev, Y.V., & Orekhov, A.N. (2012a). Mitochondrial mutations are associated with atherosclerotic lesions in the human aorta. Clinical and Developmental Immunology, 2012, 832464.

Sobenin, I.A., Sazonova, M.A., Ivanova, M.M., Zhelankin, A.V., Myasoedova, V.A., Postnov, A.Y., Nurbaev, S.D., Bobryshev, Y.V., & Orekhov, A.N. (2012b). Mutation C3256T of mitochondrial genome in white blood cells: novel genetic marker of atherosclerosis and coronary heart disease. PLoS ONE, 7, e46573.

Sobenin, I.A., Sazonova, M.A., Postnov, A.Y., Bobryshev, Y.V., & Orekhov, A.N. (2013a). Changes of mitochondria in atherosclerosis: possible determinant in the pathogenesis of the disease. Atherosclerosis, 227, 283–288.

Sobenin, I.A., Sazonova, M.A., Postnov, A.Y., Salonen, J.T., Bobryshev, Y.V., & Orekhov, A.N. (2013b). Association of mitochondrial genetic variation with carotid atherosclerosis. PLoS One, 8, e68070.

Sobenin, I.A., Chistiakov, D.A., Bobryshev, Y.V., Postnov, A.Y., & Orekhov, A.N. (2013c). Mitochondrial mutations in atherosclerosis: new solutions in research and possible clinical applications. Current Pharmaceutical Design, 19, 5942–5953.

Strand, H., Ingebretsen, O.C., & Nilssen, O. (2008). Real-time detection and quantification of mitochondrial mutations with oligonucleotide primers containing locked nucleic acid. Clinica et Chimica Acta, 390, 126–133.

Sudo, A., Honzawa, S., Nonaka, I., & Goto, Y. (2004). Leigh syndrome caused by mitochondrial DNA G13513A mutation: frequency and clinical features in Japan. Journal of Human Genetics, 49, 92–96.

Tarnopolsky, M.A., Baker, S.K., Myint, T., Maxner, C.E., Robitaille, J., & Robinson, B.H. (2004). Clinical variability in maternally inherited Leber Hereditary Optic Neuropathy with the G14459A mutation. American Journal of Medical Genetics, 124A, 372–376.

Taylor, R.W., & Turnbull, D.M. (2005). Mitochondrial DNA mutations in human disease. Nature Reviews Genetics, 6, 389–402.

Trifunovic, A., Hansson, A., Wredenberg, A., Rovio, A.T., Dufour, E., Khvorostov, I., Spelbrink, J.N., Wibom, R., Jacobs, H.T., & Larsson, N.G. (2005). Somatic mtDNA mutations cause aging phenotypes without affecting reactive oxygen species production. Proceedings of the National Academy of Sciences of the United States of America, 102, 17993–17998.

Valente, L., Piga, D., Lamantea, E., Carrara, F., Uziel, G., Cudia, P., Zani, A., Farina, L., Morandi, L., Mora, M., Spinazzola, A., Zeviani, M., & Tiranti, V. (2009). Identification of novel mutations in five patients with mitochondrial encephalomyopathy. Biochimica et Biophysica Acta, 1787, 491–501.

Wallace, D.C. (1992). Diseases of the mitochondrial DNA. Annual Review of Biochemistry, 61, 1175–1212.

Wallace, D.C. (2010). Mitochondrial DNA mutations in disease and aging. Environmental and Molecular Mutagenesis, 51, 440–450.

Wang, Y.C., Lee, W.C., Liao, S.C., Lee, L.C., Su, Y.J., Lee, C.T., & Chen, J.B. (2011). *Mitochondrial DNA copy number correlates with oxidative stress and predicts mortality in nondiabetic hemodialysis patients. Journal of Nephrology, 24, 351–358.*

Weakley, S.M., Jiang, J., Kougias, P., Lin, P.H., Yao, Q., Brunicardi, F.C., Gibbs, R.A., & Chen, C. (2010). *Role of somatic mutations in vascular disease formation. Expert Review of Molecular Diagnostics, 10, 173–185.*

Wong, L.J., Chen, T.J., & Tan, D.J. (2004). *Detection of mitochondrial DNA mutations using temporal temperature gradient gel electrophoresis. Electrophoresis, 25, 2602–2610.*

Wu, L.L., Chiou, C.C., Chang, P.Y., & Wu, J.T. (2004). *Urinary 8-OHdG: a marker of oxidative stress to DNA and a risk factor for cancer, atherosclerosis and diabetics. Clinica et Chimica Acta, 339, 1–9.*

Yakes, F.M., & Van Houten, B. (1997). *Mitochondrial DNA damage is more extensive and persists longer than nuclear DNA damage in human cells following oxidative stress. Proceedings of the National Academy of Sciences of the United States of America, 94, 514–519.*

Yarham, J.W., Elson, J.L., Blakely, E.L., McFarland, R., & Taylor, R.W. (2010). *Mitochondrial tRNA mutations and disease. Wiley Interdisciplinary Reviews RNA, 1, 304–324.*

Zaragoza, M.V., Fass, J., Diegoli, M., Lin, D., Arbustini, E. (2010). *Mitochondrial DNA variant discovery and evaluation in human cardiomyopathies through next-generation sequencing. PLoS One, 5, e12295.*

The Roles of Thiamine in Myocardial Infarction Possible Genetic and Cellular Signaling Mechanisms

Khanh vinh quốc Lương
Vietnamese American Medical Research Foundation
Westminster, California, United States

Lan Thi Hoàng Nguyễn
Vietnamese American Medical Research Foundation
Westminster, California, United States

1   Introduction

The relationship between thiamine and myocardial infarction (MI) has been previously reported in the literature. In thiamine-deficient (TD) rats, electrocardiograms (ECGs) showed marked bradycardia as well as T wave and ST-segment changes. These changes usually disappear within a few hours of thiamine administration (Weiss *et al.*, 1938). Beriberi heart disease is a very rare disease caused by thiamine deficiency. Bello *et al.* (2011) described two patients who presented with fatal cardiac beriberi, an acute MI and extensive colliquative myocytolisis. Another beriberi heart patient presented with chest discomfort, diffuse ST-segment depression in the ECG with ST-segment elevation in a VR, and rapidly evolving congestive heart failure leading to cardiogenic shock. An emergency coronary angiogram was performed that showed normal coronary arteries. Right heart catheterization showed a high-output state with elevated filling pressures suggesting high-output heart failure. The echocardiography confirmed normal left and right ventricular contraction. After a single dose of intravenous thiamine (100 mg), the patient's hemodynamic status dramatically improved within minutes, allowing for rapid discontinuation of hemodynamic support. Subsequent ECGs showed complete resolution of ST-segment abnormalities. Serial lactate measurements, red blood cell transketolase (*Tk*) activity, and the thiamine pyrophosphate (TPP) response test were concordant with thiamine deficiency (Loma-Osorio *et al.*, 2011). In addition, beriberi heart patients also demonstrated ST-segment elevation and myocardial damage without coronary artery stenosis, and they improved rapidly after thiamine was administered (Ito *et al.*, 2002; Kawano *et al.*, 2005a). Daly and Dixon (2009) described a patient who presented acutely with Wernicke's encephalopathy, chest pain, ST-segment elevation, and congestive cardiac failure associated with hypotension. Coronary angiography demonstrated no abnormalities. The patient's hemodynamics improved significantly in the short-term following intravenous thiamine replacement, with complete resolution of all ST-segment abnormalities and normalization of left ventricular function at the six-week follow-up. Interstitial fibrosis and a variation in the size of the myocardial fibers were the main findings after thiamine treatment in these patients (Kawano *et al.*, 2005b). An electron microscopy study on myocardial lesions in TD rats revealed changes in the heart muscle, including a decrease in electron density of the mitochondrial matrix, swelling and rupture of the mitochondria, reduction and derangement of cristae, mitochondrial degeneration, enlargement and destruction of cisternae of the sarcoplasmic reticulum, appearance of large vacuoles, and disappearance of cross striation in myofibrils (Suzuki, 1967). Tylicki *et al.* (2008) observed the effects of $MnCl_2$ and TPP changes on EEG and pyruvate dehydrogenase complex (PDC) enzyme activity in the hearts of rats after MI induction. TPP also plays the important role of the positive regulatory effector of pig heart PDC (Strumilo *et al.*, 1999). In isoprenaline-induced MI rats, male rats developed much more severe myocardial necrosis than female rats and concomitantly exhibited significantly greater reduction in myocardial thiamine during acute ischemia compared with female subjects (Wexler and Lutmer, 1973). Two hours before the start of the experiment, thiamine administration (200 mg/kg) substantially reduced the myocardial ischemic lesion in a rat model of experimental MI (Vinogradov *et al.*, 1991). Benfotiamine, a fat-soluble thiamine analog, accelerated the healing of ischemia in the limbs of diabetic mice (Gadau *et al.*, 2006) and improved the functional recovery of the infarcted heart via activation of the pro-survival glucose-6-phosphate dehydrogenase/Akt signaling pathway and modulation of the neurohormonal response (Katare *et al.*, 2010). Thiamine has a cyto-protective effect on cultured neonatal rat cardio-myocytes under hypoxic insult, and it also protects the cardio-myocytes against hypoxia-induced apoptosis (Shin *et al.*, 2004). A single thiamine administration yielded a marked anti-ischemic protective effect on the heart (Shneĭder, 1991). The beneficial effects of TPP were demonstrated in the treatment of experimental MI in dogs and rats. There were beneficial hemodynamic changes, including significantly decreased heart rate, increased stroke volume, decreased systemic vascular resistance, and decreased myocardial O_2 consumption, in the MI group compared with the control group (Larrieu et al., 1987a & 1987b). Thiamine also has a cardiovascular effect. High doses of thiamine in the dog decreased the mean peripheral pressure by up to 25%, left ventricular pressure by up to 15%,, coronary sinus blood flow by up to 31%, and myocardial oxygen consumption by up to 45% (Freye et al., 1976). These findings suggest that thiamine may play a role in MI. In this paper, we further discuss the potential role of thiamine in MI, along with the possible genetic and cell signaling mechanisms involved.

2   The Genomic Role of Thiamine in Myocardial Infarction

2.1   Diabetes Mellitus (DM)

DM increases the risk of cardiovascular disease (CVD) (Bornfeldt and Tabas, 2011). In a systematic review and meta-analysis study, stress hyperglycaemia with MI is associated with an increased risk of in-hospital mortality in patients with and without diabetes (Capes et al., 2000). According to the Cooperative Cardiovascular Project, higher glucose levels are associated with a greater risk of mortality in patients without known diabetes compared with diabetics (Kosiborod et al., 2005). In addition, the relationship between thiamine and DM has been previously reported in the literature. Acute TD was reported in a child with diabetic ketoacidosis (Clark et al., 2006). In addition, plasma thiamine levels are decreased by 76% in type 1 diabetic patients and 75% in type 2 diabetic patients and are associated with increased renal clearance and fractional excretion of thiamine (Thornalley et al., 2007). Furthermore, the thiamine transporter protein concentration has been shown to be increased in the erythrocyte membranes of type 1 and type 2 diabetic patients. Therefore, changes in thiamine levels may be masked by an increase in thiamine transporter expression. The dysfunction of endothelial cells has been known to play a major role in both micro- and macro-vascular complications of DM. Diabetic cardiomyopathy can progress to overt heart failure with increased mortality. Thiamine repletion prevented diabetes-induced cardiac fibrosis in an experimental model of diabetes (Kohda et al., 2008). High-dose benfotiamine rescued cardiomyocyte contractile dysfunction in streptozotocin-induced DM (Ceylan-Isik et al., 2006). Additionally, thiamine reversed hyperglycemia-induced dysfunction in cultured endothelial cells (Ascher et al., 2001). Thiamine and benfotiamine have been demonstrated in vitro to counteract the damaging effects of hyperglycemia on cultured vascular cells (Beltramo et al., 2004). In addition, thiamine has been reported to improve endothelial vasodilatation in patients with hyperglycemia (Arora et al., 2006). Benfotiamine and fenofibrate ameliorated the diabetes-induced vascular endothelial dysfunction and nephropathy in rats (Balakumar et al., 2009). Benfotiamine also attenuated nicotine- and uric acid-induced vascular endothelial dysfunction in rats (Balakumar et al., 2008). The daily intake of thiamine was positively correlated with the circulating level of endothelial progenitor cells and vascular endothelial function in type 2 diabetic patients (Wong et al., 2008). Treatment with benfotiamine prevented sodium arsenite-induced vascular endothelial dysfunction and oxidative stress (Verma et al., 2010) and counteracted smoking-induced vascular dysfunction in healthy smokers (Stirban et al., 2012).

2.2   The Renin-Angiotensin System (RAS)

The primary function of the RAS is to maintain fluid homeostasis and regulate blood pressure. The angiotensin-converting enzyme (ACE) is a key enzyme in the RAS that converts angiotensin (AT) I to the potent vasoconstrictor AT II (Johnston, 1994). The activation of the RAS plays a critical role in the pathophysiology of MI by inducing the up-regulation of angiotensin II type 1 receptor, ACE, and collagen I mRNAs (Qi *et al.*, 2012). Elevated baseline plasma renin activity (PRA) is associated with cardiac morbidity and mortality in CAD patients who otherwise have normal left ventricular function and no previous MI or heart failure (Muhlestein *et al.*, 2010). RAS blockade with ACE inhibitors or angiotensin receptor blockers (ARBs) improves cardiac remodeling and outcomes in patients (White *et al.*, 2005). Impaired post-infarction cardiac remodeling in chronic kidney disease is due to an excessive renin release (Ogawa *et al.*, 2012). The inhibition of brain angiotensin III, one of the main effector peptides of the RAS in the brain, attenuates sympathetic hyperactivity and cardiac dysfunction in rat post-MI (Huang *et al.*, 2012). A direct renin inhibitor (DRI), aliskiren, when combined with ACE inhibitors (ACEIs) or angiotensin II type 1 receptor blockers (ARBs), improved the extent of myocardial salvage after AMI compared with an ACEI or ARB alone and was associated with a decrease in circulating $CD14^+CD16^-$ monocytes (Ozaki *et al.*, 2012). In a hypertensive rat model subjected to experimental MI, ejection fraction (EF) and left ventricular end-diastolic pressure (LVEDP), key functional indices of heart failure, were improved by treatment with a combination of ACE and direct renin inhibition compared with either agent used alone (Connelly *et al.*, 2013). The RAS activity may be modified by variants of the genes that code for the functional proteins in this pathway. A combination of three common polymorphisms of RAS genes (*ACE Ins/Del*, *angiotensin receptor type 1 [AGT1R] A1166C,* and *angiotensinogen [ATG] M235T*) are linked to adverse events in patients with CAD (Dzielińska *et al.*, 2011). There were significant differences in the distribution of genotypes for the *AGT Thr174Met* polymorphism between patients with ST-elevation myocardial infarction (STEMI) and healthy subjects. The most powerful predictor of STEMI was the *Thr/Met* genotype and the *Met174* allele of the *AGT Thr174Met* gene polymorphism (Konopka *et al.*, 2011). The *DD* genotype of *ACE* may be a genetic risk factor for cardiovascular events in hypertensive patients in Japan (Kato *et al.*, 2011). There was a significant association between the *AGT* gene polymorphism and the extent of CAD in Greek patients with a history of MI (Karayannis *et al.*, 2010). Men who carry the *ACE DD* genotype and have high total cholesterol, high LDL cholesterol, and low HDL cholesterol levels may be predisposed to the development of more severe CAD (Borzyszkowska *et al.*, 2012). An interaction between thiamine and the RAS has been observed. Thiamine attenuates hypertension and metabolic abnormalities in spontaneously hypertensive rats (SHRs). Thiamine repletion down-regulates the expression of angiotensinogen (-80%), ACE (-77%), and angiotensin type 1 receptor (-72%) mRNAs in SHRs (Tanaka *et al* 2007). In addition, oxidative DNA damage induced by angiotensin II was completely prevented by benfotiamine (Schmid *et al.*, 2008). These observations suggest that thiamine affects ACE activity in MI patients.

2.3   The Reduced Form of the Nicotinamide Adenine Dinucleotide Phosphate (NADPH) Oxidase (NOX) Enzyme Complex

NOX mediates critical physiological and pathological processes, including cell signaling, inflammation, and mitogenesis, by generating reactive oxygen species (ROS) from molecular oxygen. NOX family enzymes are the major sources of ROS that are implicated in the pathophysiology of many cardiovascular diseases. An increase in NOX2, NOX4, $p22^{phox}$, and $p67^{phox}$ mRNAs was also found in mice post-MI

(Doerries *et al.*, 2007; Looi *et al.*, 2008; Zhao *et al.*, 2009). NOX5 expression is increased in intra-myocardial blood vessels and cardiomyocytes after AMI in humans (Hahn *et al.*, 2012). Furthermore, NOX4 mRNA and protein levels were up-regulated in peripheral muscles after hindlimb ischemia in mice (Craige *et al.*, 2011). Taken together, the aforementioned studies indicate that NOX isoforms are up-regulated at the mRNA level. NOX generated large amounts of ROS, which have direct cytotoxic effects (Elahi *et al.*, 2009; Griendling and FitzGerald, 2003). NOX can also indirectly cause damage by enhancing the inflammatory response (Cave *et al.*, 2006). Specific knock-down of Nox4 mRNA by siRNA caused a decrease in ROS production and a decrease in NOX activity. Moreover, Nox4 silencing decreased PAI-1 expression, release, and activity; p38 MAPK pathways activation; and NFκB activation (Jaulmes *et al.*, 2009). A variant of *p22^phox*, which is involved in the generation of ROS in the vessel wall, is associated with the progression of coronary atherosclerosis (Cahilly *et al.*, 2000). Goliasch *et al.* (2011) demonstrated a protective association between the *-930A>G* promoter polymorphism in the *p22^phox* gene and the development of MI in young individuals ($\leq$ 40 years). The expression of Nox4 is significantly down-regulated by benfotiamine treatment under both normo- and hyper-glycemic conditions (Frazer *et al.*, 2012). Taken together, these results indicate that thiamine may have a beneficial role in MI by suppressing NOX expression.

2.4 Poly (ADP-ribose) Polymerases (PARPs)

PARPs comprise a family of enzymes that share a conserved catalytic domain and support mono- or poly (ADP-ribosyl) transferase activity using NAD^+ as a donor of ADP-ribosyl units. PARPs are involved in a wide range of molecular and cellular processes, including maintenance of genome stability, regulation of chromatin structure, transcription, cell proliferation, and apoptosis (Krishnakumar and Kraus, 2010). AMI-induced increases in plasma tumor necrosis factor-alpha (TNF-α) and interleukin-10 (IL-10) are associated with the activation of PARP-1 in circulating mononuclear cells (Yao *et al.*, 2008). The activation of PARP-1 was demonstrated in circulating leukocytes during MI and was inhibited by the administration of the pharmacologic PARP inhibitor INO-1001 in rats (Murthy *et al.*, 2004; Tóth-Zsámboki *et al.*, 2006). Excessive PARP-1 activation is an important cause of infarction and contractile dysfunction in heart tissue during interruptions of blood flow. A strong association between PARP-1 hyper-activation and impairment of mitochondrial respiratory chain complex I function was demonstrated in reperfused mouse hearts (Zhou *et al.*, 2006). Treatment with the PARP inhibitor PJ34 began 1 week after the onset of diabetes. PJ34 restored normal vascular responsiveness and significantly improved cardiac dysfunction, despite the persistence of severe hyperglycemia. The beneficial effects of PARP inhibition persisted even after several weeks of treatment discontinuation (Pacher *et al.*, 2002). These findings suggest a role of PARP-1 activation in the development of myocardial and endothelial dysfunction in diabetes. PARP-1 contributes to the development of MI in diabetic rats and regulates the nuclear translocation of apoptosis-inducing factor (Xiao *et al.*, 2004). In a rat model of MI, suppression of PARP-1 activation by 3-aminobenzamide demonstrated long-term, beneficial morphological and functional effects in reperfused myocardium (Liaudet *et al.*, 2001). Myocardial post-ischemic injury is reduced by *PARP-1* gene disruption (Pieper *et al.*, 2000). In addition, the suppression of TNF-α, IL-10, and nitric oxide (NO) production was found in the absence of functional PARP (Yang *et al.*, 2000). These findings provide direct evidence that PARP activation participates in the development of delayed cell injury and delayed mediator production in myocardial reperfusion injury. Furthermore, thiamine has a cyto-protective effect on cultured neonatal rat cardio-myocytes under hypoxic insult, and it also inhibits PARP cleavage and DNA fragmentation (Shin *et al.*, 2004). Benfotiamine prevents bacterial endotoxin-induced inflammation and PARP cleavage in mouse macrophage cell lines (Yaday *et al.*, 2010). Adenosine thiamine triphosphate (ATTP), a new thiamine derivative, has been identified in small amounts in the mouse brain, heart, skeletal muscle, liver, and kidneys (Frédérich *et al.* 2009), and it has been shown to inhibit PARP-1 activity (Tanaka *et al.*, 2011). These findings suggest that thiamine may have a protective role in MI by down-regulating PARP.

2.5   The Advanced Glycation End Products (AGEs)

AGEs are a heterogeneous group of macromolecules formed by the non-enzymatic glycation of proteins, lipids, and nucleic acids. Receptors for AGEs (RAGEs) are multi-ligand receptors, and their ligands are also likely to recognize several receptors that mediate their biological effects (Bierhaus *et al.*, 2006). AGEs act through receptor-independent and -dependent mechanisms to promote vascular damage, fibrosis, and inflammation associated with accelerated atherogenesis. Diabetic RAGE transgenic mice that overexpress RAGE in vascular cells exhibited exacerbation of the indices of nephropathy and retinopathy, which was prevented by inhibiting AGE formation (Yonekura *et al.*, 2005). Diabetic RAGE-null mice were significantly protected from the adverse impact of I/R injury in the heart (Bucciarelli *et al.*, 2008). These findings demonstrate both novel and key roles for RAGE in I/R injury in the diabetic heart. An inverse association between cardiac troponin-I and soluble RAGEs was demonstrated in patients with NSTEMI (McNair *et al.*, 2009 & 2011). Plasma levels of soluble RAGEs are associated with endothelial function and predict cardiovascular events in non-diabetic patients (Chiang *et al.*, 2009), cardiovascular mortality in patients with end-stage renal disease (Koyama *et al.*, 2007), restenosis following percutaneous coronary intervention (McNair *et al.*, 2010), and the development of post-infarction heart failure (Raposeiras-Roubin *et al.*, 2012). The *-374T/A RAGE* polymorphism is an independent protective factor for cardiac events in both non-diabetic and diabetic patients with CAD (Falcone *et al.*, 2008; Picheth *et al.*, 2007; dos Santos *et al.*, 2005). The *-429 T/C* and *-374 T/A* polymorphisms of the *RAGE* gene are not risk factors for coronary artery disease in a Slovene population with type 2 diabetes and in Chinese patients with diabetic nephropathy (Kirbis *et al.*, 2004; Poon *et al.*, 2010). The *RAGE Gly82Ser* polymorphism is not associated with cardiovascular disease in the Framingham offspring study (Hofmann *et al.*, 2005). Furthermore, thiamine and a benfotiamine supplement prevented tissue accumulation and increased the urinary excretion of protein glycation and oxidation and nitration adducts associated with experimental diabetes (Karachalias *et al.*, 2010). Karachalias *et al.* (2005) reported that, in streptozotocin-induced (STZ) diabetic rats, the hydroimidazolone of AGE residues derived from glyoxal and methylglyoxal (G-H1 and MG-H1, respectively) increased by 115 and 68%, respectively, and thiamine and benfotiamine normalized these residues. However, in diabetic-induced rats, N-carboxymethyl-lysine (CML) and N-carboxyethyl-lysine (CEL) residues increased by 74 and 118%, respectively, and only thiamine normalized these residues. Serum markers of endothelial dysfunction, oxidative stress, and AGE increased after a meal high in AGE content, and benfotiamine significantly reduced these effects (Stirban *et al.*, 2006). The addition of benfotiamine enhanced T*k* activity and decreased the expression of AGE and RAGE in a peritoneal dialysis model of uremic rats (Kihm *et al.*, 2011). The combined administration of thiamine and vitamin B6 to patients with diabetic nephropathy decreased DNA glycation in leukocytes; however, vitamin B6 alone did not have such an effect (Polizzi *et al.*, 2012). Taken together, these findings suggest that thiamine may have a role in MI by modulating AGEs

3   The Non-genomic Role of Thiamine in Myocardial Infarction

3.1   Matrix Metalloproteinases (MMPs)

MMPs are proteolytic enzymes that are responsible for remodeling the extracellular matrix and regulating leukocyte migration through the extracellular matrix. This migration is an important step in inflammatory and infectious pathophysiology. MMPs are produced by many cell types, including lymphocytes, granulocytes, astrocytes, and activated macrophages. There is growing evidence that MMPs play an important role in the pathogenesis of MI. In patients with STEMI, circulating levels of MMP-2, measured early and even before reperfusion therapy, are strongly associated with infarct size and LV dysfunction (Nilsson *et al.*, 2012). Increased plasma levels of MMP-9 predict future coronary revascularization in AMI patients (Wang *et al.*, 2013). The MMP-9 and myeloperoxidase (MPO) values in patients with non-obstructive CAD were significantly higher than in patients with no coronary plaque. The levels of MMP-9 and MPO were significantly correlated with the Framingham risk score (Hou *et al.*, 2013). Serum levels of MMP-1, MMP-9, and IL-6 were elevated in patients with CAD and, to a greater extent, in patients with acute coronary syndromes. MMP-1, MMP-9, and IL-6 are associated with more extensive and severe CAD (Tanindi *et al.*, 2011). The *MMP-2-1575* (*rs243866*) gene polymorphism is associated with a risk of developing MI in Mexican individuals (Pérez-Hernández *et al.*, 2012). There is a trend of the MMP-1 and MMP-12 polymorphisms toward the prediction of future clinical events in patients with CAD (Jguirim-Souissi *et al.*, 2011). In an Indian population, serum MMP-3 levels were significantly elevated at the presentation of acute MI compared with controls (36.8%) and were more associated with the *6A* genotype (Shalia *et al.*, 2010). A systematic review and meta-analysis provided strong evidence regarding the association of the *MMP-3* and *MMP-9* genes with the development of CAD (Wang *et al.*, 2011; Niu and Qi, 2012). However, MMP-9 has also been shown to be up-regulated in the TD mouse brain (Calingasan and Gibson, 2000; Beauchesne *et al.*, 2009). Thiamine prevents diabetes-induced cardiac fibrosis and decreases MMP-2 activity in the heart of diabetic rats (Kohda *et al.*, 2008). Moreover, thiamine and benfotiamine correct the increase in MMP-2 activity that results from high glucose levels in human retinal pericytes, while increasing TIMP-1 (Tarallo *et al.*, 2010). Together, these studies suggest that thiamine may play an important role in the pathological processes of MI by down-regulating the levels of MMPs and regulating the levels of TIMPs.

3.2   The Mitogen-Activated Protein Kinase (MAPK) Pathways

MAPK provide a key link between the membrane-bound receptors that receive these cues and the changes in gene expression patterns, including the extracellular signal-regulated kinase (ERK) cascade, stress-activated protein kinases/c-jun N-terminal kinase (SAPK/JNK) cascade, and p38 MAPK/RK/HOG cascade (Hipskind and Bilbe, 1998). Myocardial ischemia activates a number of kinases, including members of the p38 MAPK family (p38s) (Tanno *et al.*, 2003; Kumphune *et al.*, 2010). Compared with the control group, levels of p-ERK1/2, p-JNK, and p38 were significantly increased in the isoproterenol-induced, AMI-treated group (Guo *et al.*, 2012). In the minutes after experimental MI, ERK1/2, JNK1/2, and p38α MAPK are all activated in both the ischemic myocardium and unaffected portions of the left ventricle of mice and rats (Ren *et al.*, 2005; Yoshida *et al.*, 2001). Treatment with SB203580, a p38α and p38β inhibitor, resulted in reduced myocardial fibrosis, reduced TNF-α and collagen I levels, and increased LV contractile function (Yin *et al.*, 2008). MAPKs also have a role in atherosclerotic development. When mouse peritoneal macrophages were treated with oxLDL, ERK1/2, p38α MAPK, and JNK1/2 were activated within 15 minutes (Rahaman *et al.*, 2006). oxLDL-induced foam cell formation in the J774 macrophage cell line was found to be blocked by administration of the p38 MAPK inhibitor SB203580 (Zhao *et al.*, 2002). Macrophages lacking JNK2 displayed suppressed foam cell formation caused by defective uptake and degradation of modified lipoproteins and exhibited an increased binding of the modified lipoproteins (Ricci *et al.*, 2004). Moreover, benfotiamine was shown to modulate the macrophage response to bacterial endotoxin-induced inflammation by preventing the activation of p38 MAPK and stress-activated kinases (SAPK/JNK) (Yadav *et al.*, 2010).

3.3   Prostaglandins (PGs)

PGs play a role in inflammatory processes. Cyclooxygenase (COX) participates in the conversion of arachidonic acid into PGs. Plasma 8-iso-PG F2α levels, markers of oxidative stress, were significantly elevated in patients with AMI compared with patients with stable CAD and patients with no significant CAD (Elesber *et al.*, 2006). Following reperfusion by primary percutaneous coronary intervention in AMI, oxidative stress and an inflammatory response are induced immediately. A rise in 8-iso-PG F2α during ischemia indicates that ROS generation may also take place during severely reduced coronary blood flow and hypoxia (Berg *et al.*, 2005). COX-2 has been found to be up-regulated in atherosclerotic plaques (Kuge *et al.*, 2007). Selective COX-2 inhibition protects against myocardial damage in experimental acute ischemia (Carnieto *et al.*, 2009). MI size in celecoxib-treated rats was significantly reduced compared with the control group (Lada-Moldovan *et al.*, 2009). However, COX-2 inhibitors recently were reported to be associated with MI and cardiovascular risk (Canon and Canon, 2012; Schjerning Olsen *et al.*, 2011), which refecoxib was withdrawn from the U.S. market. Pharmacological activation of the PGE2 receptor EP4 improves cardiac function after myocardial I/R injury (Hishikari *et al.*, 2009). Reduced cardiac remodeling and function was observed in cardiac-specific EP4 receptor knockout mice with MI (Qian *et al.*, 2008). Deletion of microsomal PG synthetase-1 leads to eccentric cardiac myocyte hypertrophy, LV dilation, and impaired LV contractile function after AMI (Degousee *et al.*, 2008). The *CC* genotype of the *prostacyclin synthase* (*PGIS*) gene (*CYP8A1*) or the *-765CC genotype* of *PGIS2* is associated with MI (Lemaitre *et al.*, 2009; Xie *et al.*, 2009). The *COX-2* gene has been associated with ischemic heart disease and stroke risk (Cipollone *et al.*, 2004; Orbe *et al.*, 2006). The Helsinki sudden death study demonstrated that the *COX-2* gene promoter polymorphism was associated with coronary artery disease in middle-aged men. Men carrying the minor *C* allele had larger areas of complicated lesions and a higher number of coronary arteries that had over 50% stenosis compared with men representing the common *GG* genotype (Huuskonen *et al.*, 2008). Moreover, the expression of *COX-2* mRNA and PGE$_2$ was selectively increased in vulnerable regions during the symptomatic stages of TD encephalopathy in animal models (Gu *et al.*, 2008). Up-regulation of 15-hydroxyprostaglandin dehydrogenase (15-PGDH) expression was observed in breast cancer cell lines transfected with the thiamine transporter (*ThTr2*) gene, and down-regulation was observed after the suppression of *ThTr2* with siRNA vectors (Liu *et al.*, 2004). Over-expression of 15-PGDH inhibited IL-1β-induced COX-2 expression (Tai *et al.*, 2007). In murine macrophages, benfotiamine also blocked the expression of COX-2 and its product, PGE$_2$, by LPS-induced cytotoxicity (Yaday *et al.*, 2009). In addition, benfotiamine significantly prevented LPS-induced macrophage death and monocyte adhesion to endothelial cells (Yaday *et al.*, 2010). These anti-inflammatory effects of benfotiamine are mediated through the regulation of the arachidonic acid pathway in macrophages (Shoeb and Ramana, 2012). These findings suggest that thiamine may play a role in modulating the inflammatory process in MI.

3.4   Reactive Oxygen Species (ROS)

ROS are produced by activated phagocytes as part of their microbicidal activities. A decrease in the blood supply to the heart caused by atherosclerosis or thrombosis is known to induce MI. Following ischemia, ROS are produced during the reperfusion phase (Espat and Nelton, 2000). Antioxidants decrease reperfusion-induced arrhythmias in MI with ST elevation (Hicks *et al*, 2007). During ischemia and reperfusion, ROS can be produced by both endothelial cells and circulating phagocytes. The sources of ROS in cardio-myocytes could be the mitochondrial electron transport chain, nitric oxide synthase (NOS), NOX, xanthine oxidase, lipoxygenase/COX, and/or the auto-oxidation of various substances, particularly catecholamines (Misra *et al.*, 2009). MI was reported secondary to unintentional ingestion of hydrogen peroxide in a case study of a 60-year-old woman (Islamoglu *et al.*, 2012). SOD1 over-expression in the paraventricular nucleus improves post-infarct myocardial remodeling and ventricular function (Gao *et al.*, 2012). Antioxidant vitamins reduce oxidative stress and ventricular remodeling in patients with AMI (Gasparetto *et al.*, 2005). The inhibition of ROS production reduced adverse remodeling and improved LV contractile function, and it may therefore hold therapeutic potential for the treatment of chronic heart failure following AMI (Grieve *et al.*, 2004). Cardiac oxidative stress is involved in heart failure that is induced by thiamine deprivation in rats (Gioda *et al.*, 2010). *In vitro,* thiamine inhibits lipid peroxidation in rat liver microsomes and free radical oxidation of oleic acid (Lukienko *et al.*, 2000). Benfotiamine promotes a reduction in ROS that is induced by advanced glycated albumin in macrophages (de Souza Pinto *et al.*, 2012). In primary human peritoneal mesothelial cells and in a rat model of peritoneal dialysis, the addition of benfotiamine enhanced T*k* activity and decreased the expression of AGEs and their receptors (Kihm *et al.*, 2011). These data suggest that benfotiamine protects the peritoneal membrane and remnant kidney in a rat model of peritoneal dialysis and uremia. Thiamine rescues hepatocytes from iron-catalyzed oxidative stress by decreasing lipid peroxidation, mitochondrial damage, protein damage, and DNA oxidation (Mehta *et al.*, 2011). These findings suggest that thiamine modulates oxidative stress in MI.

3.5   Nitric Oxide Synthase (NOS)

NOS is an enzyme that is involved in the synthesis of nitric oxide (NO), which regulates a variety of important physiological responses, including cell migration, the immune response, and apoptosis. Endothelial nitric oxide synthase (eNOS) and NO may play an important role in attenuating cardiac remodeling and apoptosis after MI. There is a close relationship between eNOS activity and the development of insulin resistance and macro-vascular disease in AMI patients (Li *et al.*, 2012). eNOS-deficient mice developed more severe LV dysfunction and remodeling after MI than wild-type mice (Scherrer-Crosbie *et al.*, 2001), whereas endothelial overexpression of eNOS has been shown to attenuate LV dysfunction in mice after MI (Jones *et al.*, 2003). Deficiency in NOS-3 resulted in coronary artery hypoplasia in fetal mice and spontaneous MI in postnatal hearts (Liu *et al.*, 2012). Inhibition of MAPK signaling by e*NOS* gene transfer improves ventricular remodeling after MI through the reduction of inflammation (Chen *et al.*, 2010). There is a significant association between the *eNOS T-786C* polymorphism, CAD, and coincident putative risk factors in type 2 DM individuals of the South Indian population (Narne *et al.*, 2012). The *E298D* polymorphism of the *eNOS* gene is associated with MI occurrence in the Greek population (Dafni *et al.*, 2010). Increased brain eNOS expression was demonstrated in TD animals (Kruse *et al.*, 2004). In murine macrophages, benfotiamine also blocks the expression of iNOS by LPS-induced cytotoxicity (Yaday *et al.*, 2009). Benfotiamine reduces oxidative stress and activates eNOS to enhance the generation and bioavailability of NO, and it subsequently improves the integrity of vascular endothelium to prevent sodium arsenite-induced experimental vascular endothelial dysfunction (Verma *et al.*, 2010).

4   Conclusions

This paper reviewed the relationship between thiamine and MI. Genetic studies provide opportunities to determine which proteins link thiamine to MI pathology. Thiamine is also able to act through numerous non-genomic mechanisms, including protein expression, oxidative stress, inflammation, and cellular metabolism. These findings suggest that thiamine may play an important role in MI. Therefore, further investigation of thiamine in MI patients is warranted.

References

Arora S, Lidor A, Abularrage CJ, Weiswasser JM, Nylen E, et al. (2006). Thiamine (vitamin B1) improves endothelium-dependent vasodilatation in the presence of hyperglycemia. Ann Vasc Surg, 20, 653-658.

Ascher E, Gade PV, Hingorani A, Puthukkeril S, Kallakuri S, et al. (2001). Thiamine reverses hyperglycemia-induced dysfunction in cultured endothelial cells. Surgery, 130:851-858.

Balakumar P, Sharma R & Singh M. (2008). Benfotiamine attenuates nicotine and uric acid-induced vascular endothelial dysfunction in the rat. Pharmacol Res, 58, 356-363.

Balakumar P, Chakkarwar VA & Singh M. (2009). Ameliorative effect of combination of benfotiamine and fenofibrate in diabetes-induced vascular endothelial dysfunction and nephropathy in the rat. Mol Cell Biochem, 320, 149-162.

Beauchesne É, Desjardins P, Hazell AS & Butterworth RF. (2009). eNOS gene deletion restores blood-brain barrier integrity and attenuates neurodegeneration in the thiamine-deficient mouse brain. J Neurochem, 111:452-459.

Bello S, Neri M, Riezzo I, Othman MS, Turillazzi E & Fineschi V. (2011). Cardiac beriberi: morphological findings in two fatal cases. Diagn Pathol, 6, 8.

Beltramo E, Berrone E, Buttiglieri S & Porta M. (2004). Thiamine and benfotiamine prevent increased apoptosis in endothelial cells and pericytes cultured in high glucose. Diabetes Metab Res Rev, 20, 330-336.

Berg K, Jynge P, Bjerve K, Skarra S, Basu S & Wiseth R. (2005). Oxidative stress and inflammatory response during and following coronary interventions for acute myocardial infarction. Free Radic Res, 39, 629-636.

Bierhaus A, Humpert PM, Morcos M, Wendt T, Chavakis T, et al. (2005). Understanding RAGE, the receptor for advanced glycation end products. J Mol Med (Berl), 83, 876-886.

Bornfeldt KE & Tabas I. (2011). Insulin resistance, hyperglycemia, and atherosclerosis. Cell Metab, 14, 575-585.

Borzyszkowska J, Stanislawska-Sachadyn A, Wirtwein M, Sobiczewski W, Ciecwierz D, et al. (2012). Angiotensin converting enzyme gene polymorphism is associated with severity of coronary artery disease in men with high total cholesterol levels. J Appl Genet, 53, 175-182.

Bucciarelli LG, Ananthakrishnan R, Hwang YC, Kaneko M, Song F, et al. (2008). RAGE and modulation of ischemic injury in the diabetic myocardium. Diabetes, 57, 1941-1951.

Cahilly C, Ballantyne CM, Lim DS, Gotto A & Marian AJ. (2000). A variant of p22(phox), involved in generation of reactive oxygen species in the vessel wall, is associated with progression of coronary atherosclerosis. Circ Res, 86, 391-395.

Cannon CP & Cannon PJ.(2012). Physiology. COX-2 inhibitors and cardiovascular risk. Science, 336, 1386-1387.

Calingasan NY & Gibson GE. (2000). Dietary restriction attenuates the neuronal loss, induction of heme oxygenase-1 and blood-brain barrier breakdown induced by impaired oxidative metabolism. Brain Res, 885, 62-69.

Capes SE, Hunt D, Malmberg K & Gerstein HC. (2000). Stress hyperglycemia and increased risk after myocardial infarction in patients without diabetes: A systematic overview. Lancet, 355. 773 -778.

Carnieto A Jr, Dourado PM, Luz PL & Chagas AC. (2009). Selective cyclooxygenase-2 inhibition protects against myocardial damage in experimental acute ischemia. Clinics (Sao Paulo). 64, 245-252.

Cave AC, Brewer AC, Narayanapanicker A, Ray R, Grieve DJ. et al. (2006). NADPH oxidases in cardiovascular health and disease. Antioxid Redox Signal, 8, 691-728.

Ceylan-Isik AF, Wu S, Li Q, Li SY & Ren J. (2006). High-dose benfotiamine rescues cardiomyocyte contractile dysfunction in streptozotocin-induced diabetes mellitus. J Appl Physiol, 100, 150-156.

Chen LL, Zhu TB, Yin H, Huang J, Wang LS, et al. (2010). Inhibition of MAPK signaling by eNOS gene transfer improves ventricular remodeling after myocardial infarction through reduction of inflammation. Mol Biol Rep, 37, 3067-3072.

Chiang KH, Huang PH, Huang SS, Wu TC, Chen JW & Lin SJ. (2009). Plasma levels of soluble receptor for advanced glycation end products are associated with endothelial function and predict cardiovascular events in nondiabetic patients. Coron Artery Dis, 20, 267-273.

Cipollone F, Toniato E, Martinotti S, Fazia M, Iezzi A, et al. (2004). A polymorphism in the cyclooxygenase-2 gene as an inherited protective factor against myocardial infarction and stroke. J Am Med Assoc, 291, 2221–2228.

Clark JA, Burny I, Sarnaik AP & Audhya TK. (2006). Acute thiamine deficiency in diabetic ketoacidosis: Diagnosis and management. Pediatr Crit Care Med, 7, 595-599.

Connelly KA, Advani A, Advani S, Zhang Y, Thai K, et al. (2013). Combination Angiotensin Converting Enzyme and Direct Renin Inhibition in Heart Failure following Experimental Myocardial Infarction, 31, 84-91.

Craige SM, Chen K, Pei Y, Li C, Huang X, et al. (2011). NADPH oxidase 4 promotes endothelial angiogenesis through endothelial nitric oxide synthase activation. Circulation, 124, 731-740.

Dafni C, Drakoulis N, Landt O, Panidis D, Reczko M & Cokkinos DV. (2010). Association of the eNOS E298D polymorphism and the risk of myocardial infarction in the Greek population. BMC Med Genet, 11, 133.

Daly MJ& Dixon LJ. (2009). A case of ST-elevation and nystagmus--when coronary thrombosis is not to blame. QJM, 102, 737-739.

Degousee N, Fazel S, Angoulvant D, Stefanski E, Pawelzik SC, et al. (2008). Microsomal prostaglandin E2 synthase-1 deletion leads to adverse left ventricular remodeling after myocardial infarction. Circulation, 117, 1701-1710.

de Souza Pinto R, Castilho G, Paim BA, Machado-Lima A, Inada NM. et al.(2012). Inhibition of macrophage oxidative stress prevents the reduction of ABCA-1 transporter induced by advanced glycated albumin. Lipids, 47, 443-450.

Doerries C, Grote K, Hilfiker-Kleiner D, Luchtefeld M, Schaefer A, et al. (2007). Critical role of the NAD(P)H oxidase subunit p47phox for left ventricular remodeling/dysfunction and survival after myocardial infarction. Circ Res, 100, 894-903.

dos Santos KG, Canani LH, Gross JL, Tschiedel B, Pires Souto KE & Roisenberg I. (2005). The -374A allele of the receptor for advanced glycation end products gene is associated with a decreased risk of ischemic heart disease in African-Brazilians with type 2 diabetes. Mol Genet Metab, 85, 149-156.

Dzielińska Z, Małek LA, Roszczynko M, Szperl M, Demkow M, et al. (2011). Combined renin-angiotensin system gene polymorphisms and outcomes in coronary artery disease - a preliminary report. Kardiol Pol, 69, 688-695.

Elahi MM, Kong YX & Matata BM. (2009). Oxidative stress as a mediator of cardiovascular disease. Oxid Med Cell Longev, 2, 259-269.

Elesber AA, Best PJ, Lennon RJ, Mathew V, Rihal CS, et al. (2006). Plasma 8-iso-prostaglandin F2alpha, a marker of oxidative stress, is increased in patients with acute myocardial infarction. Free Radic Res, 40, 385-391.

Espat NJ & Nelton WS. (2000). Oxygen free radicals, oxidative stress, and antioxidants in critical illness. Support Line, 22, 11–20.

Falcone C, Geroldi D, Buzzi MP, Emanuele E, Yilmaz Y, et al. (2008). The -374T/A RAGE polymorphism protects against future cardiac events in nondiabetic patients with coronary artery disease. Arch Med Res, 39, 320-325.

Fraser DA, Hessvik NP, Nikolić N, Aas V, Hanssen KF, et al. (2012). Benfotiamine increases glucose oxidation and down-regulates NADPH oxidase 4 expression in cultured human myotubes exposed to both normal and high glucose concentrations. Genes Nutr, 7,459-469.

Frédérich M, Delvaux D, Gigliobianco T, Gangolf M, Dive G, et al. (2009). Thiaminylated adenine nucleotides. FEBS J, 276, 3256–3268.

Freye E. (1976). Cardiovascular effects of high doses of thiamine (vit B1) in the dog with special reference to myocardial oxygen consumption. Basic Res Cardiol, 71, 192-198.

Gadau S, Emanueli C, Van Linthout S, Graiani G, Todaro M, et al. (2006). Benfotiamine accelerates the healing of ischaemic diabetic limbs in mice through protein kinase B/Akt-mediated potentiation of angiogenesis and inhibition of apoptosis. Diabetologia, 49, 405-420.

Gao J, Zhong MK, Fan ZD, Yuan N, Zhou YB, et al. (2012). SOD1 overexpression in paraventricular nucleus improves post-infarct myocardial remodeling and ventricular function. Pflugers Arch, 463, 297-307.

Gasparetto C, Malinverno A, Culacciati D, Gritti D, Prosperini PG, et al. (2005). Antioxidant vitamins reduce oxidative stress and ventricular remodeling in patients with acute myocardial infarction. Int J Immunopathol Pharmacol, 18, 487-496.

Gioda CR, de Oliveira Barreto T, Primola-Gomes TN, de Lima DC, Campos PP, et al. (2010). Cardiac oxidative stress is involved in heart failure induced by thiamine deprivation in rats. Am J Physiol Heart Circ Physiol, 298, H2039-H2045.

Goliasch G, Wiesbauer F, Grafl A, Ponweiser E, Blessberger H, et al. (2011). The effect of p22-PHOX (CYBA) polymorphisms on premature coronary artery disease (≤ 40 years of age). Thromb Haemost, 105, 529-534.

Griendling KK & FitzGerald GA. (2003). Oxidative stress and cardiovascular injury: Part I: basic mechanisms and in vivo monitoring of ROS. Circulation, 108, 1912-1916.

Grieve DJ, Byrne JA, Cave AC& Shah AM. (2004). Role of oxidative stress in cardiac remodelling after myocardial infarction. Heart Lung Circ, 13,132-138.

Gu B, Desjardins P, & Butterworth RF. (2008). Selective increase of neuronal cyclooxygenase-2 (COX-2) expression in vulnerable brain regions of rats with experimental Wernicke's encephalopathy: effect of numesulide. Metab Brain Dis, 23, 175-187.

Guo J, Li HZ, Wang LC, Zhang WH, Li GW, et al. (2012). Increased expression of calcium-sensing receptors in atherosclerosis confers hypersensitivity to acute myocardial infarction in rats. Mol Cell Biochem, 366, 345-354.

Hahn NE, Meischl C, Kawahara T, Musters RJ, Verhoef VM, et al. (2012). NOX5 expression is increased in intramyocardial blood vessels and cardiomyocytes after acute myocardial infarction in humans. Am J Pathol, 180, 2222-2229.

Hicks JJ, Montes-Cortes DH, Cruz-Dominguez MP, Medina-Santillan R & Olivares-Corichi IM. (2007). Antioxidants decrease reperfusion induced arrhythmias in myocardial infarction with ST-elevation. Front Biosci, 12, 2029-2037.

Hipskind RA & Bilbe G. (1998). MAP kinase signaling cascades and gene expression in osteoblasts. Front Biosci, 3,d804-816.

Hishikari K, Suzuki J, Ogawa M, Isobe K, Takahashi T, et al. (2009). Pharmacological activation of the prostaglandin E2 receptor EP4 improves cardiac function after myocardial ischaemia/reperfusion injury. Cardiovasc Res, 81, 123-132.

Hofmann MA, Yang Q, Harja E, Kedia P, Gregersen PK, et al. (2005). The RAGE Gly82Ser polymorphism is not associated with cardiovascular disease in the Framingham offspring study. Atherosclerosis, 182, 301-305.

Hou ZH, Lu B, Gao Y, Cao HL, Yu FF, et al. (2013). Matrix Metalloproteinase-9 (MMP-9) and Myeloperoxidase (MPO) Levels in Patients with Nonobstructive Coronary Artery Disease Detected by Coronary Computed Tomographic Angiography. Acad Radiol, 20, 25-31.

Huang BS, Ahmad M, White RA, Marc Y, Llorens-Cortes C & Leenen FH. (2013). Inhibition of brain angiotensin III attenuates sympathetic hyperactivity and cardiac dysfunction in rats post myocardial infarction. Cardiovasc Res, 97, 424-431.

Huuskonen KH, Kunnas TA, Tanner MM, Mikkelsson J, Ilveskoski E, et al. (2008). COX-2 gene promoter polymorphism and coronary artery disease in middle-aged men: the Helsinki sudden death study. Mediators Inflamm, 2008, 289453.

Islamoglu Y, Cil H, Atilgan Z, Elbey MA, Tekbas E & Yazici M. (2012). Myocardial infarction secondary to unintentional ingestion of hydrogen peroxide. Cardiol J, 19, 86-88.

Ito M, Tanabe Y, Suzuki K, Kumakura M & Aizawa Y. (2002). Shoshin beriberi with vasospastic angina pectoris possible mechanism of mid-ventricular obstruction: possible mechanism of mid-ventricular obstruction. Circ J, 66,1070-1072.

Jaulmes A, Sansilvestri-Morel P, Rolland-Valognes G, Bernhardt F, Gaertner R, et al. (2009). Nox4 mediates the expression of plasminogen activator inhibitor-1 via p38 MAPK pathway in cultured human endothelial cells. Thromb Res, 124, 439-446.

Johnston CI. (1994). Tissue angiotensin converting enzyme in cardiac and vascular hypertrophy, repair, and remodeling. Hypertension, 23, 258-268.

Jones SP, Greer JJ, van Haperen R, Duncker DJ, de Crom R & Lefer DJ. (2003). Endothelial nitric oxide synthase overexpression attenuates congestive heart failure in mice. Proc Natl Acad Sci U S A, 100, 4891-4896

Jguirim-Souissi I, Jelassi A, Slimani A, Addad F, Hassine M, et al. (2011). Matrix metalloproteinase-1 and matrix metalloproteinase-12 gene polymorphisms and the outcome of coronary artery disease. Coron Artery Dis, 22, 388-393.

Karachalias N, Babaei-Jadidi R, Kupich C, Ahmed N & Thornalley PJ. (2005). High-dose thiamine therapy counters dyslipidemia and advanced glycation of plasma protein in streptozotocin-induced diabetic rats. Ann N Y Acad Sci 1043, 777-783.

Karachalias N, Babaei-Jadidi R, Rabbani N & Thornalley PJ. (2010). Increased protein damage in renal glomeruli, retina, nerve, plasma and urine and its prevention by thiamine and benfotiamine therapy in a rat model of diabetes. Diabetologia, 53, 1506-1516.

Karayannis G, Tsezou A, Giannatou E, Papanikolaou V, Giamouzis G & Triposkiadis F. (2010). Polymorphisms of renin-angiotensin system and natriuretic peptide receptor A genes in patients of Greek origin with a history of myocardial infarction. Angiology, 61,737-743.

Katare R, Caporali A, Emanueli C & Madeddu P. (2010). Benfotiamine improves functional recovery of the infarcted heart via activation of pro-survival G6PD/Akt signaling pathway and modulation of neurohormonal response. J Mol Cell Cardiol, 49, 625-638.

Kato N, Tatara Y, Ohishi M, Takeya Y, Onishi M, et al. (2011). Angiotensin-converting enzyme single nucleotide polymorphism is a genetic risk factor for cardiovascular disease: a cohort study of hypertensive patients. Hypertens Res, 34, 728-734.

Kawano H, Koide Y, Toda G & Yano K. (2005a). ST-segment elevation of electrocardiogram in a patient with Shoshin beriberi. Intern Med, 44, 578-585.

Kawano H, Hayashi T, Koide Y, Toda G & Yano K. (2005b). Histopathological changes of biopsied myocardium in Shoshin beriberi. Int Heart J, 46, 751-759.

Kihm LP, Müller-Krebs S, Klein J, Ehrlich G, Mertes L, et al. (2011). Benfotiamine protects against peritoneal and kidney damage in peritoneal dialysis. J Am Soc Nephrol, 22, 914-926.

Kirbis J, Milutinović A, Steblovnik K, Teran N, Terzić R & Zorc M. (2004). The -429 T/C and -374 T/A gene polymorphisms of the receptor of advanced glycation end products gene (RAGE) are not risk factors for coronary artery disease in Slovene population with type 2 diabetes. Coll Antropol, 28, 611-616.

Kohda Y, Shirakawa H, Yamane K, Otsuka K, Kono T, et al. (2008). Prevention of incipient diabetic cardiomyopathy by high-dose thiamine. J Toxicol Sci, 33, 459-472.

Konopka A, Szperl M, Piotrowski W, Roszczynko M & Stępińska J.(2011). Influence of renin-angiotensin system gene polymorphisms on the risk of ST-segment-elevation myocardial infarction and association with coronary artery disease risk factors. Mol Diagn Ther, 15, 167-176.

Kosiborod M, Rathore SS, Inzucchi SE, Masoudi FA, Wang Y, et al. (2005). Admission glucose and mortality in elderly patients hospitalized with acute myocardial infarction: Implications for patients with and without recognized diabetes. Circulation, 111, 3078-3086.

Koyama H, Shoji T, Fukumoto S, Shinohara K, Shoji T, et al. (2007). Low circulating endogenous secretory receptor for AGEs predicts cardiovascular mortality in patients with end-stage renal disease. Arterioscler Thromb Vasc Biol, 27, 147-153.

Krishnakumar R & Kraus WL. (2010). The PARP side of the nucleus: molecular actions, physiological outcomes, and clinical targets. Mol Cell, 39, 8–24.

Kruse M, Navarro D, Desjardins P & Butterworth RF. (2004). Increased brain endothelial nitric oxide synthase expression in thiamine deficiency: relationship to selective vulnerability. Neurochem Int, 45, 49-56.

Kumphune S, Bassi R, Jacquet S, Sicard P, Clark JE, et al. (2010). A chemical genetic approach reveals that p38alpha MAPK activation by diphosphorylation aggravates myocardial infarction and is prevented by the direct binding of SB203580. J Biol Chem, 285, 2968-2975.

Kuge Y, Takai N, Ishino S, Temma T, Shiomi M & Saji H. (2007). Distribution profiles of membrane type-1 matrix metalloproteinase (MT1-MMP), matrix metalloproteinase-2 (MMP-2) and cyclooxygenase-2 (COX-2) in rabbit atherosclerosis: comparison with plaque instability analysis. Biol Pharm Bull, 30,1634–1640.

Lada-Moldovan L, Kaloustian S, Bah TM, Girard SA, Déry MA & Rousseau G. (2009). Chronic pretreatment with celecoxib reduces infarct size. J Cardiovasc Pharmacol, 54, 31-37.

Larrieu AJ, Yazdanfar S, Redovan E, Eftychiadis A, Kao R, et al. (1987a). Beneficial effects of cocarboxylase in the treatment of experimental myocardial infarction in dogs. Am Surg, 53, 721-725.

Larrieu AJ, Kao RL, Yazdanfar S, Redovan E, Silver J, et al. (1987b). Preliminary evaluation of cocarboxylase on myocardial protection of the rat heart. Ann Thorac Surg, 43, 168-171.

Lemaitre RN, Rice K, Marciante K, Bis JC, Lumley TS, et al. (2009). Variation in eicosanoid genes, non-fatal myocardial infarction and ischemic stroke. Atherosclerosis, 204, e58-63.

Li JL, Yang Z, Wu S & Kong J. (2012). Relationship between endothelial nitric oxide synthase, insulin resistance and macrovascular disease in patients with acute myocardial infarction. J Int Med Res, 4, 687-693.

Liaudet L, Szabó E, Timashpolsky L, Virág L, Cziráki A & Szabó C. (2001). Suppression of poly (ADP-ribose) polymerase activation by 3-aminobenzamide in a rat model of myocardial infarction: long-term morphological and functional consequences. Br J Pharmacol, 133, 1424-1430.

Liu S, Stromberg A, Tai HH & Moscow JA. (2004). Thiamine transporter gene expression and exogenous thiamine modulate the expression of genes involved in drug and prostaglandin metabolism in breast cancer cells. Mol Cancer Res, 2, 477-487.

Liu Y, Lu X, Xiang FL, Poelmann RE, Gittenberger-de Groot AC, et al. (2012). Nitric oxide synthase-3 deficiency results in hypoplastic coronary arteries and postnatal myocardial infarction. Eur Heart J, 2012 Oct 9. [Epub ahead of print]

Loma-Osorio P, Peñafiel P, Doltra A, Sionis A & Bosch X. (2011). Shoshin beriberi mimicking a high-risk non-ST-segment elevation acute coronary syndrome with cardiogenic shock: when the arteries are not guilty. J Emerg Med, 41,e73-77.

Looi YH, Grieve DJ, Siva A, Walker SJ, Anilkumar N, et al. (2008). Involvement of Nox2 NADPH oxidase in adverse cardiac remodeling after myocardial infarction. Hypertension, 51, 319-325.

Lukienko PI, Mel'nichenko NG, Zverinskii IV & Zabrodskaya SV. (2000). Antioxidant properties of thiamine. Bull Exp Biol Med, 130,874-876.

McNair ED, Wells CR, Qureshi AM, Basran RS, Pearce C, et al. (2009). Low levels of soluble receptor for advanced glycation end products in non-ST elevation myocardial infarction patients. Int J Angiol, 18, 187-192.

McNair ED, Wells CR, Mabood Qureshi A, Basran R, Pearce C, et al. (2010). Soluble receptors for advanced glycation end products (sRAGE) as a predictor of restenosis following percutaneous coronary intervention. Clin Cardiol, 33, 678-685.

McNair ED, Wells CR, Qureshi AM, Pearce C, Caspar-Bell G & Prasad K. (2011). Inverse Association between Cardiac Troponin-I and Soluble Receptor for Advanced Glycation End Products in Patients with Non-ST-Segment Elevation Myocardial Infarction. Int J Angiol, 20, 49-54.

Mehta R, Dedina L & O'Brien PJ. (2011). Rescuing hepatocytes from iron-catalyzed oxidative stress using vitamins B1 and B6. Toxicol In Vitro, 25, 111411-22.

Misra MK, Sarwat M, Bhakuni P, Tuteja R & Tuteja N. (2009) Oxidative stress and ischemic myocardial syndromes. Med Sci Monit, 15, RA209-219.

Muhlestein JB, May HT, Bair TL, Prescott MF, Horne BD, et al. (2010). Relation of elevated plasma renin activity at baseline to cardiac events in patients with angiographically proven coronary artery disease. Am J Cardiol, 106, 764-769.

Murthy KG, Xiao CY, Mabley JG, Chen M & Szabó C. (2004). Activation of poly(ADP-ribose) polymerase in circulating leukocytes during myocardial infarction. Shock, 21, 230-234.

Narne P, Ponnaluri KC, Singh S, Siraj M & Ishaq M. (2013). Association of the genetic variants of endothelial nitric oxide synthase gene with angiographically defined coronary artery disease and myocardial infarction in South Indian patients with type 2 diabetes mellitus. J Diabetes Complications, 27, 255-261.

Nilsson L, Hallén J, Atar D, Jonasson L & Swahn E. (2012) Early measurements of plasma matrix metalloproteinase-2 predict infarct size and ventricular dysfunction in ST-elevation myocardial infarction. Heart, 98, 31-36.

Niu W & Qi Y. (2012). Matrix metalloproteinase family gene polymorphisms and risk for coronary artery disease: systematic review and meta-analysis. Heart, 98, 1483-1491.

Ogawa M, Suzuki J, Takayama K, Senbonmatsu T, Hirata Y, et al. (2012). Impaired post-infarction cardiac remodeling in chronic kidney disease is due to excessive renin release. Lab Invest, 92, 1766-1776.

Orbe J, Beloqui O, Rodriguez JA, Belzunce MS, Roncal C, et al. (2006). Protective effect of the G-765C COX-2 polymorphism on subclinical atherosclerosis and inflammatory markers in asymptomatic subjects with cardiovascular risk factors. Clin Chim Acta, 368, 138–143.

Ozaki Y, Imanishi T, Tanimoto T, Kashiwagi M, Tsujioka H, et al. (2012). Effect of direct renin inhibitor, aliskiren, on peripheral blood monocyte subsets and myocardial salvage in patients with primary acute myocardial infarction. Circ J, 76. 1461-1468.

Pacher P, Liaudet L, Soriano FG, Mabley JG, Szabó E & Szabó C. (2002). The role of poly(ADP-ribose) polymerase activation in the development of myocardial and endothelial dysfunction in diabetes. Diabetes, 51, 514-521.

Pérez-Hernández N, Vargas-Alarcón G, Martínez-Rodríguez N, Martínez-Ríos MA, Peña-Duque MA, et al. (2012). The matrix metalloproteinase 2-1575 gene polymorphism is associated with the risk of developing myocardial infarction in Mexican patients. J Atheroscler Thromb, 19, 718-727.

Picheth G, Costantini CO, Pedrosa FO, Leme da Rocha Martinez T & Maltempi de Souza E. (2007). The -374A allele of the receptor for advanced glycation end products (RAGE) gene promoter is a protective factor against cardiovascular lesions in type 2 diabetes mellitus patients. Clin Chem Lab Med, 45, 1268-1272.

Pieper AA, Walles T, Wei G, Clements EE, Verma A, et al. (2006). Myocardial postischemic injury is reduced by poly-ADPribose polymerase-1 gene disruption. Mol Med, 6, 271-282

Polizzi FC, Andican G, Cetin E, Civelek S, Yumuk V & Burçak G. (2012). *Increased DNA-Glycation in Type 2 Diabetic Patients: The Effect of Thiamine and Pyridoxine Therapy.* Exp Clin Endocrinol Diabetes, 120, 329-334.

Poon PY, Szeto CC, Chow KM, Kwan BC & Li PK. (2010). *Relation between polymorphisms of receptor for advanced glycation end products (RAGE) and cardiovascular diseases in Chinese patients with diabetic nephropathy.* Clin Nephrol, 73, 44-50.

Qi Y, Li H, Shenoy V, Li Q, Wong F, et al. (2012). *Moderate cardiac-selective overexpression of angiotensin II type 2 receptor protects cardiac functions from ischaemic injury.* Exp Physiol, 97, 89-101.

Qian JY, Harding P, Liu Y, Shesely E, Yang XP & LaPointe MC. (2008). *Reduced cardiac remodeling and function in cardiac-specific EP4 receptor knockout mice with myocardial infarction.* Hypertension, 51, 560-566.

Rahaman SO, Lennon DJ, Febbraio M, Podrez EA, Hazen SL & Silverstein RL. (2006). *A CD36-dependent signaling cascade is necessary for macrophage foam cell formation.* Cell Metab, 4, 211-221.

Raposeiras-Roubín S, Rodiño-Janeiro BK, Paradela-Dobarro B, Grigorian-Shamagian L, García-Acuña JM, et al. (2012). *Predictive value of advanced glycation end products for the development of post-infarction heart failure: a preliminary report.* Cardiovasc Diabetol, 11, 102.

Ren J, Zhang S, Kovacs A, Wang Y & Muslin AJ. (2005). *Role of p38alpha MAPK in cardiac apoptosis and remodeling after myocardial infarction.* J Mol Cell Cardiol, 38, 617-263.

Ricci R, Sumara G, Sumara I, Rozenberg I, Kurrer M, et al. (2004). *Requirement of JNK2 for scavenger receptor A-mediated foam cell formation in atherogenesis.* Science, 306, 1558-1561.

Scherrer-Crosbie M, Ullrich R, Bloch KD, Nakajima H, Nasseri B, et al. (2001). *Endothelial nitric oxide synthase limits left ventricular remodeling after myocardial infarction in mice.* Circulation, 104, 1286-1291.

Schjerning Olsen AM, Fosbøl EL, Lindhardsen J, Folke F, Charlot M, et al. (2011). *Duration of treatment with nonsteroidal anti-inflammatory drugs and impact on risk of death and recurrent myocardial infarction in patients with prior myocardial infarction: a nationwide cohort study.* Circulation, 123, 2226-2235.

Schmid U, Stopper H, Heidland A & Schupp N. (2008). *Benfotiamine exhibits direct antioxidative capacity and prevents induction of DNA damage in vitro.* Diabetes Metab Res Rev, 24, 371-377.

Shalia KK, Shah VK, Mashru MR, Soneji SL, Vasvani JB, et al. (2010). *Matrix metalloproteinase-3 (MMP-3) -1612 5A/6A promoter polymorphism in coronary artery disease in Indian population.* Indian J Clin Biochem, 25, 133-140.

Shin BH, Choi SH, Cho EY, Shin MJ, Hwang KC, Cho HK, et al. (2004). *Thiamine attenuates hypoxia-induced cell death in cultured neonatal rat cardiomyo-cytes.* Mol Cells, 18, 133–140.

Shneĭder AB. (1991). *[Anti-ischemic heart protection using thiamine and nicotinamide].* Patol Fiziol Eksp Ter, (1), 9-10. [Article in Russian]

Shoeb M & Ramana KV. (2012). *Anti-inflammatory effects of benfotiamine are mediated through the regulation of the arachidonic acid pathway in macrophages.* Free Radic Biol Med, 52, 182-190.

Stirban A, Negrean M, Stratmann B, Gawlowski T, Horstmann T, et al. (2006). *Benfotiamine prevents macro- and microvascular endothelial dysfunction and oxidative stress following a meal rich in advanced glycation end products in individuals with type 2 diabetes.* Diabetes Care, 29, 2064-2071.

Stirban A, Nandrean S, Kirana S, Götting C, Veresiu IA & Tschoepe D.(2012). *Benfotiamine counteracts smoking-induced vascular dysfunction in healthy smokers.* Int J Vasc Med, 2012, 968761.

Strumilo S, Czerniecki J & Dobrzyn P. (1999). *Regulatory effect of thiamin pyrophosphate on pig heart pyruvate dehydrogenase complex.* Biochem Biophys Res Commun, 256, 341-345.

Suzuki T. (1967). *Electron microscopic study on myocardial lesions in thiamine-deficient rats.* Tohoku J Exp Med, 91, 249-259.

Tai HH, Tong M & Ding Y. (2007). *15-hydroxyprostaglandin dehydrogenase (15-PGDH) and lung cancer.* Prostaglandins Other Lipid Mediat, 83, 203-208.

Tanaka T, Sohmiya K, Kono T, Terasaki F, Horie R, et al. (2007). Thiamine attenuates the hypertension and metabolic abnormalities in CD36-defective SHR: uncoupling of glucose oxidation from cellular entry accompanied with enhanced protein O-GlcNAcylation in CD36 deficiency. Mol Cell Biochem, 299, 23–35.

Tanaka T, Yamamoto D, Sato T, Tanaka S, Usui K, et al. (2011). Adenosine thiamine triphosphate (AThTP) inhibits poly(ADP-ribose) polymerase 1 (PARP-1) activity. J Nutr Sci Vitaminol, 57,192–196.

Tanindi A, Sahinarslan A, Elbeg S & Cemri M. (2011). Relationship Between MMP-1, MMP-9, TIMP-1, IL-6 and Risk Factors, Clinical Presentation, Extent and Severity of Atherosclerotic Coronary Artery Disease. Open Cardiovasc Med J, 5, 110-116.

Tanno M, Bassi R, Gorog DA, Saurin AT, Jiang J, et al. (2003). Diverse mechanisms of myocardial p38 mitogen-activated protein kinase activation: evidence for MKK-independent activation by a TAB1-associated mechanism contributing to injury during myocardial ischemia. Circ Res, 93, 254-261.

Tarallo S, Beltramo E, Berrone E, Dentelli P & Porta M. (2010). Effects of high glucose and thiamine on the balance between matrix metalloproteinases and their tissue inhibitors in vascular cells. Acta Diabetol, 47,105-111.

Thornalley PJ, Babaei-Jadidi R, Al Ali H, Rabbani N, Antonysunil A, et al. (2007). High prevalence of low thiamine concentration in diabetes linked to a marker of vascular disease. Diabetologia, 50, 2164-2170.

Tóth-Zsámboki E, Horváth E, Vargova K, Pankotai E, Murthy K, et al. (2006). Activation of poly(ADP-ribose) polymerase by myocardial ischemia and coronary reperfusion in human circulating leukocytes. Mol Med, 12, 221-228.

Tylicki A, Czerniecki J, Godlewska A, Kieliszek M, Zebrowski T, et al. (2008). Changes in ECG and enzyme activity in rat heart after myocardial infarction: effect of TPP and MnCl2. J Physiol Biochem, 64, 93-101.

Verma S, Reddy K& Balakumar P. (2010). The defensive effect of benfotiamine in sodium arsenite-induced experimental vascular endothelial dysfunction. Biol Trace Elem Res, 137, 96-109.

Vinogradov VV, Shneider AB & Senkevich SB. (1991). Thiamine cardiotropism. Cor Vasa, 33, 254-262.

Wang J, Xu D, Wu X, Zhou C, Wang H, et al. (2011). Polymorphisms of matrix metalloproteinases in myocardial infarction: a meta-analysis. Heart, 97, 1542-1546.

Wang KF, Huang PH, Chiang CH, Hsu CY, Leu HB, et al. (2013). Usefulness of plasma matrix metalloproteinase-9 level in predicting future coronary revascularization in patients after acute myocardial infarction. Coron Artery Dis, 24, 23-28.

Weiss S, Haynes FW & Zoll PP. (1938). Electrocardiographic manifestations and the cardiac effect of drugs in vitamin B-1 deficiency in rats. Amer Heart J, 15, 206-220.

Wexler BC & Lutmer RF.(1973). Changes in myocardial thiamine in arteriosclerotic and non-arteriosclerotic rats subjected to isoprenaline induced myocardial infarction. Br J Exp Pathol, 54, 479-491.

White HD, Aylward PE, Huang Z, Dalby AJ, Weaver WD, et al. (2005). Mortality and morbidity remain high despite captopril and/or valsartan therapy in elderly patients with left ventricular systolic dysfunction, heart failure, or both after acute myocardial infarction: results from the Valsartan in Acute Myocardial Infarction Trial (VALIANT). Circulation, 112, 3391-3399.

Wong CY, Qiuwaxi J, Chen H, Li SW, Chan HT, et al. (2008). Daily intake of thiamine correlates with the circulating level of endothelial progenitor cells and the endothelial function in patients with type II diabetes. Mol Nutr Food Res, 52, 1421-1427.

Xiao CY, Chen M, Zsengellér Z & Szabó C. (2004). Poly(ADP-ribose) polymerase contributes to the development of myocardial infarction in diabetic rats and regulates the nuclear translocation of apoptosis-inducing factor. J Pharmacol Exp Ther, 310, 498-504.

Xie X, Ma YT, Fu ZY, Yang YN, Ma X, et al. (2009). Association of polymorphisms of PTGS2 and CYP8A1 with myocardial infarction. Clin Chem Lab Med, 47, 347-352.

Yaday UC, Subramanyam S & Ramana KV. (2009). Prevention of endotoxin-induced uveitis in rats by benfotiamine, a lipophilic analogue of vitamin B1. Invest Ophthalmol Vis Sci, 50, 2276-2282.

Yaday UC, Kalariya NM, Srivastava SK & Ramana KV. (2010). Protective role of benfo-tiamine, a fat soluble vitamin B1 analogue, in the lipopolysaccharide-induced cytotoxic signals in murine macrophages. Free Radic Biol Med, 48, 1423–1434.

Yang Z, Zingarelli B & Szabó C. (2000). Effect of genetic disruption of poly (ADP-ribose) synthetase on delayed production of inflammatory mediators and delayed necrosis during myocardial ischemia-reperfusion injury. Shock, 13, 60-66.

Yao L, Huang K, Huang D, Wang J, Guo H & Liao Y. (2008). Acute myocardial infarction induced increases in plasma tumor necrosis factor-alpha and interleukin-10 are associated with the activation of poly(ADP-ribose) polymerase of circulating mononuclear cell. Int J Cardiol, 123, 366-368.

Yin H, Zhang J, Lin H, Wang R, Qiao Y, et al. (2008). p38 mitogen-activated protein kinase inhibition decreases TNFalpha secretion and protects against left ventricular remodeling in rats with myocardial ischemia. Inflammation, 31, 65-73.

Yonekura H, Yamamoto Y, Sakurai S, Watanabe T & Yamamoto H. (2005). Roles of the receptor for advanced glycation endproducts in diabetes-induced vascular injury. J Pharmacol Sci, 97, 305-311.

Yoshida K, Yoshiyama M, Omura T, Nakamura Y, Kim S, et al. (2001). Activation of mitogen-activated protein kinases in the non-ischemic myocardium of an acute myocardial infarction in rats. Jpn Circ J, 65, 808-814.

Zhao M, Liu Y, Wang X, New L, Han J & Brunk UT. (2002). Activation of the p38 MAP kinase pathway is required for foam cell formation from macrophages exposed to oxidized LDL. APMIS, 110, 458-468.

Zhao W, Zhao D, Yan R & Sun Y. (2009). Cardiac oxidative stress and remodeling following infarction: role of NADPH oxidase. Cardiovasc Pathol, 18, 156-166.

Zhou HZ, Swanson RA, Simonis U, Ma X, Cecchini G & Gray MO. (2006). Poly(ADP-ribose) polymerase-1 hyperactivation and impairment of mitochondrial respiratory chain complex I function in reperfused mouse hearts. Am J Physiol Heart Circ Physiol, 291, H714-H723.

Approach to Vascular Therapy for the Lower Legs: A Special Reference to Vascular Remodeling

Yasutaka Baba, Sadao Hayashi, Shunichiro Ikeda, Masayuki Nakajo
Department of Radiology
Kagoshima University, Japan

1   Introduction

We present our experiences with the diagnosis and endovascular treatment of lower leg arterial and venous diseases. First, we focus on the diagnosis and endovascular treatment of atherosclerotic disease. In particular, we discuss the therapeutic results for femoropopliteal arterial diseases, comparing bypass surgery and endovascular treatment, and examine the possibility of endovascular treatment for Trans-Atlantic Inter-Society Consensus (TASC) II C and D lesions, which are ordinarily contraindicated for endovascular treatment. Next, we present cases of iliofemoral venous disease. Differing from arterial diseases, venous disorders involve problems associated with venous valves and remodeling. We therefore discuss in detail the iliofemoral veno-occlusive diseases from the perspective of vascular remodeling and therapeutic options.

2   Artery

2.1   Pathogenesis of Arteriosclerotic Vascular Disease (AVD)

Atherosclerotic vascular lesions of the legs are related not only to ischemic damage to the leg tissue but also to a predisposition toward lethal systemic conditions, such as septicemia and acute embolic syndrome. Therefore, understanding the etiology of atherosclerotic vascular lesions is important. Hypertension, diabetes mellitus (DM), and hyperlipidemia, the so-called chronic adult diseases, are currently considered to represent risk factors for atherosclerotic vascular lesions. The underlying pathogenesis of atherosclerosis is an imbalance in lipid metabolism (Hansson & Hermansson, 2011), a maladaptive immune response, and chronic inflammation of the arterial wall. The main cause of the disrupted equilibrium among the accumulation (Hansson & Hermansson, 2011) and clearance of lipids and the immune responses is mediated by macrophage- (Moore & Tabas, 2011), neutrophil- (Zernecke, et al., 2008), T-cell- (Hansson & Hermansson, 2011) and dendritic cell-driven (Weber et al., 2008) pathways, and homeostasis is governed by chemokines and their receptors.

First, the absence of a confluent luminal elastin layer and the exposure of proteoglycans (Kwon et al., 2008; Weber & Noels, 2011) in the artery could induce the accumulation of LDL (low density lipoprotein). Second, an elevated level of circulating cholesterol transported by apolipoprotein B100 (ApoB100)-containing LDL generates atherosclerosis (Hansson & Hermansson, 2011). Third, LDA is exposed to oxidative modification, leading to chemokine secretion from endothelial cells (Weber & Noels, 2011). Fourth, the immune interaction among macrophages, neutrophils, T cells and dendrite cells leads to the accumulation of apoptotic cells, debris and cholesterol necrosis (Weber & Noels, 2011). Finally, fibroatheromatous plaques are composed of collagen and smooth muscle cells infiltrated by T cells and mast cells, creating a place where several inflammatory changes can occur (Weber & Noels, 2011) and resulting in atherosclerosis in the arterial wall.

2.2   Endovascular Treatment of ASD: Update

Endovascular treatment of atherosclerotic vascular lesions has been developing along with revolutionary advances in medical equipment. For common iliac or external iliac arterial lesions, endovascular treatments, including percutaneous transluminal angioplasty (or balloonplasty) and stent deployment, play major roles in restoring blood flow to the legs (Ichihashi, Higashiura et al., 2011; Mwipatayi, Thomas et al., 2011). However, controversy remains regarding the efficacy of endovascular treatment for vascular lesions below the inguinal ligament (Conrad, Crawford *et al.*, 2011; Baril, Chaer *et al.*, 2010). To date, many comparative studies have examined balloon angioplasty (BAP) versus stent deployment (SD) (Chalmers, Walker *et al.*, 2012) and BAP versus the use of a cutting balloon catheter (Canaud, Alric *et al.*, 2008; Poncyljusz, Falkowski *et al.*, 2013; Cardon, Jan *et al.*, 2008; Cotroneo, Pascali *et al.*, 2008; Garvin and Reifsnyder, 2007). Chalmers *et al.* (2012) reported that at 12-month follow-up, there was no statistically significant difference in restenosis (stenting and PTA: 40.8 %; PTA: 46.7 % (p = 0.68)) for a long superficial femoral artery stenosis. There were fewer target lesion revascularizations in the patients randomized to stenting, but this result did not reach statistical significance (12.5 vs. 20.8 %, p = 0.26). There was no difference in the rate of amputation. Patients in both groups reported an improved quality of life. Therefore, Chalmers et al. could not demonstrate the superiority of PTA plus stenting compared to PTA alone. Poncyljusz (Poncyljus *et al.*, 2013) reported that in the intention-to-treat analysis, the restenosis rates for superficial femoral artery stenosis at 2-month follow-up were 9 of 30 (30 %) in the PTA group and 4 of 30 (13 %) in the cutting balloon angioplasty (CBA) group (p = 0.117), and the ABI values at 12 months between the PTA and CBA groups were 0.77 +/- 0.11 versus 0.82 +/- 0.12, respectively (p = 0.039). Poncyliusz (Poncyljusz *et al.*, 2013) could not demonstrate the superiority of CBT compared to PTA alone. Although techniques and devices for endovascular treatment have been developed, the promising results published previously do not yet appear to be sufficient to confirm the superiority of BAP and associated procedures over bypass surgery.

2.3   Comparison of the Mid-term Results between Endovascular Treatment and Bypass Surgery

Al-Nouri reported that failed intervention for superficial femoral artery occlusive disease has an impact on the preservation of ischemic limbs (Al-Nouri, Krezalek *et al.*, 2012). Therefore, treating superficial femoral arterial lesions is important in salvaging critically ischemic legs. Among the previously reported comparative studies for BAP, the BASIL study only revealed proof of superiority or even efficacy of BAP over bypass surgery for infra-inguinal vascular disease (Bradbury, Adam *et al.*, 2010; Moxey, Brownrigg *et al.*, 2012). According to a randomized study comparing bypass surgery and endovascular treatment for superficial femoral arterial lesions, BAP appears superior to bypass surgery with artificial grafts in terms of patency of the superficial femoral vascular lesions (Bradbury, Adam *et al.*, 2010). Meanwhile, our retrospective study comparing PTA and saphenous vein bypass surgery (Figures 1, 2; Tables 1, 2, unpublished data) revealed that the results for endovascular treatment of femoropopliteal TASCII C/D lesions showed that the 1-year patency rates were between 65 and 77% in the PTA and 73 and 75% in the PTA plus stent deployment groups, compared to bypass surgery.

There was no statistically significant difference in the survival (PTA: 79.3 % at 2 years, bypass: 72.6% at 2 years, P=0.94) and patency (PTA: 70%, bypass: 78.1%, P=0.29) rates between PTA and bypass surgery in patients with TASCII C/D femoropopliteal lesions. In addition, there was a statistically significant difference in the limb salvage rates between endovascular treatment and bypass surgery in patients with TASCII C/D femoropopliteal lesions (PTA: 76.9 %, bypass: 96.8%, P=0.039). There was no statistically significant difference in the run off scores (ROSs) between the limb salvage and non-limb salvage subgroups (limb salvage: median 7.0, non-salvage: median 3.75, P=0.44) in the endovascular treatment group (Table 2).

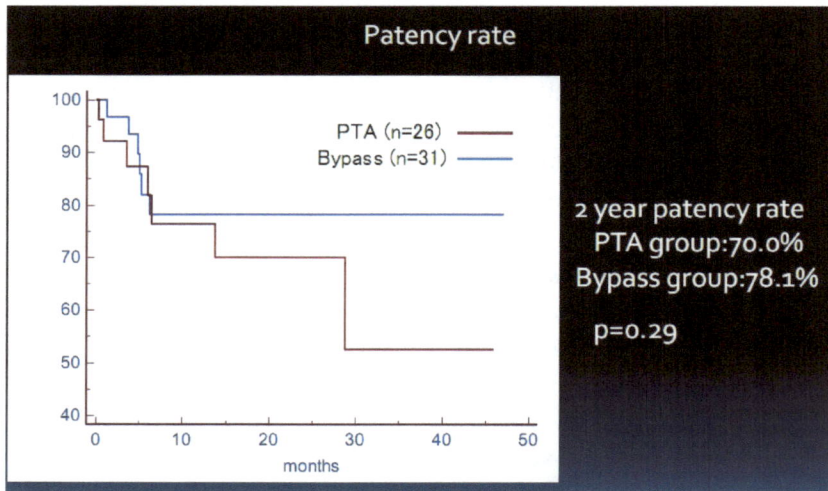

Figure 1: Comparison of the patency rates between the PTA and bypass surgery groups

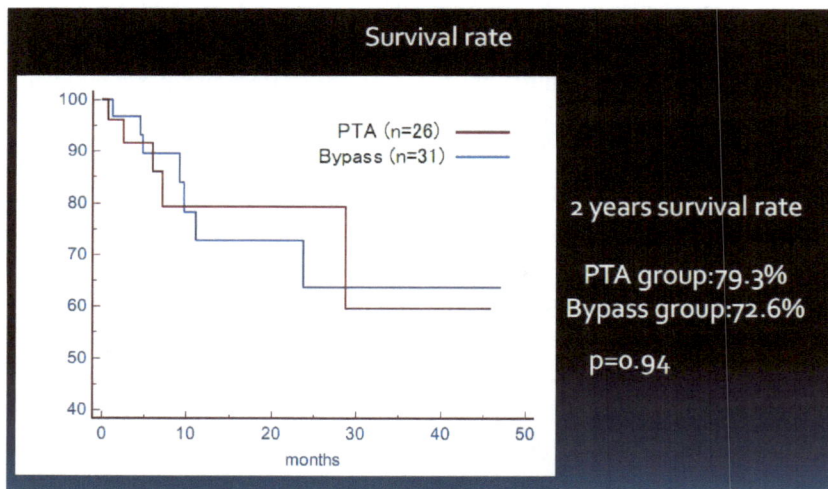

Figure 2: Comparison of the survival rates between the PTA and bypass surgery groups

		Total	PTA	Bypass
Patients		57	26	31
Age		70.3	74.1	67.1
Male		45	18	27
Female		12	8	4
Fontaine				
	II	8	4	4
	III	18	7	11
	IV	31	15	16
TASC				
	B	1	1	0
	C	12	12	0
	D	44	13	31
ROS				
	Average		4.5	4.02
	Median		4	4
Technical Success rate			25 (96.1%)	31 (100%)
Average follow-up periods (month)			13.4 (0.7 - 45.9)	14.7 (1.2 - 47.1)

Table 1: Patient characteristics

	Limb salvage rate
Non Limb Salvage cases	
PTA group	6/26 (limb salvage rate: 76.9%)
Bypass group	1/31 (limb salvage rate: 96.8%)
	$p = 0.039$
ROS	
PTA group	
Limb salvage cases	average value: 6.91 (3 - 10)
	median value: 7.0
Non limb salvage cases	average value: 3.59 (1 - 7)
	median value: 3.75

Table 2: Results of Limb Salvage Rates

2.4   Treatment of Peripheral Arterial Lesions below the Knee

For peripheral arterial lesions below the knee, the efficacy of endovascular treatment is more controversial than for infrainguinal arterial lesions. However, a recent study (Iida, Soga et al. , 2013) of 884 patients with infrapopliteal arterial lesions, showed that with balloon angioplasty, freedom from major adverse limb events (MALE)+perioperative death (POD) was 82 +/- 1% and 74 +/- 2% at 1 and 5 years, respectively. The risk factors associated with MALE+POD were age >/=80 years (adjusted hazard ratio [HR], 0.4; P < .001), non-ambulatory status (HR, 2 0; P < .001), albumin <3.0 g/dL (HR, 1.4; P < .0001), Rutherford 6 (HR, 2.2; P < .001), C-reactive protein >/=3.0 mg/dL (HR, 2.1; P < .001), and below-the-ankle disease (HR, 2.0; P < .001) (Iida, Soga et al., 2013). The 1- and 5-year amputation-free survival rates were 71 +/- 2% and 38 +/- 3%, respectively (Iida, Soga *et al.*, 2013). These data could support the usefulness of endovascular treatment for infrapopliteal arterial lesions. The cutting balloon catheter (Canaud, Alric *et al.* 2008) and subintimal arterial flossing with antegrade-retrograde intervention (SAFARI)(Zhuang, Tan *et al.*, 2011; Spinosa, Harthun *et al.*, 2005; Gandini, Pipitone *et al.*, 2007) have the potential to improve the patency rate compared to simple balloon angioplasty.

3   Vein

3.1   Iliofemoral Veno-occlusive Disease: Definition

Iliofemoral veno-occlusive disease (IVD) is manifested by varicose veins, venous ulceration, edema, venous eczema, and lipodermatosclerosis. The main cause of the above manifestations is venous hypertension as a result of venous stasis with secondary inflammation. In an experimental study using venous hypertension caused by arteriovenous fistulae, Takase et al. found that the venous valve leaflets were occupied with granulocytes, monocytes, T-lymphocytes, and endothelial cells expressing high levels of P-secretin and intercellular adhesion molecule 1 (ICAM-1) (Takase, Pascarella *et al.*, 2004). These data suggest that venous hypertension and the sequential degeneration of the venous valves generate IVD through apoptosis of the venous valves (Takase, Pascarella *et al.*, 2004).

3.2   Mechanism of Venous Valve Movement (Figure 3)

Venous valves are moved by venous pressure rather than blood flow, so complete closure of the venous valves is required to prevent valve degeneration (Qui, Quijano *et al.*, 1995; Lurie, Kistner *et al.*, 2003). Venous flow is usually pulsatile, and 20 cycles of valve movement per minute occur during standing (Bergan, Schmid-Schonbein *et al.*, 2006). In addition, the venous leaflets do not touch the vascular sinus wall when the venous valves are completely open (Bergan, Schmid-Schonbein *et al.*, 2006). This characteristic is responsible for preventing venous sclerosis through shear stress and the cytokine cascade. Considering the dynamic movement of the venous valves, Lurie *et al.* (Lurie., *et al.*, 2003) reported that the valve cusps move in four phases constituting the valve cycle. The vortical stream behind the valve cusps plays a role in valve function and prevents stasis inside the valve pocket (Lurie, Kistner *et al.*, 2003). Thus, the central jet may facilitate outflow (Lurie, Kistner *et al.*, 2003).

Close   Open

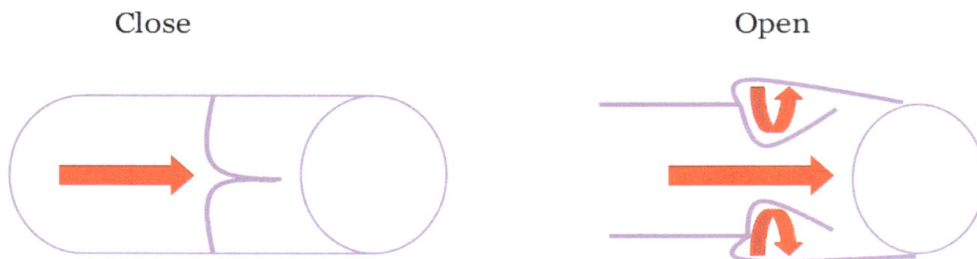

Figure 3: Mechanism of venous valve movement. Venous flow: Normally pulsatile; Venous valves open and close with movement; 20 times per minute; When the valve leaflets are fully open, they do not touch the sinus wall. All surfaces of the valve are exposed to shear stress.

3.3   Shear Stress (Figure 4 and 5)

Shear stress is generated and mediated in endothelial cells by a network of signaling pathways that can promote gene expression. A lack of shear stress on the venous sinus leaflets generates inflammation and thrombotic conditions. A strong correlation exists between endothelial cell dysfunction and areas of low mean shear stress and oscillatory flow with flow reversal (Traub and Berk, 1998). Disturbed flow and the associated low-shear stress generally upregulate endothelial cell genes and proteins that promote atherogenesis (Chiu and Chien, 2011). In the venous system, disturbed flow resulting from reflux, outflow obstruction, and/or stasis leads to venous inflammation and thrombosis and hence the development of CVD (Chiu and Chien, 2011).

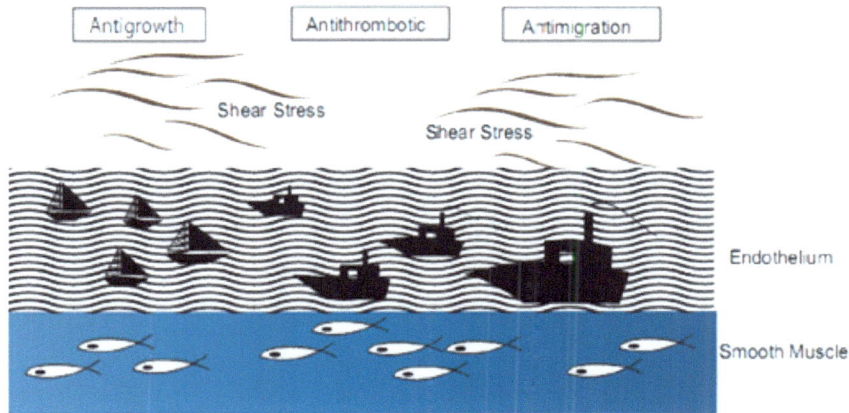

Figure 4: Normal Shear Stress. Under shear stress due to stable venous flow, there is a release of factors from endothelial cells that inhibit coagulation, leukocyte migration, and smooth muscle proliferation.

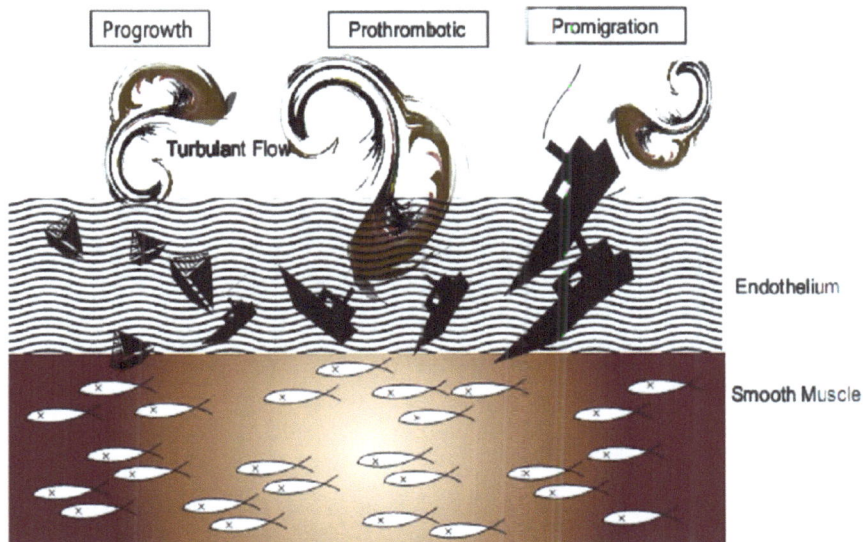

Figure 5: Shear Stress and Static Flow. Meanwhile, under opposite shear stress, some factors promote the growth of smooth muscle and the activation of leukocyte factors.

3.4   Classification of Venous Disease

Venous disease can be classified by the CEAP. CEAP stands for Clinical severity, Etiology, Anatomy, and Pathophysiology. Clinical signs in the affected legs are categorized into seven classes, designated C0 to C6 (Table 3). Leg symptoms associated with CVD include aching, heaviness, swelling, and skin irritation. Limbs categorized in any clinical class may be symptomatic (S) or asymptomatic (A). CVD encompasses the full spectrum of signs and symptoms associated with classes C0 to C6, whereas the term "chronic venous insufficiency" is generally restricted to disease of greater severity (i.e., classes C4-C6). Thus, varicose veins in the absence of skin changes are not indicative of chronic venous insufficiency (Porter and Moneta, 1995; Eklof, Rutherford et al., 2004).

C_0	No visible of palpable signs of venous disease.
C_1	Telangiectasies of reticular veins
C_2	Varicose veins: distinguished from reticular veins by a diameter of 3 mm or more
C_3	Edema
C_4	Changes in skin and subcutaneous tissue secondary to CVD, now divided into 2 subclassers to better define the differing severity of venous disease:
C_{4a}	Pigmentation or eczema
C_{4b}	Lipodermatoscierosis or atrophie blanche
C_5	Healed venous ulcer
C_6	Active venous ulcer

Table 3: Refinement of C classes in CEAP. CEAP classes C_5 and C_6 has been likened to the impairment associated with heart failure.

3.5   Current Topics in Venous Ulceration Associated with Chronic Venous Disease

Among the complications associated with chronic venous disease, a venous ulcer on the lower extremity is a major problem due to difficulty in managing infections, inflammation, and pain (Mosti, 2013). As for familial heredity, Serra et al. (Serra *et al.*, 2012) performed a genetic study in patients with chronic venous insufficiency and verified that varicose veins (saphenofemoral junction reflux) were linked to the candidate marker D16S520 on chromosome 16q24, which may account for the linkage to FOXC2. Previous studies have reported that matrix metalloproteinases (MMP) and neutrophil gelatinase-associated lipocalin (NGAL) might have a role in the healing process in patients with chronic venous ulcers (Rayment *et al.*, 2008; Pukstad *et al.*, 2010). In a biochemistry study for venous ulcer patients, Serra *et al.* (Serra, *et al.*, 2013) reported that enzyme-linked immunosorbent assay (ELISA) tests revealed significantly higher levels of MMP-9 and NGAL in the plasma and wounds from patients with ulcers compared to patients without ulcers ($p < 0.01$). In addition, Serra reported that Western blot analysis demonstrated increased expression of MMP-9 and NGAL from biopsies from patients with ulcers compared to patients without ulcers ($p < 0.01$). Therefore, Serra speculated that MMP-9 and NGAL have a role as biomarkers for healing in patients with a venous ulcer (Serra *et al.*, 2013). In addition, Serra reported that subantimicrobial doses of doxycycline seem to generate chronic venous leg ulcer healing through the inhibition of MMP-9, NGAL and VEGF (Serra *et al.*, 2013).

Hyperhomocysteinemia (HHc) is a factor associated with cardiovascular and cerebrovascular disease (Vollset *et al.*, 2001; De Bree *et al.*, 2002; Boysen *et al.*, 2003). Sam et al. (Sam *et al.*, 2003) described the relationship between chronic venous ulceration and HHc as a thrombophilic disorder. Additionally, de Franciscis *et al.* (de Franciscis *et al.*, 2013) found that homocysteine-lowering therapy with folic acid improved wound healing in patients with chronic venous leg ulcers. They also reported that low molecular weight heparin has a role in chronic venous ulcer healing, possibly due to the antithrombotic and anticoagulant effects (Serra *et al.*, 2013; Serra *et al.*, 2011).

3.6   Endovascular Treatment for Chronic Venous Occlusive Disease

Standard anticoagulation decreases the risk of pulmonary embolism and thrombus propagation, but does not treat the occlusion itself. Up to half of all patients with an iliofemoral DVT treated by anticoagulation alone subsequently develops post-thrombotic syndrome (PTS) (Kahn *et al.*, 2008; Baldwin *et al.*, 2013). PTS is associated with significant morbidity (leg swelling, pain, and ulceration), resulting in poor quality of life and lifelong socioeconomic implications (Kahn *et al.*, 2008; Baldwin *et al.*, 2013).

Endovascular treatment with catheter-directed thrombolysis is a good treatment option for not only restoring the occluded vein but preventing the occurrence of PTS. A Cochrane review suggested a significant reduction in the rate of PTS from 65 to 48 percent with any thrombolysis (Watson & Armon, 2004), and a more recent systematic review reported that systemic thrombolysis reduced PTS from 57 percent to 27 percent with CDT (Alesh *et al.*, 2007).

Stent deployment for a residual stenotic lesion after catheter-directed fibrinolytic therapy is controversial (Park *et al.*, 2013). May-Turner syndrome is characterized by left common iliac vein stenosis due to extrinsic compression by the left common iliac artery. After catheter-directed thrombolysis is performed, residual stenosis in May-Turner syndrome is a good indication for stent deployment to prevent the recurrence of deep vein thrombosis (Park *et al.*, 2013). Warner *et al.* reported that functional outcomes, including pain relief, edema, and return to work, can improve after CDI and stent deployment in patients with an iliofemoral deep vein thrombosis (Warner *et al.*, 2013). However, for DVTs located below the inguinalis, CDT and stent deployment cannot always improve the long-term patency and prevent the occurrence of PTS (Jackson *et al.*, 2005).

Therefore, the indications for endovascular treatment for patients with DVT in our institute are as follows: DVT due benign or malignant disease; recent (within 2 weeks) occurrence of symptoms related to a DVT; no contraindication to thrombolysis, such as brain lesions, previous cerebrovascular attack, and recent surgical procedure; stent deployment for residual stenosis of the common/iliac vein after CDT; stent deployment for lesions below the inguinal level.

In the prone position, venographies via a popliteal vein catheter revealed thrombosis from the left popliteal vein to the external iliac vein and various collateral pathways (a-c). We performed fibrinolytic therapy using urokinase (120.000 units/day via an indwelling catheter) and anticoagulation therapy (10.000 units via the dorsal pedal vein).

The day after treatment, restoration of the vein was observed, but stenosis of the common femoral vein was seen (arrow in d). Balloon dilation was attempted, but residual stenosis was still seen (arrow in f). Five days after treatment, venography showed thrombotic occlusion of the left superficial vein (g and h) and residual stenosis of the left common iliac vein (arrow in i). Residual stenosis of the common femoral vein could have driven the relapse of thrombotic occlusion of the superficial vein. On clinical follow-up, this patient was taking warfarin to prevent the development of thrombosis. No leg swelling was noted after the procedure.

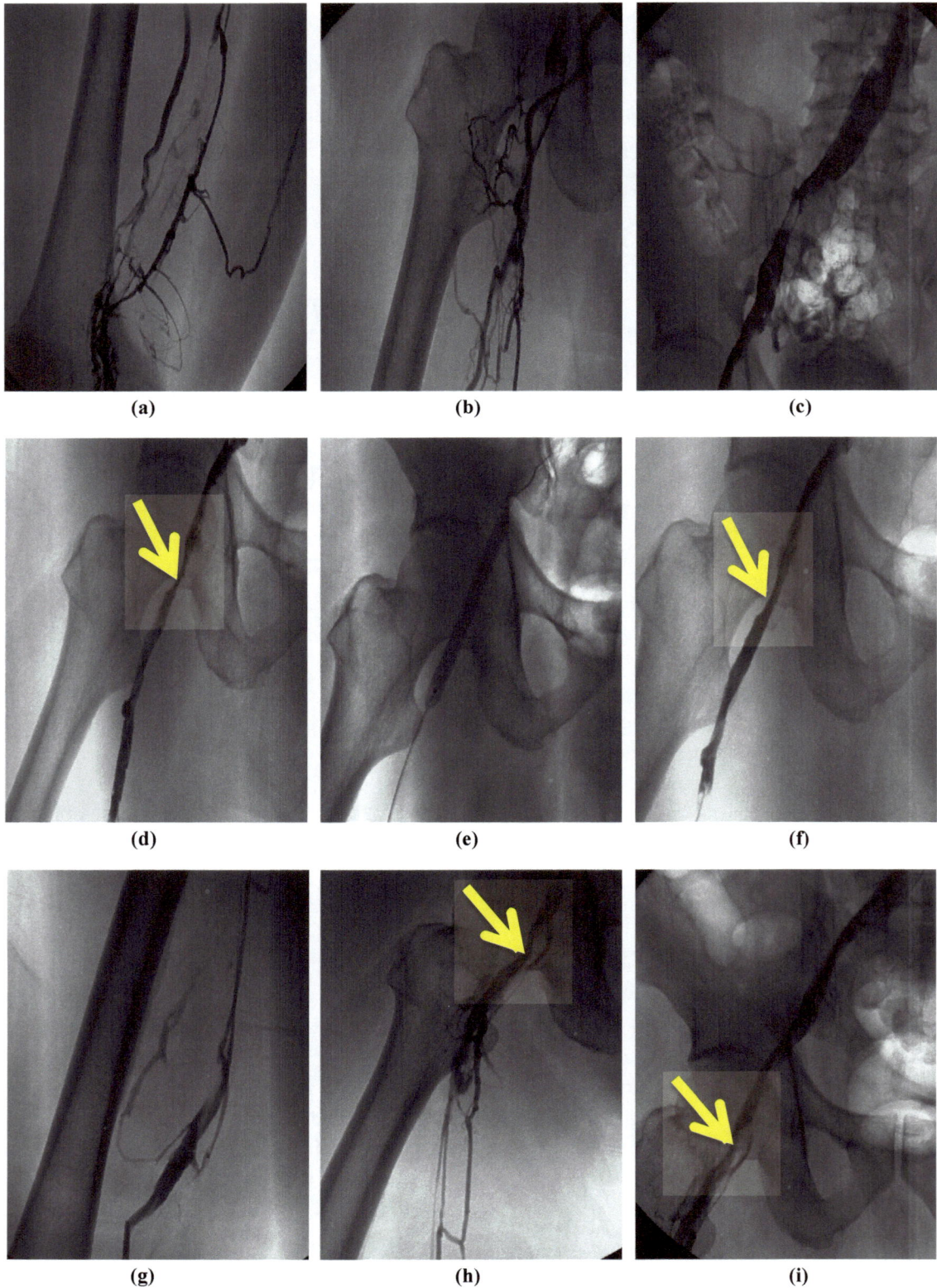

Figure 6: 72-year-old man with a left leg DVT (1): CEAP C3

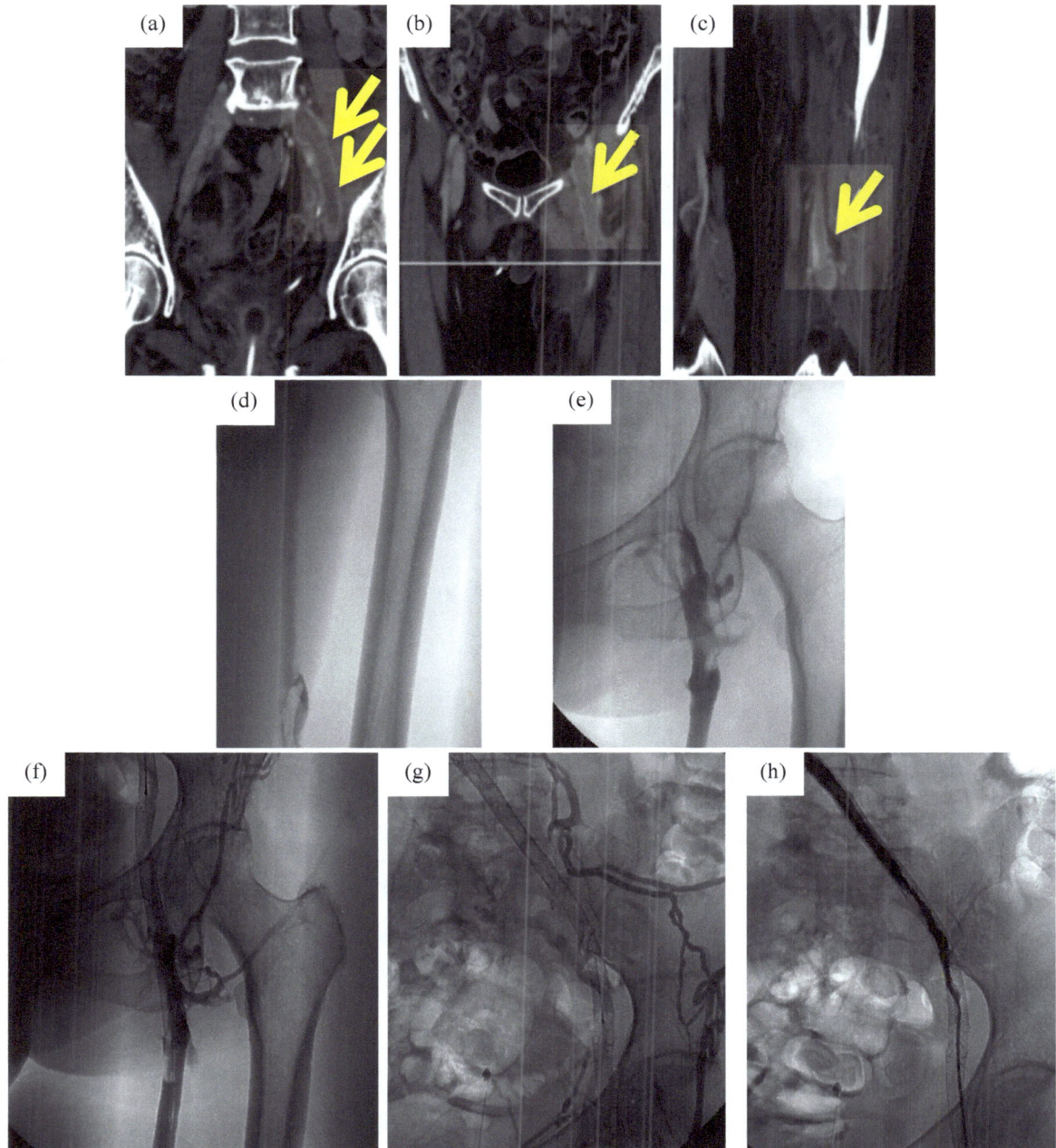

Figure 7: 64-year-old woman with a DVT due to inguinal lymph node removal for melanoma (1): CEAP C3.Contrast-enhanced CT images showed thrombotic occlusion of the left lower leg from the left common iliac vein above the popliteal vein (arrows in all of the images). Venography in the supine position showed flow in the superficial vein (d), but severe stenosis was observed in the common iliac vein (e). We tried to perform fibrinolytic and anticoagulant therapies, but restoration of the iliac vein could not be achieved (f, g). Balloon dilation and stent deployment were not effective, resulting in the recurrence of thrombotic occlusion of the left iliac vein (h). On clinical follow-up, this patient was taking warfarin to prevent the further development of thrombosis. No leg swelling was noted after the procedure until the patient eventually died from melanoma.

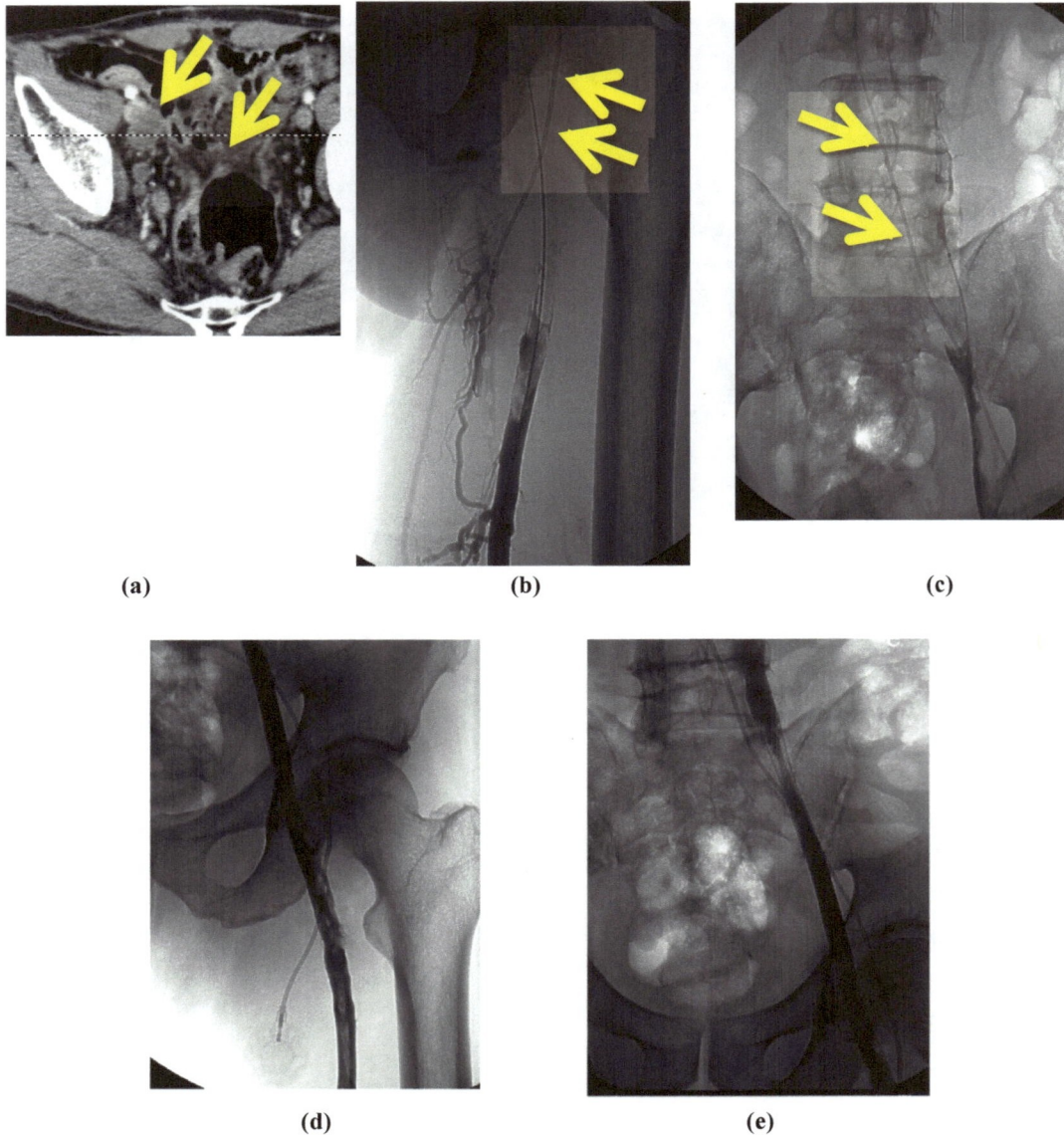

Figure 8: 66-year-old man with metastatic lymph nodes from colon cancer that compressed the right external iliac vein: CEAP C4a. CT (a) showed a bulky metastatic lymph node compressing the right external iliac vein (arrow in a). Venography in the prone position showed thrombotic occlusion of the right common iliac and superficial veins. An indwelling catheter for metastatic liver disease was also seen (yellow arrows in the b and c images). Nine days after fibrinolytic and anticoagulant treatment, restoration of the occluded veins was achieved (d). Stent deployment at the stenotic site was performed to prevent the recurrence of a thrombotic occlusion of the iliac vein (e).

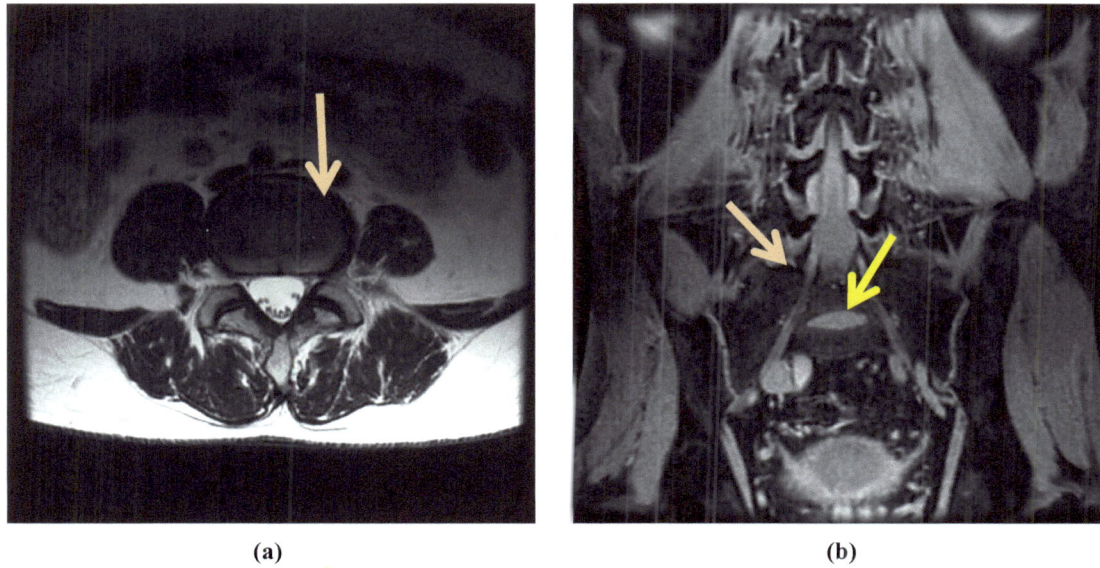

(a)   (b)

Figure 9: 58-year-old man with intractable right sciatic pain. On the MRI images, the left common iliac vein was compressed by the right common iliac artery (arrow in a and b), and the sacral nerve root (white arrow in b) was compressed by a varicose vein (yellow arrow in b). Varicose formation was driven by compression of the left common iliac vein. The intractable right sciatic pain may have been induced by direct compression of the sciatic nerve by the varicose vein (Hu and Wu et al., 2010).

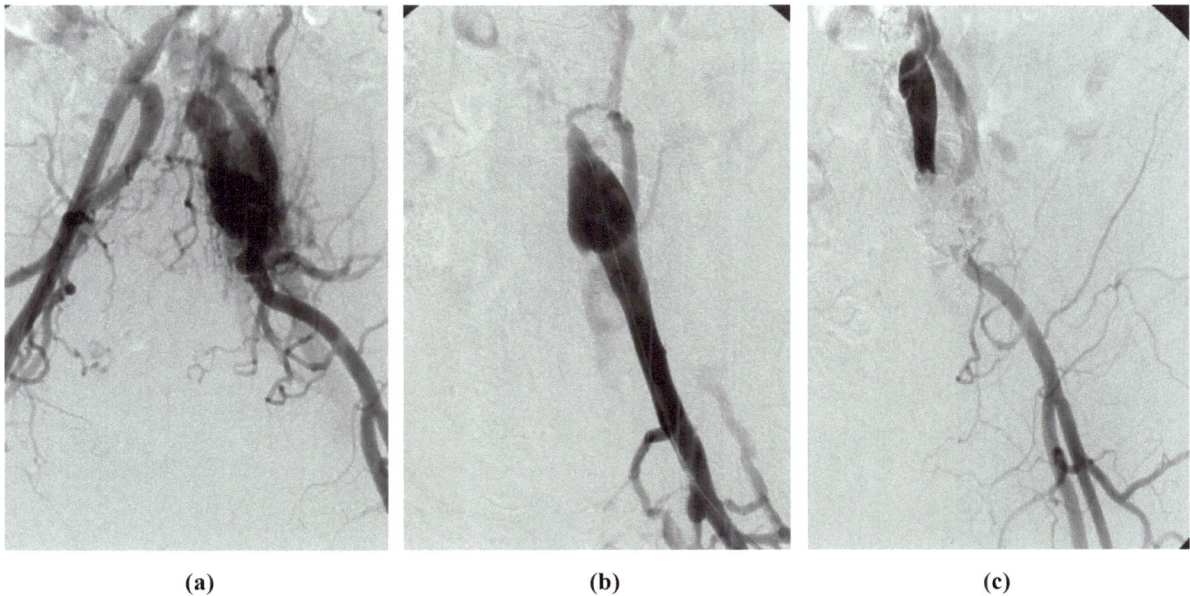

(a)   (b)   (c)

Figure 10: 70-year-old woman with an arteriovenous fistula and May-Turner syndrome: CEAP C4a. (a) Aortography showed fine vessel proliferation around the left iliac artery and early visualization of the left iliac veins. (b)Venography showed an occlusion of the left common iliac vein. (c) Left common iliac arteriography showed no fine vessel proliferation or early venous drainage. However, deep vein thrombosis occurred after arterial embolization. Therefore, we speculate that venous stasis after shunt occlusion led to DVT formation.

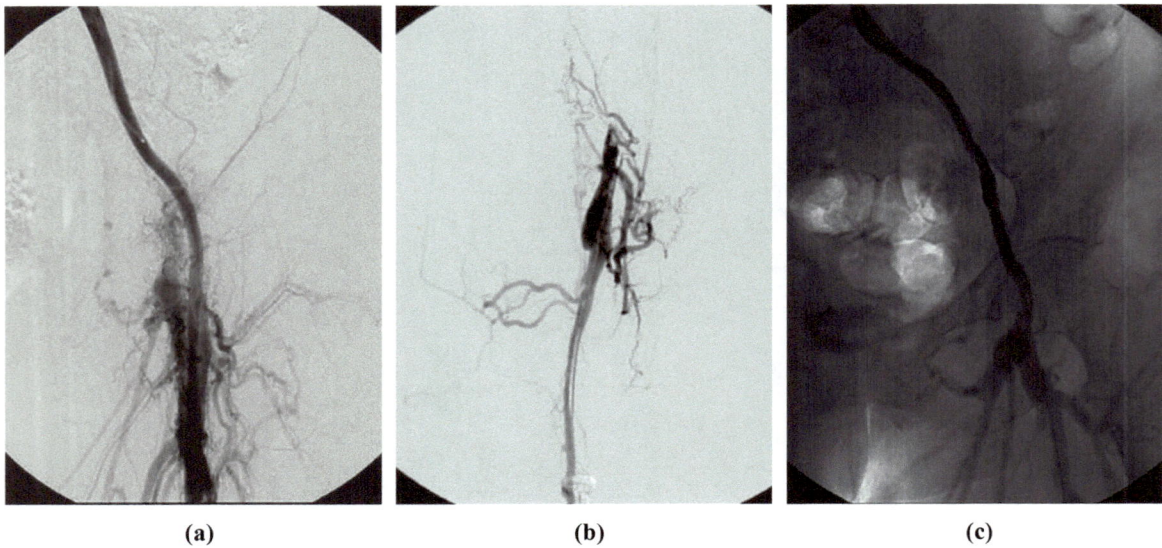

(a)   (b)   (c)

Figure 11: 77-year-old woman with an arteriovenous fistula and with DVT (1): CEAP C5. (a) Left common iliac arteriography showed fine vessel proliferation around the left inguinal region and early visualization of the left common iliac vein. Occlusion of the left common iliac vein was also observed. (b)Venography via the left popliteal vein showed an occlusion of the left common iliac vein. (c) After treatment, venography showed recanalization of the left common iliac vein.

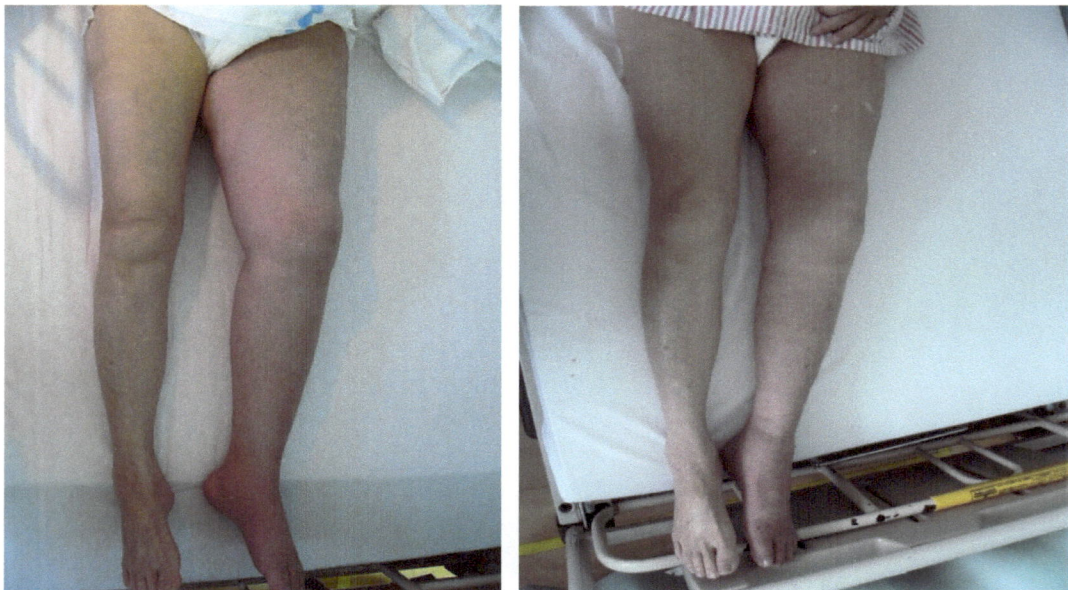

The photos before (left) and after (right) treatment for DVT show that the swollen left lower leg shrank significantly. Skin pigmentation was noted after treatment (right).

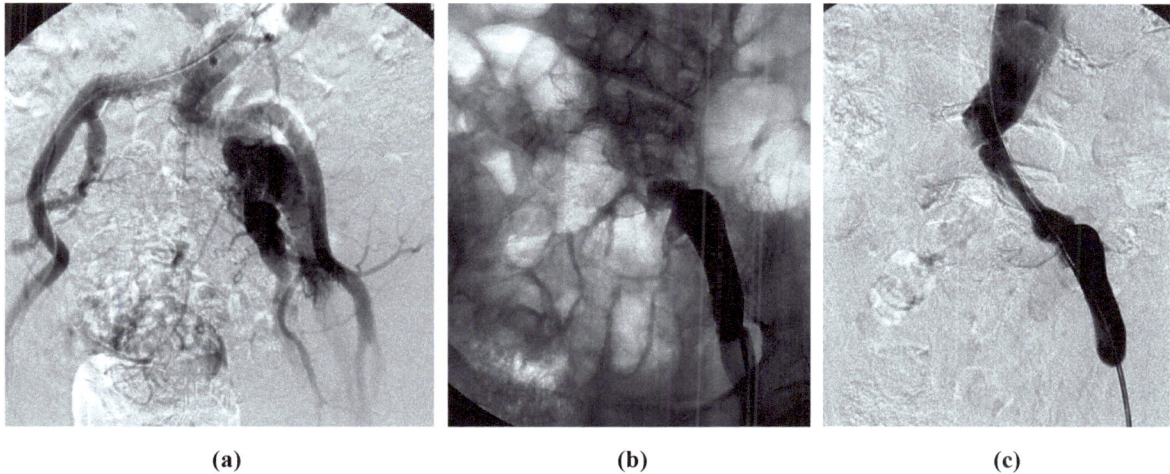

(a)   **(b)**   **(c)**

Figure 12: 88-year-old woman with an arteriovenous fistula and DVT (1): CEAP C6. Aortography showed fine vessel proliferation around the left internal iliac artery and early visualization of the left iliac vein. (b) Venography showed an occlusion of the left common iliac vein. (c) After balloon PTA and stent deployment, venography showed recanalization of the left common iliac vein.

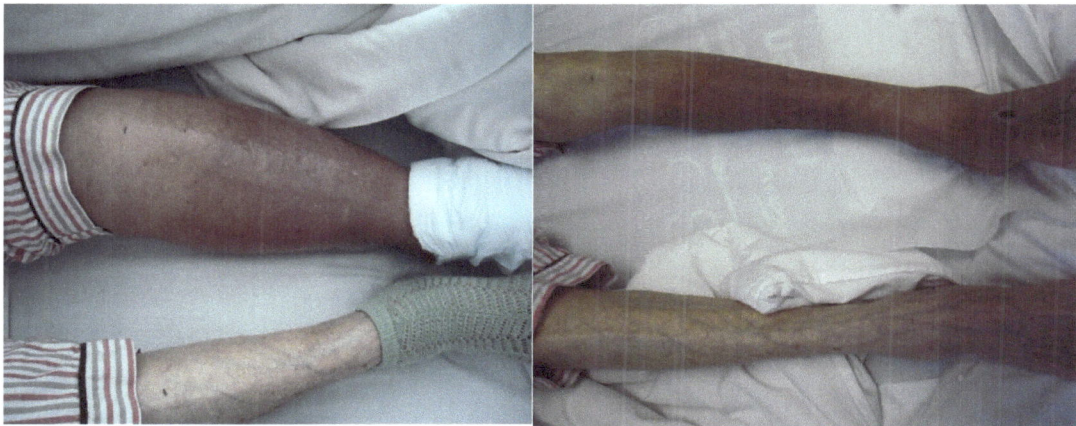

Figure 13: The photos before (left) and after (right) treatment for DVT show that the swollen left lower leg shrank significantly. Skin pigmentation and a healing skin ulcer were noted after treatment (right).

4   Summary

Vascular approach to lower legs is now challenging and developing treatment option for restoring both the occluded arterial or venous peripheral disease. On peripheral arteriosclerosis disease, endovascular therapy including PTA(percutaneous transluminal angioplasty) and stent deployment seem to be effective at the above knee. However, endovascular treatment for below the knee is not sufficient to reach the outcome of long term patency results of bypass surgery. Meanwhile, on peripheral venous disease including deep vein thrombosis, anticoagulant and conservative therapies have a major role of treating venous disease. On view of preventing post thrombotic syndrome, catheter directed therapy seem to be effective to restore the occluded venous disease despite high level evidence of revealing the effectiveness of catheter directed therapy has not been verified.

Acknowledgement

Special thanks to Yukiko Baba for illustrating the figures.

References

Al-Nouri, O., Krezalek, M., Hershberger, R., Halandras, P., Gassman, A., Aulivola, B., & Milner, R.(2012). Failed superficial femoral artery intervention for advanced infrainguinal occlusive disease has a significant negative impact on limb salvage. J Vasc Surg, 56(1), 106-110. discussion 110-111.

Baril, D. T., Chaer, R. A., Rhee, R. Y., Makaroun, M. S., & Marone, L. K. (2010). Endovascular interventions for TASC II D femoropopliteal lesions. J Vasc Surg, 51(6), 1406-1412.

Bergan, J. J., Schmid-Schonbein, G. W., Smith, P. D., Nicolaides, A. N., Boisseau, M. R., & Eklof, B. (2006). Chronic venous disease. N Engl J Med, 355(5), 488-498.

Boysen, G., Brander, T., Christensen, H., Gideon, R., & Truelsen, T. (2003). Homocysteine and risk of recurrent stroke. Stroke 34 (5):1258-1261.

Bradbury, A. W., Adam, D. J. , Bell, J., Forbes, J. F., Fowkes, F. G., Gillespie, I., Ruckley, C. V., & Raab, G. M. (2010). Bypass versus Angioplasty in Severe Ischaemia of the Leg (BASIL) trial: Analysis of amputation free and overall survival by treatment received. J Vasc Surg, 51(5 Suppl), 18S-31S.

Canaud, L., Alric, P., Berthet, J. P., Marty-Ane, C., Mercier, G., & Branchereau, P. (2008). Infrainguinal cutting balloon angioplasty in de novo arterial lesions. J Vasc Surg, 48(5), 1182-1188.

Cardon, J. M., Jan, F., Vasseur, M. A., Ferdani, M., Rind, A., Francois, F., & Cardon, A.(2008). Value of cutting balloon angioplasty for limb salvage in patients with obstruction of popliteal and distal arteries. Ann Vasc Surg, 22(3), 314-318.

Chalmers, N., Walker, P. T., Belli, A. M., Thorpe, A. P., Sidhu, P. S., Robinson, G., van Ransbeeck, M., & Fearn, S. A. (2012). Randomized trial of the SMART stent versus balloon angioplasty in long superficial femoral artery lesions: the SUPER study. Cardiovasc Intervent Radiol, 36(2), 353-361.

Chiu, J. J. & Chien, S. (2011). Effects of disturbed flow on vascular endothelium: pathophysiological basis and clinical perspectives. Physiol Rev, 91(1), 327-387.

Conrad, M. F., Crawford, R. S., Hackney, L. A., Paruchuri, V., Abularrage, C. J., Patel, V. I., Lamuraglia, G. M., & Cambria, R. P. (2011). Endovascular management of patients with critical limb ischemia. J Vasc Surg, 53(4), 1020-1025.

Cotroneo, A. R., Pascali, D., & Iezzi, R. (2008). Cutting balloon versus conventional balloon angioplasty in short femoropopliteal arterial stenoses. J Endovasc Ther, 15(3), 283-291.

De Bree, A., Verschuren, W. M., Kromhout, D., Mennen, L. I., & Blom, H.J., (2002). Homocysteine and coronary heart disease: the importance of a distinction between low and high risk subjects. Int J Epidemiol 31 (6):1268-1272; author reply 1271-1262.

de Franciscis, S., De Sarro, G., Longo, P., Buffone, G., Molinari, V., Stillitano, D.M., Gallelli, L., & Serra, R. Hyperhomocysteinaemia and chronic venous ulcers. Int Wound J. Epub ahead of print.

Eklof, B., Rutherford, R. B., Bergan, J. J., Carpentier, P. H., Gloviczki, P., Kistner, R. L., Meissner, M. H., Moneta, G. L., Myers, K., Padberg, F. T., Perrin, M., Ruckley, C. V., Smith, P. C., & Wakefield, T. W. (2004). Revision of the CEAP classification for chronic venous disorders: consensus statement. J Vasc Surg, 40(6), 1248-1252.

Gandini, R., Pipitone, V., Stefanini, M., Maresca, L., Spinelli, A., Colangelo, V., Reale, C. A., Pampana, E., & Simonetti, G. (2007). The "Safari" technique to perform difficult subintimal infragenicular vessels. Cardiovasc Intervent Radiol, 30(3), 469-473.

Garvin, R. & Reifsnyder, T. (2007). Cutting balloon angioplasty of autogenous infrainguinal bypasses: short-term safety and efficacy. J Vasc Surg, 46(4), 724-730.

Hansson, G. K., & Hermansson, A. (2011). The immune system in atherosclerosis. Nat Immunol 12 (3):204-212

Hu, M. H., Wu, K. W., Jian, Y. M., Wang, C. T., Wu, I. H., & Yang, S. H. (2010) Vascular compression syndrome of sciatic nerve caused by gluteal varicosities. Ann Vasc Surg, 24(8),1134, e1-4.

Ichihashi, S., Higashiura, W. , Itoh, H., Sakaguchi, S., Nishimine, K., & Kichikawa, K. (2011). Long-term outcomes for systematic primary stent placement in complex iliac artery occlusive disease classified according to Trans-Atlantic Inter-Society Consensus (TASC)-II. J Vasc Surg, 53(4), 992-999.

Iida, O., Soga, Y., Yamauchi, Y., Hirano, K., Kawasaki, D., Yamaoka, T., Takahara, M., & Uematsu, M. (2013). Clinical efficacy of endovascular therapy for patients with critical limb ischemia attributable to pure isolated infrapopliteal lesions. J Vasc Surg, 57(4), 974-981 e1.

Kistner, R. L., Eklof, B. , & Masuda, E. M. (1996). Diagnosis of chronic venous disease of the lower extremities: the "CEAP" classification. Mayo Clin Proc, 71(4), 338-345.

Kwon, G. P., Schroeder, J. L., Amar, M.J., Remaley, A.T., & Balaban, R.S. (2008). Contribution of macromolecular structure to the retention of low-density lipoprotein at arterial branch points. Circulation 117 (22):2919-2927.

Lurie, F., Kistner, R. L., Eklof, B., & Kessler, D. (2003). Mechanism of venous valve closure and role of the valve in circulation: a new concept. J Vasc Surg, 38(5), 955-961.

Moore, K. J., & Tabas, I. Macrophages in the pathogenesis of atherosclerosis. (2011). Cell 145 (3):341-355.

Mosti, G. Wound care in venous ulcers. (2013). Phlebology 28 Suppl 1:79-85.

Moxey, P. W., Brownrigg, J., Kumar, S. S., Crate, G., Holt, P. J., Thompson, M. M., Jones, K. G., & Hinchliffe, R. J. (2012). The BASIL survival prediction model in patients with peripheral arterial disease undergoing revascularization in a university hospital setting and comparison with the FINNVASC and modified PREVENT scores. J Vasc Surg, 57(1), 1-7.

Mwipatayi, B. P., Thomas, S., Wong, J., Temple, S. E., Vijayan, V., Jackson, M., & Burrows, S. A. (2011). A comparison of covered vs bare expandable stents for the treatment of aortoiliac occlusive disease. J Vasc Surg, 54(6), 1561-1570.

Poncyljusz, W., Falkowski, A., Safranow, K., Rac, M., & Zawierucha, D. (2013). Cutting-Balloon Angioplasty Versus Balloon Angioplasty as Treatment for Short Atherosclerotic Lesions in the Superficial Femoral Artery: Randomized Controlled Trial. Cardiovasc Intervent Radiol. Apr 11. [Epub ahead of print]

Porter, J. M. & Moneta, G. L. (1995). Reporting standards in venous disease: an update. International Consensus Committee on Chronic Venous Disease. J Vasc Surg, 21(4), 635-645.

Pukstad, B. S., Ryan, L., Flo, T.H., Stenvik, J., Moseley, R., Harding, K., Thomas, D.W., and Espevik, T. (2910). Non-healing is associated with persistent stimulation of the innate immune response in chronic venous leg ulcers. J Dermatol Sci 59 (2):115-122.

Qui, Y., R. C. Quijano, Wang, S. K., & Hwang, N. H. (1995). Fluid dynamics of venous valve closure. Ann Biomed Eng, 23(6), 750-759.

Rayment, E. A., Upton, Z., & Shooter, G.K. (2008). *Increased matrix metalloproteinase-9 (MMP-9) activity observed in chronic wound fluid is related to the clinical severity of the ulcer. Br J Dermatol 158 (5):951-961.*

Sam, R. C., Burns, P. J., Hobbs, S.D., Marshall, T., Wilmink, A.B., Silverman, S.H., & Bradbury, A.W. (2003). *The prevalence of hyperhomocysteinemia, methylene tetrahydrofolate reductase C677T mutation, and vitamin B12 and folate deficiency in patients with chronic venous insufficiency. J Vasc Surg 38 (5):904-908.*

Serra, R., Buffone, G., de Franciscis, A., Mastrangelo, D., Molinari, V., Montemurro, R., & de Franciscis, S. (2012). *A genetic study of chronic venous insufficiency. Ann Vasc Surg 26 (5):636-642.*

Serra, R., Buffone, G., de Franciscis, A., Mastrangelo, D., Vitagliano, T., Greco, M., & de Franciscis, S. (2011) *Skin grafting followed by low-molecular-weight heparin long-term therapy in chronic venous leg ulcers. Ann Vasc Surg 26 (2):190-197.*

Serra, R., Buffone, G., Falcone, D., Molinari, V., Scaramuzzino, M., Gallelli, L., & de Franciscis, S. (2013) *Chronic venous leg ulcers are associated with high levels of metalloproteinases-9 and neutrophil gelatinase-associated lipocalin. Wound Repair Regen 21 (3):395-401.*

Serra, R., Buffone, G., Molinari, V., Montemurro, R., Perri, P., Stillitano, D.M., Amato, B., & de Franciscis, S.(2013). *Low molecular weight heparin improves healing of chronic venous ulcers especially in the elderly. Int Wound J. [Epub ahead of print]*

Serra, R., Gallelli, L., Buffone, G., Molinari, V., Stillitano, D.M., Palmieri, C., & de Franciscis, S. (2013). *Doxycycline speeds up healing of chronic venous ulcers. Int Wound J. [Epub ahead of print]*

Spinosa, D. J., Harthun, N. L., Bissonette, E. A., Cage, D., Leung, D. A., Angle, J. F., Hagspiel, K. D., Kern, J. A., Crosby, I., Wellons, H. A., Hartwell, G. D., & Matsumoto, A. H. (2005). *Subintimal arterial flossing with antegrade-retrograde intervention (SAFARI) for subintimal recanalization to treat chronic critical limb ischemia. J Vasc Interv Radiol, 16(1), 37-44.*

Takase, S., Pascarella, L., Bergan, J. J., Schmid-Schonbein, G. W. (2004). *Hypertension-induced venous valve remodeling. J Vasc Surg, 39(6), 1329-1334.*

Takase, S., Pascarella, L., Lerond, L., Bergan, J. J., & Schmid-Schonbein, G. W. (2004). *Venous hypertension, inflammation and valve remodeling. Eur J Vasc Endovasc Surg, 28(5), 484-493.*

Traub, O. & Berk, B. C. (1998). *Laminar shear stress: mechanisms by which endothelial cells transduce an atheroprotective force. Arterioscler Thromb Vasc Biol, 18(5), 677-685.*

Vollset, S. E., Refsum, H., Tverdal, A., Nygard, O., Nordrehaug, J.E., Tell, G.S., & Ueland, P.M. (2001). *Plasma total homocysteine and cardiovascular and noncardiovascular mortality: the Hordaland Homocysteine Study. Am J Clin Nutr 74 (1):130-136.*

Weber, C., & Noels, H. (2011). *Atherosclerosis: current pathogenesis and therapeutic options. Nat Med 17 (11):1410-1422.*

Weber, C., Zernecke, A., & Libby, P. (2008). *The multifaceted contributions of leukocyte subsets to atherosclerosis: lessons from mouse models. Nat Rev Immunol 8 (10):802-815.*

Zernecke, A., Bot, I., Djalali-Talab, Y., Shagdarsuren, E., Bidzhekov, K., Meiler, S., Krohn, R., Schober, A., Sperandio, M., Soehnlein, O., Bornemann, J., Tacke, F., Biessen, E.A., & Weber, C. (2008). *Protective role of CXC receptor 4/CXC ligand 12 unveils the importance of neutrophils in atherosclerosis. Circ Res 102 (2):209-217.*

Zhuang, K. D., Tan, S. G., Tay, K. H. (2011). *The "SAFARI" technique using retrograde access via peroneal artery access. Cardiovasc Intervent Radiol, 35(4), 927-931.*

Nanomedicine for the Diagnosis and Treatment of Cardiovascular Disease: Current Status and Future Perspective

Evren Gundogdu
Radiopharmacy Department, Faculty of Pharmacy
Ege University, Turkey

Zeynep Senyigit
Pharmaceutical Technology, Faculty of Pharmacy
Ege University, Turkey

Derya Ilem-Ozdemir
Radiopharmacy Department, Faculty of Pharmacy
Ege University, Turkey

1   Introduction

Cardiovascular disease (CVD) encompasses all pathologies of the heart or circulatory system, including coronary heart disease, peripheral vascular disease and stroke. Cardiovascular diseases are the primary morbidity and mortality cause in the world and seen among nearly 25% of adult population who are over 20 years of age, although it differs in continents and regions. The primary conditions underlying the great majority of cardiovascular diseases are dyslipidemia, atherosclerosis and hypertension.

Treatments for CVD include non-invasive therapy such as prescription medication and lifestyle alterations, or surgical therapy such as coronary artery bypass grafting and angioplasty. Effective drug treatments for heart disease can help lower blood pressure or cholesterol, prevent or dissolve blood clots, relieve and prevent angina symptoms or improve the strength or rhythm of the heart's contractions. Angiotensin-converting enzyme inhibitors, angiotensin receptor blockers, anti-clotting drugs and beta blockers are the examples of drug classes which are commonly used in CVD. Up to date, these drugs are mostly introduced into the market in conventional formulations such as tablets or capsules. During the past 20 years, with the detailed molecular level understanding of the diseases and the development of sophisticated technologies for nanoscale using, nanomedicine has undergone an explosive growth in the world. Nanomedicine is the application of nanotechnology in monitoring, diagnosing, preventing, repairing or curing diseases and damaged tissues in biological systems and it is gaining importance for the treatment of CVD. In the near future, it is considered that nanomedicine approach will enable establishment of patient-specific "personalized medicine". It is also considered that gene therapies for cardiovascular applications will have a potential usage in the field of cardiovascular applications in upcoming years. This chapter focuses on recent formulations in cardiovascular therapy with comparison of conventional dosage forms. In addition, future perspectives for the treatment of CVD with nanoparticles will be discussed in details.

2   Conventional Techniques/Methods for Diagnosis, Treatment of the CVD

2.1   Nanoparticles for Diagnostics of CVD

Since everything is made of atoms and molecules, nanotechnology is an interdisciplinary research field which cover all the branches of science and technology (Balzani, 2005; Ilem Ozdemir & Asikoglu, 2012; Linazasoro, 2008; Roco, 2003; Sahoo & Labhasetwar, 2013). Nanoscience and nanotechnologies application have a huge potential to bring benefits in information and communication technologies, electronics, transportation, the production of stronger and lighter materials, biology, medicine, pharmacy and more (Bassecoulard & Zitt, 2007; Karunaratne, 2007; Roco, 2001; Sahoo et al., 2007). Since most of these applications are centered on improving human health nanotechnology has given rise to a whole new field called nanomedicine (Karunaratne, 2007; Sahoo et al., 2007). Nanomedicine is the application of nanotechnology in preventing, monitoring, diagnosing, repairing diseases and damaged tissues in biological system (Bassecoulard & Zitt, 2007; Gupta, 2011). In the few past decades, nanomedicine has been developed into a strong multidisciplinary field, enabling prominent technological advances such as intelligent materials and substances with durable surface coating, faster electronics, responsive biosensors, targeted therapeutics nanovectors, and improved nanodiagnostics. The overall goal of nanomedicine is to diagnose as accurately and early as possible, to treat as effectively as possible with minimal side effects, and to evaluate the efficacy of treatment noninvasively (Ilem Ozdemir & Asikoglu, 2012; Roco, 2001). When medical check-up had found an indication for a disease, it is important to exclude the "false positives" by applying more specific diagnostic procedures. In this case, specific targeted agents in molecular imaging, plays a crucial role for localization and staging of a disease. The main advantage of nanomedicine is earlier detection of a disease, leading to less severe and costly therapeutic demands, and an improved clinical result.

Nanotechnology application in diagnostics can be subdivided into three areas: in vitro diagnostics, in vivo diagnostics and medical devices. In vitro diagnosis for medical applications has traditionally been a laborious task. Nanotechnology enables the development of smaller, faster and cheaper new generation medical devices (Renzo et al., 2006).

Medical imaging is an essential diagnostic too lover the last 25 years. Molecular imaging and image guided therapy are now basic tools for monitoring disease.

Since CVD have been the top killers for human beings, rapid and accurate diagnosis of CVD is critically important to save lives. Since the underlying pathological conditions such as plaque formation remain largely unclear, early diagnosis is difficult and morbidity and mortality rate is high (Biana, 2012; Hong & Kang, 2006). The imaging techniques routinely used for cardiovascular disease diagnosis are electrocardiography (ECG), chest X-ray, echocardiography, cardiac catheterization and blood tests (Kakoti et al., 2013). These imaging techniques could only detect changes in the appearance of tissues when the symptoms were relatively advanced. Today, nanotechnology based imaging applications are being refined with the goal of detecting disease as early as possible (Biana, 2012; Renzo et al., 2006).

Nanoparticles have the potential for imaging from its current anatomy based level to the molecular level. So nanoparticle imaging techniques cover advanced optical and luminescence imaging and spectroscopy, ultrasound, and X-ray imaging, magnetic resonance imaging, and nuclear imaging with radioactive tracers most of which depend on targeting agents or contrast agents that have been introduced into the body to mark the disease site (Godin et al., 2010; Renzo et al., 2006).

Fluorescent nanocrystal (also quantum dots) can be used as fluorescent markers for diagnostic purposes. Since quantum dots have unique fluorescent properties they have been studied as optical probes for cardiovascular imaging (Choi et al., 2009; Gupta, 2011; Smith et al., 2004). Quantum dots are defined as particle with physical dimension smaller than the excitation Bohr radius. Since the size, particle absorbed light at a wide range of wavelength and emits almost monochromatic light of a wavelength (Han et al., 2001; Sahoo & Labhasetwar, 2003). Due to their excellent optical properties quantum dots have been improved despite the cytotoxicity and limited clinical safety. On the other hand some research groups have reported that in vivo behavior of particles can be modified by carefully controlling of surface chemistry and particle size. Surface modified quantum dots have been developed for fluorescent imaging of vascular disease inflammatory events in mouse and rats models (Gupta, 2011; Jayagopal et al., 2007).

Ultrasound requires contrast agents to provide backscatter of sound waves to the scanner head (Renzo et al., 2006). For this purpose several contrast agents have been developed for ultrasound imaging. Ultrasound is a sonographic based imaging technique which established in diagnosis of physiological tissues. Stabilized gaseous microbubble contrast agents (~5μm in diameter) have been developed as ultrasound contrast agent. Microbubbles are generally used as imaging agent for vasculature since their size and susceptibility to destruction with clinical ultrasound imaging intensities. Takeuchi et al. have been reported microbubbles which were used for targeting to thrombi. Several researchers have demonstrated the modified bubble system by ligands for specific binding to cells and tissues. Because GPIIbIIIa-expressing fibrinogen binding activated platelets are major players in thrombosis, Alonso et al. have been developed surface modified GPIIbIIIa-specific antibody gas-filled microbubbles for molecular targeting of thrombus. Cavari *et al.* have been reported polyvinyl alcohol based bubbles for imaging vascular disease (Gupta, 2011; Wickline & Lanza, 2002).

Nanotechnology based particles have been used as computed tomography (CT) contrast agents tent to the based on high molecular atomic number elements such as gold, iron and bismuth (Cormode *et al.*, 2009; Hainfeld *et al.*, 2006; Hyafil *et al.*, 2007; Rabin *et al.*, 2006; Mukundan *et al.*, 2006). Since CT requires high contrast differences, gold nanoparticles are popular choice for CT (Kim *et al.*, 2007; Mukundan *et al.*, 2006). Gold provides unique properties like, resistant to oxidation under physiological conditions and have particularly plasmon resonance in the visible range of the electromagnetic spectrum. These properties have led to application of gold particles in various diagnostic and therapeutic areas like immuno labeling, radiotherapy and X ray image contrast enhancement. Solid iodine based nanoparticle has been demonstrated to image arteriosclerosis by Hyafil *et al* (Cormode *et al.*, 2009; Gupta, 2011).

Today, magnetically sensitive nanoparticles have become important tool in diagnostic application of detecting disease as early as possible (Gupta, 2011; Renzo *et al.*, 2006). Since reflexivity properties, paramagnetic and superparamagnetic metals linked carriers such as liposomes, micelles, dendrimers, perflurocarbon bubbles etc. are used in magnetic resonance imaging (MRI) applications (Wickline & Lanza, 2002). For this purpose, magnetically sensitive carriers made with pure metals having high magnetism (cobalt, iron etc.) or decorated with paramagnetic elements like Gadolinium (Gd). FDA has been approved Gd as a T1 relaxation paramagnetic MRI contrast agent and many research papers have been published about Gd decorated contrast agents in cardiovascular disease imaging.αvβ3is overexpressed in angiogenesis, therefore Winter *et al* demonstrated the Gd decoratedαvβ3targeted perflurocarbon nanoparticles imaging potential of vascular disease associated with angiogenic neovasculature (Li *et al.*, 2010; Maiseyeu *et al.*, 2009; Mulder *et al.*, 2006; Rensen *et al.*, 2006; Winter *et al.*, 2006).

Many research papers have been demonstrated particles which taken up by macrophage rich atherosclerotic lesions (Jaffer *et al.*, 2006; Tang *et al.*, 2009; Trivedi *et al.*, 2004). Due to Gd decorated liposomes which enriched with PS are phagocytized by macrophages, located at the site of high macrophage activity like atherosclerosis associated inflammation (Maiseyeu *et al.*, 2009). Gd loaded immunomicelles surface modified with antibodies have been reported for MRI of cardiovascular disease (Amirbekian *et al.*, 2007; 2009; Lipinski *et al.*, 2006; Mulder *et al.*, 2007;).

Superparamagnetic iron oxide has been widely used to induce contrast for T2 relaxation MRI. Gd or iron oxide can be chosen as depending on the application. Gd produce positive contrast which can easily visualized while iron oxide induced negative contrast and signal loss and because many sources of signal loss in MRI other than iron oxide it may be hard to ascribe signal loss certainly (Cormode *et al.*, 2009). Superparamagnetic iron oxide has been investigated as MRI imaging agent for atherosclerotic and thrombotic lesions (Frias *et al.*, 2004; Gupta, 2011).

Dendrimers are a class of cascade polymers which are rendered a globular confirmation. In the area of vascular disease dendrimers have been used for loading and imaging MRI etc). Fahmy *et al* have demonstrated ligand modified dendrimers as MRI imaging probes. Also radioactive Bromine encapsulated biodegradable dendrimers structures were used in positron emission tomography imaging of ischemia in mouse model (Fahmy *et al.*, 2007; Gupta, 2011; Hagooly *et al.*, 2008).

Nuclear imaging modalities like single photon emission tomography (SPECT) and PET are significant imaging techniques for early diagnose of vascular disease (Cormode *et al.*, 2009). While many radiopharmaceuticals have been developed for cardiovascular imaging, elements were labeled with a radionuclide. In recent years developing of multicomponent nanoparticles are getting popular which combine nuclear imaging probes and therapeutic agents (McCarthy, 2010). Polysaccharide coated iron oxide nanoparticles have been developed and radiolabeled with Floursne-18 radionuclide for PET imaging. The most widely use radionuclide Techntium-99m has been conjugated directly to Annexin 5 for imaging arteriosclerosis associated inflammatory events. Also Iodine-125 labeled nanoparticles were investigated as SPECT imaging agent (Chrastina & Schnitzer, 2010; Cormode et al., 2009).

Many of these reports are relatively new and ongoing research, their promising results makes nanomedicine promising in revolutionizing diagnostic modalities for vascular disease. Effective molecular, imaging contrast agents can be synthesized using nanoparticles Through the design of nanoparticle based probes, highly sensitive, highly reliable imaging techniques have been performed for diagnostic application. In future nanoscale science will play an important role in imaging modalities.

2.2   Nanoparticles for Treatment of Cardiovascular Disease

Cardiovascular disease (CVD) encompasses a class of diseases that involves the heart and vasculature. For decades, CVD has been one of the leading causes of mortality and accounts for virtually 1/3 of all deaths in the world. Therefore, there is pressing a need to develop novel techniques such as nanotechnology for the early detection and treatment of several CVD (McCarthy, 2010).

Nanotechnology offers advantages for CVD mainly in four areas:

i.   Targeted therapeutics: delivering drugs where they are needed.

ii.   Tissue engineering: building new tissues to replace defective valves, damaged heart muscle, clogged blood vessels, etc.

iii. Molecular imaging: using "smart" imaging agents that identify disease more specifically

iv.   Biosensors and diagnostics: improved diagnostic devices for the laboratory, and implantable sensors to detect problems inside the body (Arayne et al., 2007).

The most important clinical applications of nanotechnology are in area of pharmaceutical development and pharmaceutical nanoparticles have gained great importance for the treatment of CVD. In pharmaceutical technology and biomedicine, nanoparticles are typically defined as particles with diameter from 1 to 100 nm and have been exploited for both diagnostic and therapeutic purposes. The ideal size of nanoparticles used as drug delivery systems ranges from 10 to 100 nm. They can be classified into several categories, according to their structure (i.e., nanoparticles, nanospheres, nanocapsules, nanotubes and colloidal carriers such as liposomes or dendrimers), physicochemical properties (i.e., pH sensitive, magnetic, stealth nanoparticles) and the materials used for its synthesis (i.e., natural, synthetic, hybrid, or gold nanoparticles). Nanoparticles can achieve controlled drug release, targeting and increase the effectiveness or bioavailability of many diagnostic or therapeutic agents. In this section, some drugs formulated in nanoparticles for the treatment of CVD are summarized (Arayne et al., 2007; Goldberg et al., 2007).

Endothelial-selective delivery of therapeutic agents would provide a useful tool for modifying vascular function in various cardiovascular diseases and several research groups are interested in this targeting approach (Spragg et al., 1997).

Kona et al. developed a novel nanoparticulate drug delivery system that mimics platelets binding to the injured vessel wall under physiological flow conditions. Glycoprotein Ib (GPIb) was chosen as the targeting ligand and conjugated to nanoparticles because its role in platelet adhesion to the vascular wall under high shear flow conditions is well-recognized. Dexamethasone-loaded biodegradable poly-(d,l-lactic-co-glycolic acid) (PLGA) nanoparticles were formulated using a standard emulsion method. The results demonstrate that conjugation of GPIb to PLGA nanoparticles increased particle adhesion onto targeted surfaces and increased cellular uptake of these nanoparticles by activated endothelial cells under shear stresses. In addition, these nanoparticles also provided a controlled release of the model drug. Therefore, this drug-loaded, GPIb-conjugated PLGA nanoparticles could be used as a targeted and controlled drug delivery system to the site of vascular injury for treatment of cardiovascular diseases (Soujanya et al., 2012).

Restenosis, the principal complication of percutaneous transluminal coronary angioplasty is responsible for the 35–40% long-term failure rate following coronary revascularization.

Song et al. (1998) investigated the potential usefulness of biodegradable nanoparticles for the local intraluminal therapy of restenosis. NPs containing a water-insoluble anti-proliferative agent U-86983 were formulated from oil–water emulsions using biodegradable polymers such as poly-(lactic acid–co-glycolic acid) (PLGA), and specific additives after particle formation, to enhance arterial retention using either heparin, didodecylmethylammonium bromide, fibrinogen, or combinations. The in vivo studies were conducted with a new dog model for arterial angioplasty. The results support the view that modified nanoparticles along with optimized infusion conditions could enhance arterial wall drug concentrations of agents to treat restenosis.

In other studies; Fishbein and coworkers, prepared tyrphostin inhibitor containing poly (DL-lactide) (PLA) nanoparticles for intrarterial administration by spontaneous emulsification / solvent displacement technique for the treatment of restenosis (Fishbein et al., 2000). Klugherz et al. (1999) have demonstrated transcatheter local delivery of the antirestenotic agent probucol loaded PLGA particles, in rabbit iliac arteries, for enhanced retention, sustained release and increased therapeutic effects.

Winter et al. (2008) performed studies to develop a prolonged antiangiogenesis therapy regimen based on theranostic αvβ3–targeted nanoparticles. For this purpose, fumagillin was incorporated into perfluorooctylbromide nanoparticles to elicit acute antiangiogenic effects. The impetus for this study is the observation in animal models that chronically high systemic doses of a water-soluble version of fumagillin resulted in a decrease in neovascularization and plaque development, thus a targeted nanoagent may allow for localized delivery requiring decreased dosing.

Liposomes are spherical platforms that use natural lipids and/or synthetic polymers and cholesterol as building blocks to form the bilayer structure. They possess a hydrophilic core surrounded by a hydrophobic membrane and they are in size from 50 nm to several microns (Ruiz-Esparza et al., 2013). Currently, in the drug market, there is no liposomal formulation approved for the treatment of cardiovascular disease. However, several innovative examples of liposomal technologies have been developed for the treatment of cardiovascular disease and researches are going on.

Joner et al. (2008) have developed cationic liposomal nanoparticles of prednisolone that specifically bind to chondroitin sulfate proteoglycans that are expressed within the subendothelial matrix but not vascular endothelial cells. In vivo studies were conducted with atherosclerotic New Zealand white Rabbits which were implanted with bare metal stents. Results showed that site-specific targeting by this nanoparticle steroid in injured atherosclerotic areas might be a valuable and cost-effective approach for the prevention of in-stent restenosis.

Cardiovascular diseases are not as much benefited from nanotechnology in terms of drug delivery as the field of cancer and others. There are still unmet aspects of cardiovascular drug delivery that need to be worked upon.

3   New Techniques/Methods for Diagnosis, Treatment of the CVD

3.1   Therapeutic and Theranostic Nanoparticles for Cardiovascular Disease

The theranostics has been identified as recognition of heterogeneous diseases requires more personalized solutions (Espina *et al.*, 2009). Theranostics entitles to the fusion of therapy and diagnostics, with the purpose of optimizing efficacy and safety, as well as updating the process of drug development. The increasing of number of scientific inventions has made the development of theranostics possible. The theranostic agents have a number of advantages, as they potentially allow for the concomitant determination of agent localization, release, and efficacy. Whereas the use of these agents in cancer treatment has received the majority of the attention, their use in cardiovascular disease is increasing.

In the field of biology, the human genome project and the development of biomarker initiatives have improved the understanding of disease progression. Genotyping or gene expression technologies make it possible to transfer this newly needing biological knowledge into the development of diagnostic tests. Theranostics allow doctors with high medical value testing for science-driven treatment decisions; enhance patient safety by identifying patients who won't respond to a drug or who have an adverse effect; increase the efficiency of drug development, helping pharmaceutical companies by developing new drug; and positive effect on health economics, thus selecting optimal and cost effective therapy by doctors. Although such a thought on this field has much potential in improving healthcare, there are some objections that must be corrected before it offers to routine use in the clinic (Falk, 2008; Buxton, 2009; Nazem & Mansoori, 2008; Couvreur & Vauthier, 2006).

The disease elimination can be improved by using theranostic agents to perform localized cytotoxicity with little collateral damage. The control of drug dosing, location, and time is an important purpose for drug delivery development, as enhanced therapeutic effect while reducing side effects. Systems responsive to a stimulus such as temperature, pH, applied magnetic or electrical field, ultrasound, light, or enzymatic action have been proposed as triggered delivery systems (McCoy *et al.*, 2010). Recently, light has been used to release therapeutic agents from delivery systems or activate agents that produce cytotoxic effect. For instance, light-activatable agent (Visudyne) that has been approved by the food and drug administration (FDA) is widely used for the treatment of age-related macular degeneration (AMD, is the major cause of blindness among the elderly in the developed world) (Amirbekian *et al.*, 2007).

Atherosclerosis is occurring over a number of decades that often goes undetected until the onset of clinical symptoms. Atherosclerotic lesions offer a plethora of potential targets, including specific inflammatory cell types. Various nanotechnology applications are being developed for the treatment of atherosclerosis, including nanocarriers drug delivery systems and devices such as mechanical stents, possessing nanoscale components. Targets for imaging of atherosclerotic plaques contain endothelia, macrophages, fibrin, collagen III, and markers of angiogenesis (Botnar *et al.*, 2004; Cyrus *et al.*, 2006). Along with the development of novel strategies for treatment of CVDs, efforts are being spent to apply nanotechnologies for ex-vivo and in vivo detection of CVD signals. The awareness of precursor signal of CVD reduces the many fatalities associated with the diseases.

The main nanocarrier classes researched as therapeutic and 'theranostic' agents for atherosclerosis are liposomes with different surface characteristics, polymeric nanoparticles and micelles, perfluorocarbon nano-emulsions and cross-linked iron oxide (CLIO) particles conjugated to therapeutic molecules (Danenberg *et al.*, 2002; Stephan *et al.*, 1997; Hecman *et al.*, 2003; Lanza *et al.*, 2006) For example, a prolonged anti-angiogenesis therapy was reported using theranostic avb3-integrin-targeted paramagnetic nanoparticles in hyperlipidemic animals (Winter *et al.*, 2006; 2008) MRI data showed that the neovascular signal has reduced for 3 weeks with histological evaluation, pointing toward the potential of this strategy for efficient antiangiogenic therapy and simultaneously evaluating plaque stability. Another example for angiogenesis therapy is fibrincoated perfluorocarbon nanoparticles. These nanoparticles can also be used for acoustic or MRI imaging with targeted thrombolysis (Marsh *et al.*, 2007). Hua *et al.* (2010) have developed the targeting perfluoropropane-containing liposomes to activated platelets via a peptide (RGDS) derived from the α-chain of fibrinogen. Initially, the peptide and rtPA were each modified with distinct fluorescent labels to obtain tracking of the microbubbles and thrombolytic drug. When injected into healthy rabbits, the thrombolytic drug was visualized within the liver by using ultrasound imaging. This may demonstrate the additive effect of microbubble rupture on the ultimate lysis of clots. There is also a disadvantage about the nanoparticles. They can affect the walls of blood vessel. The vascular endothelium could be a barrier and unwanted target for nanoparticles to be delivered to other organs (Lukyanenko, 2007). In this respect, the transport of nanoparticles across vessel walls, organelle-targeted delivery of nanoparticles, and other effects of nanoparticles on vessel cells may affect the CVDs. These factors should be considered in future for nanomedicine research.

3.2   Biomarkers in Cardiovascular Disease

Biomarkers are an important tool in clinical practice, helping to improve patient care. For example, biomarkers have showed that a significant impact in early detection of sub-clinical disease (*e.g.*, prostate-specific antigen screening for prostate cancer), diagnosis of acute or chronic syndromes (*e.g.*, B-type natriuretic peptide in heart failure), risk stratification (*e.g.*, cardiac troponin in acute coronary syndromes), and monitoring of disease or therapy (*e.g.*, hemoglobin A1c in diabetes mellitus) (Catalona *et al.*, 1991; Maisel *et al.*, 2002; Anderson *et al.*, 2007 Goldstein *et al.*, 2004).

Local inflammation in the vessel wall plays a key role in the development of atherosclerosis (Hansson, 2005). Therefore, inflammatory biomarker could be prognostic biomarkers in CVD. Epidemiological and clinical studies have shown strong and consistent relationship between biomarkers of inflammation, evaluated by high sensitivity C-reactive protein (HsCRP), and risk of cardiovascular events in patients with cardiovasculary especially ischemic heart disease (Harutyunyan *et al.*, 2011; Mathiasen *et al.*, 2010; Mygind *et al*). However, when HsCRP is used in general population studies, HsCRP does not always seem to have a significant prognostic value in detecting future cardiovascular disease (Olsen *et al.*, 2007).

YKL-40 is an acute phase protein and a new potential biomarker of inflammation in CVD patients, which is expressed by several cell types of the immune system (Johansen, 2006). Macrophages in atherosclerotic plaques express YKL-40, and the highest expression was found in macrophages in early atherosclerotic lesions. Some studies have showed that serum YKL-40 is increased in patients with acute myocardial infarction YKL-40 is associated with both early and late phases in the development of atherosclerosis. It has been demonstrated that YKL-40 stimulates the maturation of monocytes to macrophages and then is hidden by macrophages during the late stages of differentiation (Johansen, 2006; Rehli *et al.*, 2003).

The role of the activation of the sympathetic system and the renin-angiotensin-aldosterone system (RAAS) in the development of CV diseases has been extensively explored. Renin is the first limiting step of the RAAS and plays an important role in CVD. There are new progresses in pharmacological inhibition of RAAS by using angiotensin-converting enzyme (ACE) inhibitors or Angiotensin Receptor Blockers (ARBs). However, whether plasma renin has a direct prognostic role in predicting CVD risk, it can be offered as a biomarker to improve CV risk stratification which is a topic of discussion.

Starting from the observations, an association between increased rennin levels and CV risk has been supported. Bruner *et al.* (1972) indicated that hypertensive patients with low renin activities protected when compared to those patients with high rennin and suggested that renin could be a potential risk factor for the development of CVD. Although rennin has shown the positive effect on CVD according to literatures, rennin does not completely satisfy the criteria suggested by the American Heart Association criteria for the evaluation of novel biomarkers (Hlatky *et al.*, 2009).

4   The Comparison of Conventional Formulation and New Nanomedicine Therapy of Cardiovascular Disease

This review identified a significant number of nanomedicine products approved for CVDs in-human use. It is difficult to extrapolate these numbers directly, because growth in medical industries is so heavily influenced by swings in the economy and regulatory processes. However, some definite trends related to the future of nanomedicine. The most prominent theme throughout is the relative adolescence of the field. Although all the applications identified represent significant technological advancements, they are only scratching the surface of the potential available, and the continued refinement and combination of these technologies will lead to the truly transformative capabilities envisioned for nanomedicine.

One of the major concerns regarding the use of nanotechnology in the body is the question of persistence. Conventional therapeutics are generally processed by the body and the metabolites are excreted soon after administration, but some nanoparticles have demonstrated persistent in vivo deposits for months or years. Examination of the in vivo applications and products identified demonstrates a much higher prevalence of "soft" (157 applications and products) versus "hard" (30 applications and products) nanostructures (Goel *et al.*, 2009; Rx Media, 2013; Walkey & Chan, 2011). Some samples of conventional formulations and nanomedicines in the market were shown in Table 1.

5   Future Perspectives

The ability to detect and treat CVD is the main concern of clinical medicine. With the advantage of nanotechnology, and the generation of multifunctional agents, it becomes possible to perform both actions simultaneously. There are many advantages to this approach, such as ability to determine agent localization, release, or efficacy.

Nanomedicine approaches keep great promise in revolutionizing therapeutic and diagnostic modalities in the clinical treatment of CVD. The previous review and studies have attempted to emphasize the various nanomedicine fabrication and formulation strategies in this area. Many of these reports are still based on in vitro or preclinical small animal model in vivo investigations. Further studies will certainly help to test its clinical usefulness in predicting cardiovascular events.

References

Amirbekian V. et al. Detecting and assessing macrophages in vivo to evaluate atherosclerosis noninvasively using molecular MRI. Proc. Natl. Acad. Sci. U S A. 2007; 104: 961–966.

Drugs	Conventional formulation	Nanomedicines
Lipid increasing drug *-Isosorbit monohydrate*	Monoket long retard tablet 40 mg (Adeka, Turkey) Monodur tablet 60 mg (Astra Zeneca, Canada)	Monolong SR microepllet capsule 40 mg (Ali Raif, Turkey) Mono corax micropellet capsule 60 mg (corax, Germany) Monisol micropellet capsule 60 mg (Zorka, Russia) Monitan micropellet capsule 60 mg (Wyeth, Canada)
Antihypertensive drug *-Diltiazem hydrochlorure*	Diltiazem ampoule 25 mg (Mustafa Nevzat, Turkey).	Altiazem SR micropellet 60 mg (Nobel, Turkey) Dilatam SR micropellet 60 mg (Abic, Israel) Coramil SR micropellet 60 mg (Sanofi, Sweden)
Lipid increasing drug *-Phenofibrate*	Lipidil tablet 200 mg (Fournier, Germany, Canada) Lipofene tablet 200 mg (Teofarma, Italy)	Feno-micro micropellet 250 mg (Apotex, Hungary) Lipofene SR micropellet 250 mg (Nobel, Turkey)

Table 1: Conventional formulations and new nanomedicines for CVD theraphy (90).

Amirbekian V., Lipinski MJ., Briley-Saebo KC., Amirbekian S., Aguinaldo JG., Weinreb DB. et al. Detecting and assessing macrophages in vivo to evaluate atherosclerosis noninvasively using molecular MRI. Proc Natl Acad Sci. USA 2007;104:961-6.

Amirbekian V., Lipinski MJ., Frias JC., Amirbekian S., Briley-Saebo KC., Mani V. et al. MR imaging of human atherosclerosis using immuno micelles molecularly targeted to macrophages. J Cardiovasc Magn Reson. 2009;11(Supplement 1):83.

Anderson JL., Adams CD., Antman EM. et al. ACC/AHA 2007 guidelines for the management of patients with unstable angina/non ST-elevation myocardial infarction. Circulation. 2007;116: 148-304.

Arayne MS., Sultana N., Qureshi F. Nanoparticles in delivery of cardiovascular drugs. Pak J Pharm Sci 2007; 20(4): 340-348.

Arayne MS., Sultana N., Qureshi F. Nanoparticles in delivery of cardiovascular drugs, Pak. J. Pharm. Sci., 2007, 20(4): 340-348.

Balzani V., Small, 1, 278, 2005.

Bassecoulard E., Zitt AL., Scientometrics, 70, 859, 2007.

Biana G., Mauro F., Cardiovascular Nanomedicine: A Posse Ad Esse. MDCVJ. 2012, 8:1.

Botnar RM. et al. In vivo magnetic resonance imaging of coronary thrombosis using a fibrin-binding molecular magnetic resonance contrast agent. Circulation. 2004; 110:1463–1466.

Buxton DB. Current status of nanotechnology approaches for cardiovascular disease: a personal perspective, Wiley Interdiscip Rev Nanomed Nanobiotechnol. 2009; 1:149–155.

Catalona WJ., Smith DS., Ratliff TL. et al. Measurement of prostatespecific antigen in serum as a screening test for prostate cancer. N Engl J Med. 1991;324:1156-61

Choi HS. ,Ipe BI.,Misra P.,Lee JH.,Bawendi MG., Frangioni JV. Tissue and organ-selective biodistribution of NIR-fluorescentquantumdots. NanoLetters. 2009;9:2354-9.

Chrastina A., Schnitzer JE. Iodine-125 radiolabeling of silver nanoparticles for in vivo SPECT imaging. Int J Nanomed 2010;5:653-9.

Cormode DP., Skajaa T., Zahi A., Willem JM. Nanotechnology in Medical Imaging: Probe Design and Applications. 2009;29;992-1000.

Couvreur P., Vauthier C. Nanotechnology: intelligent design to treat complex disease, Pharm Res. 2006; 23:1417–1450.

Cyrus T. et al. MR three-dimensional molecular imaging of intramural biomarkers with targeted nanoparticles. J Cardiovasc Magn Reson. 2006; 8: 535–541.

Danenberg HD. et al. Macrophage depletion by clodronatecontaining liposomes reduces neointimal formation after balloon injury in rats and rabbits. Circulation. 2002;106: 599–605.

Espina V., Liotta LA., Petricoin EF. Reverse-phase protein microarrays for theranostics and patient tailored therapy. Methods Mol Biol. 2009; 520: 89–105.

Fahmy TM., Fong PM., Park J., Constable T., Saltzman WM. Nanosystems for simultaneous imaging and drug delivery to T cells. The AAPS Journal. 2007;9: 171-80.

Falk J. Epigenetics & sequencing — gene expression systems' second international meeting. Chromatin methylation to disease biology & theranostics, Drugs 2008;11: 650–652.

Fishbein I., Chorny M., Rabinovich L., Banai S., Gati I., Golomba G. Nanoparticulate delivery system of a tyrphostin for the treatment of restenosis. Journal of Controlled Release. 2000; 65: 221–229.

Frias JC., Williams KJ., Fisher EA., Fayad ZA. Recombinant HDL-like nanoparticles: a specific contrast agent for MRI of atherosclerotic plaques. J Am Chem Soc. 2004;126:16316-7.

Godin B., Sakamoto JH., Serda RE., Grattoni A., Bouamrani A., Ferrari M., Emerging applications of nanomedicine for the diagnosis and treatment of cardiovascular diseases. Trends in Pharm Sci. 2010; 31(5).

Goel R., Shah N., Visaria R., Paciotti GF., Bischof JC. Biodistribution of TNF-alpha-coated gold nanoparticles in an in vivo model system. Nanomedicine 2009; 4 (4):401–410.

Goldberg M., Langer R., Jia X. Nanostructured materials for applications in drug delivery and tissue engineering. Biomater Sci Polym Ed. 2007 ; 18(3): 241–268.

Goldstein DE., Little RR., Lorenz RA. et al. Tests of glycemia in diabetes. Diabetes Care. 2004;27:1761-73.

Gupta AS., Nanomedicine approaches in vasculardisease: a review. Nanomedicine: NanotechBiolMed. 2011;7:763–779.

Hagooly A., Almutairi A., Rossin R., Shokeen M., Ananth A., Anderson C. et al. Evaluation of a RGD-dendrimer labeled with [76]Br in hind limbischemia mouse model. J Nucl Med 2008;49(Suppl 1):184.

Hainfeld JF., Slatkin DN., Focella TM., Smilowitz HM. Gold nanoparticles: a new X-ray contrastagent. Brit J Radiol. 2006;79:248–253.

Han M. et al. Quantum-dot-taggedmicrobeadsformultiplexedopticalcoding of biomolecules. Nat. Biotechnol. 2001; 19: 631–635.

Hansson GK. Inflammation, atherosclerosis, and coronary artery disease. N Engl J Med. 2005;352 (16): 1685–1695.

Harutyunyan MJ., Mathiasen AB., Winkel P., Gøtze JP., Hansen JF., Hildebrandt P., Jensen GB., Hilden J., Jespersen CM., Kjøller E., Kolmos HJ., Gluud C., Kastrup J. High-sensitivity C-reactive protein and N-terminal pro- B-type natriuretic peptide in patients with stable coronary artery disease: a prognostic study within the CLARICOR Trial. Scand J Clin Lab Invest. 2011; 71 (1): 52–62.

Hedman M. et al. Safety and feasibility of catheter-based local intracoronary vascular endothelial growth factor gene transfer in the prevention of postangioplasty and in-stent restenosis and in the treatment of chronic myocardial ischemia: phase II results of the Kuopio Angiogenesis Trial (KAT). Circulation. 2003; 107: 2677–2683.

Hlatky MA., Greenland P., Arnett DK., Ballantyne CM., Criqui MH., Elkind MS. et al. Criteria for evaluation of novel markers of cardiovascular risk: a scientific statement from the American heart association. Circulation. 2009; 119(17):2408-16.

Hong B., Kang KA., Biocompatible, nanogold-particle fluorescence enhancer for fluorophore mediated, optical immunosensor. Biosens Bioelectron. 2006, 21(7): 1333-1338.

Hua X., Liu P., Gao YH., Tan KB., Zhou LN., Liu Z., Li X., Zhou SW., Gao YJ. Construction of thrombus-targeted microbubbles carrying tissue plasminogen activator and their in vitro thrombolysis efficacy: a primary research. J Thromb Thrombolysis. 2010;30: 29–35.

Hyafil F., Cornily JC., Feig JE., Gordon R., Vucic E., Amirbekian V., Fisher EA., Fuster V., Feldman LJ., Fayad ZA. Noninvasive detection of macrophages using a nanoparticulate contrast agent for computed tomography. Nat Med. 2007;13:636–641.

Ilem Ozdemir D.,Asikoglu M. Radio imaging and diagnostic applications. Ed. Senyigit T.,Ozcan I., Ozer O., Nanotechnology in Progress: Pharmaceutical Applications, 2012.

Jaffer FA., Nahrendorf M., Sosnovik D., Kelly KA., Aikawa E., Weissleder R. Cellular imaging of inflammation in atherosclerosis using magnet fluorescent nanomaterials. Mol Imaging 2006;5:85-92.

Jayagopal A., Russ PK., Haselton FR. Surfaceengineering of quantumdotsfor in vivovascularimaging. Bioconjugate Chem. 2007;18:1424-33.

Johansen D., Studies on serum YKL-40 as a biomarker in diseases with inflammation, tissue remodelling, fibroses and cancer. Dan Med Bull. 2006; 53 (2):172–209.

Joner M., Morimoto K., Kasukawa H., Steigerwald K., Merl S., Nakazawa G., John MC., Finn AV., Acampado E., Kolodgie F.D., Gold HK., Virmani R. Site-specific targeting of nanoparticle prednisolone reduces in-stent restenosis in a rabbit model of established atheroma. Arterioscler Thromb Vasc Biol. 2008;28: 1960–1966.

Kakoti A., Goswami P., Hearttypefattyacidbinding protein: Structure, functionandbiosensingapplicationsforearlydetection of myocardialinfarction. Biosens Bioelectron. 2013;43:400-11.

Karunaratne DN., J. Natn. Sci. Foundation Sri Lanka, 35, 149, 2007.

Kim D., Park S., Lee JH., Jeong YY., Jon S. Antibiofouling polymer-coated gold nanoparticles as a contrast agent for in vivo x-ray computed tomography imaging. J Am Chem Soc. 2007;129:7661–7665.

Klugherz BD., Meneveau N., Chen W., Wade WF., Papandreou G., Levy R. Sustained intramural retention and regional redistribution following local vascular delivery of Polylactic-coglycolic acid and liposomal nanoparticulate formulations containing probucol. J Cardiovasc Pharmacol Ther. 1999;4:167-74.

Lanza GM. et al. Nanomedicine opportunities for cardiovascular disease with perfluorocarbon nanoparticles. Nanomedicine. 2006; 1: 321–329.

Li D., Patel AR., Klibanov AL., Kramer CM., Ruiz M., Kang BY. et al. Molecular imaging of atherosclerotic plaques targeted to oxidized LDL receptor LOX-1by SPECT/CT and Magnetic Resonance. Circ Cardiovasc Imaging. 2010;3:464-72.

Linazasoro G., ParkinsonismRelatDisord, 14, 383, 2008.

Lipinski MJ., AmirbekianV., Frias JC., Aguinaldo JGS., Mani V., Briley Saebo KC. et al. MRI todetect atherosclerosis with Gadolinium containing immunomicelles targeting themacrophages cavenger receptor. Magn Reson Med 2006;56:601-10.

Lukyanenko V. Delivery of nano-objects to functional subdomains of healthy and failing cardiac myocytes. Nanomedicine. 2007; 2: 831–846.

Maisel AS., Krishnaswamy P., Nowak RM. et al. Rapid measurement of B-type natriuretic peptide in the emergency diagnosis of heart failure. N Engl J Med 2002;347:161-7.

Maiseyeu A., Mihai G., Kampfrath T., Simonetti OP., Sen CK., Roy S. et al. Gadolinium-containing phosphatidylserine liposomes for molecular imaging of atherosclerosis. J Lipid Res 2009;50:2157-63.

Maiseyeu A., Mihai G., Kampfrath T., Simonetti OP., Sen CK., Roy S. et al. Gadolinium-containing phosphatidyl serine liposomes for molecular imaging of atherosclerosis. J Lipid Res. 2009;50: 2157-63.

Marsh JN. et al. Fibrin-targeted perfluorocarbon nanoparticles for targeted thrombolysis. Nanomedicine. 2007; 2: 533–543.

Mathiasen AB., Henningsen KM., Harutyunyan MJ., Mygind ND., Kastrup J. YKL-40: a new biomarker in cardiovascular disease? Biomarkers Med. 2010; 4: 591–600.

McCarthy JR. Multifunctional agents for concurrent imaging and therapy in cardiovascular disease. Adv Drug Del Rev 2010;62:1023-30.

McCarthy JR. Multifunctional agents for concurrent imaging and therapy in cardiovascular disease. Advanced Drug Delivery Reviews 2010; 62: 1023–1030.

McCoy CP., Brady C., Cowley JF., McGlinchey SM., McGoldrick N., Kinnear DJ., Andrews GP., Jones DS. Triggered drug delivery from biomaterials. Expert Opin Drug Deliv 2010;7: 605–616.

Mukundan S., Ghaghada KB., Badea CT., Kao CY., Hedlund LW., Provanzale JM., Johnson GA., Chen E., Bellamkonda RV., Annapragada A. A liposomal nanoscale contrast agent for preclinical CT in mice. AJR. 2006;186:300–307.

Mulder WJM., Douma K., Koning GA., Zandvoort MA., Lutgens E., Daemen MJ., et al. Liposome-enhanced MRI of neointimallesions in the ApoE-KO mouse. Magn Reson Med 2006;55:1170-4

Mulder WJM., Strijker GJ., Briley-Saboe KC., Frias JC., Aguinaldo JGS., Vucic E. et al. Molecular imaging of macrophages in atherosclerotic plaques using biomodal PEG-micelles. Magn Reson Med. 2007;58:1164-70.

Mygind ND., Harutyunyan MJ., Mathiasen AB., Ripa RS., Thune JJ., Gøtze JP., Johansen JS., Kastrup J. The influence of statin treatment on the inflammatory biomarkers YKL-40 and HsCRP in patients with stable coronary artery disease. Inflamm. Res. (Epub ahead of print).

Nazem A., Mansoori G.A., Nanotechnology solutions for Alzheimer's disease: advances in research tools, diagnostic methods and therapeutic agents. J Alzheimers Dis. 2008;13:199–223.

Olsen MH., Hansen TW., Christensen MK. N-terminal pro-brain natriuretic peptide, but not high sensitivity C-reactive protein, improves cardiovascular risk prediction in the general population. Eur Heart J. 2007; 28 (11): 1374–1381.

Rabin O., Perez JM., Grimm J., Wojtkiewicz G., Weissleder R. An X-ray computed tomography imaging agent based on long-circulating bismuthsulphide nanoparticles. Nat Mater. 2006;5:118–122.

Rehli M., Niller HH., Ammon C. Transcriptional regulation of CHI3L1 a marker gene for late stages of macrophage differentiation. J Biol Chem. 2003;278 (45): 44058–44067.

Rensen PC., Gras JC., Lindfors EK., VanDijk KW., Jukema JW., Berkel TJ. Et al. Selective targeting of liposome stomacrophages using a ligand with high affinity for the macrophages cavenger receptor class A. Current Drug Discov Technol 2006;3:135-44.

Renzo T., Uta F., Oliver P., Nanomedicine: nanotechnology for health. Eur Tech Plat Strat Res Agen for Nanomed. 2006;1-39.

Roco MC., Curr. Opin. Biotechnol., 14, 337, 2003.

Roco MC., SocietalImplications of Nanoscience and Nanotechnology. W.S. Bainbridge (Ed.), Kluwer, Boston, 129, 2001.

Ruiz-Esparza GU., Flores-Arredondo JH., Segura-Ibarra V., Torre-Amione G., Ferrari M., Blanco E., Serda RE. The physiology of cardiovascular disease and innovative liposomal platforms for therapy. International Journal of Nanomedicine. 2013;8: 629–640.

Rx MediaPharma interactive drug information resource, 2013.

Sahoo SK., Labhasetwar V. Drug DiscoveryToday, 8, 1112, 2003,

Sahoo SK., Labhasetwar V. DrugDiscoveryToday, 2003, 8, 1112-1120

Sahoo SK., Parveen S., Panda JJ., Nanomedicine, 3, 20, 2007.

Smith AM., Gao X., Nie S., Quantum dotnanocrystalsfor in vivo molecular and cellular imaging. Photochem Photobiol. 2004;80:377-85.

Song C., Labhasetwara V., Cui X., Underwood T., Levy RJ. Arterial uptake of biodegradable nanoparticles for intravascular local drug delivery: Results with an acute dog model. Journal of Controlled Release. 1998;54:201–211.

Soujanya K., Jing-Fei D., Yaling L., Jifu T., Kytai TN. Biodegradable nanoparticles mimicking platelet binding as a targeted and controlled drug delivery system. International Journal of Pharmaceutics. 2012; 423:516– 524.

Spragg DD., Alford DR., Greferath R., Larsen CE., Lee K., Gurtner GC., Cybulsky MI., Tosi PF., Nicolau C., Gimbrone MA. Immuno targeting of liposomes to activated vascular endothelial cells: A strategy for site-selective delivery in the cardiovascular system, Proc. Natl. Acad. Sci. USA, 1997; 94: 8795–8800.

Stephan D. et al. Direct gene transfer in the rat kidney in vivo. Arch Mal Coeur Vaiss. 1997; 90: 1127–1130.

Tang TY., Muller KH., Graves MJ., Li ZY., Walsh SR., Young V. et al. Iron oxide particles for atheroma imaging. Arterioscler Thromb Vasc Biol. 2009;29:1001-8.

Trivedi RA., U-King-Im JM., Graves MJ., Cross JJ., Horsley J., Goddard MJ. Et al.Invivo detection of macrophages in human carotidatheroma: Temporal dependence of ultra small super paramagnetic particles of ironoxide-enhanced MRI. Stroke 2004;35:1631-5.

Walkey CD., Chan WCW. Understanding and controlling the interaction of nanomaterials with proteins in a physiological environment. Chem Soc Rev 2011; 41: 2780–2799.

Wickline SA., Lanza GM. Molecular Imaging, Targeted Therapeutics and Nanoscience. Journal of Cellular Biochemistry Supplement. 2002;39:90–97.

Winter PM. et al. Antiangiogenic synergism of integrintargeted fumagillin nanoparticles and atorvastatin in atherosclerosis. JACC Cardiovasc Imaging. 2008; 1: 624–634.

Winter PM. et al. Endothelial alpha (v) beta3 integrin-targeted fumagillin nanoparticles inhibit angiogenesis in atherosclerosis. Arterioscler Thromb Vasc Biol. 2006; 26: 2103–2219.

Winter PM., Caruthers SD., Zhang H., Williams TA., Wickline SA., Lanza GM. Antiangiogenic Synergism of Integrin-Targeted Fumagillin Nanoparticles and Atorvastatin in Atherosclerosis. JACC Cardiovasc Imaging. 2008 ; 1(5): 624–634.

Winter PM., Neubauer AM., Caruthers SD., Harris TD., Robertson JD., Williams TA., Schmieder AH., Hu G., Allen JS., Lacy EK., Zhang HY., Wickline SA., Lanza GM. Endothelial alpha (v) beta(3) integrin-targeted fumagillin nanoparticles inhibit angiogenesis in atherosclerosis. Arterioscler Thromb Vasc Biol. 2006;26:2103–2109

Cardiogenic Shock

Milovan Petrovic, Bojan Vujin, Gordana Panic
Nada Cemerlic Adjic, Slobodan Dodic
Clinic of Cardiology Institute of Cardiovascular Diseases Vojvodina
University of Novi Sad, Serbia

1   Prolog

Shock is a life-threatening condition that occurs due to circulatory insufficiency which leads to inadequate tissue perfusion with cellular metabolism disorders. Cardiogenic shock is a major, and frequently fatal, complication of a variety of acute and chronic disorders that impair the ability of the heart to maintain adequate tissue perfusion (Sharma *et al.*, 2005). Cardiogenic shock may be divided in to four major groups: myopathic (damaged myocardial contractility), arrhythmogenic (serious cardiac arrhythmias lead to shock), mechanical (valvular regurgitation) and obstructive lesions (mitral and aortic stenosis, tumor and thrombus in the left atrium, the artificial valve dysfunction, hypertrophic obstructive cardiomyopathy). Miscellaneous group of cardiogenic shock include cardiac tamponade, constrictive pericarditis, pulmonary embolism and aortic dissection. This paper will outline the causes, diagnosis, pathophysiology, and treatment of cardiogenic shock with a focus on CS complicating myocardial infarction (MI). Cardiogenic shock (CS) occurs in ≈5% to 8% of patients hospitalized with ST-elevation myocardial infarction (STEMI), but it can also be caused by mechanical complications, such as acute mitral regurgitation or rupture of either the ventricular septal or free walls. However, any cause of acute, severe left or right ventricular dysfunction may lead to CS. Early revascularization for CS improves survival substantially and new mechanical approaches to treatment are available. The mortality rate remains high (≈50%) despite intervention, and half of the deaths occur within the first 48 hours. The 3- and 6-year survival rates with the early revascularization are 41.4% and 32.8% with persistence of treatment benefit (Reynolds & Hochman, 2008). Mortality can range from 10% to 80% depending on demographic, clinical, and hemodynamic factors. These factors include age, clinical signs of peripheral hypoperfusion, anoxic brain damage, left ventricle ejection fraction (LVEF), and stroke work. Hemodynamic data are predictive of short-term but not long-term mortality. Revascularization provides benefit at every level of risk. Among CS patients undergoing percutaneous coronary intervention (PCI), age, time from symptom onset to PCI, and post-PCI TIMI (Thrombolysis in Myocardial Infarction) flow grade are independent predictors of mortality (Reynolds & Hochman, 2008).

2   Incidence

After decades of remarkable stability in the incidence of CS, it appears that the incidence is on the decline in parallel with increasing rates of use of primary PCI for acute MI. CS continues to complicate approximately 5% to 8% of STEMI (Fox, *et al.*, 2007; Babaev *et al.*, 2005) and 2.5% of non-STEMI cases (Hasdai *et al.*, 2000). This translates to 40 000 to 50 000 cases per year in the United States (Thom *et al.*, 2006).

3   Etiology

MI with left ventricle (LV) failure remains the most common cause of CS. It is critical to exclude complicating factors that may cause shock in MI patients. Chief among these are the mechanical complications: ventricular septal rupture, contained free wall rupture, and papillary muscle rupture. Mechanical complications must be strongly suspected in patients with CS complicating nonanterior MI, particularly a first MI. Any cause of acute, severe LV or right ventricle (RV) dysfunction may lead to CS. Acute my-opericarditis, tako-tsubo cardiomyopathy, and hypertrophic cardiomyopathy may all present with ST elevation, release of cardiac markers, and shock in the absence of significant coronary artery disease. Stress-induced cardiomyopathy, also known as apical ballooning or tako-tsubo cardiomyopathy, is a syndrome of acute LV dysfunction after emotional or respiratory distress that leads to CS in 4.2% of cases (Gianni et al., 2006). Idiopathic dilated cardiomyopathy presenting in CS is more common. Acute valvular regurgitation, typically caused by endocarditis or chordal rupture due to trauma or degenerative disease, may also cause CS. Aortic dissection may lead to CS via acute, severe aortic insufficiency or MI. Acute stress in the setting of aortic or mitral stenosis can also cause shock. Cardiac tamponade or massive pulmonary embolism can present as cardiogenic shock without associated pulmonary congestion. Also sustained arrhythmia may be included in etiology of cardiogenic shock.

4   Pathophysiology

Cardiogenic shock is characterized by systolic and diastolic dysfunction. Patients who develop cardiogenic shock from acute myocardial infarction consistently have evidence of progressive myocardial necrosis with infarct extension. Decreased coronary perfusion pressure and increased myocardial oxygen demand play a role in the vicious cycle that leads to cardiogenic shock. Patients suffering from cardiogenic shock often have multivessel coronary artery disease with limited coronary blood flow reserve. Ischemia remote from the infarcted zone is an important contributor to shock. Myocardial diastolic function is also impaired, because ischemia causes decreased myocardial compliance, thereby increasing left ventricular filling pressure, which may lead to pulmonary edema and hypoxemia.

Cardiogenic shock is the result of temporary or permanent derangements in the entire circulatory system. Left ventricle pump failure is the primary insult in most forms of CS, but other parts of the circulatory system contribute to shock with inadequate compensation or additional defects. Many of these abnormalities are partially or completely reversible, which may explain the good functional outcome in most survivors. Tissue hypoperfusion, with consequent cellular hypoxia, causes anaerobic glycolysis, the accumulation of lactic acid, and intracellular acidosis. Also, myocyte membrane transport pumps fail which decreases transmembrane potential and causes intracellular accumulation of sodium and calcium, resulting in myocyte swelling. If ischemia is severe and prolonged, myocardial cellular injury becomes irreversible and leads to myonecrosis, which includes mitochondrial swelling, the accumulation of denatured proteins and chromatin, and lysosomal breakdown. These events induce fracture of the mitochondria, nuclear envelopes, and plasma membranes. Additionally, apoptosis (programmed cell death) may occur in peri-infarcted areas and may contribute to myocyte loss. The activation of inflammatory cascades, oxidative stress, and stretching of the myocytes produces mediators that overpower inhibitors of apoptosis, thus activating the apoptosis (Figure 1).

4.1   Left Ventricles

Compensatory mechanisms activated when cardiac output is reduced include sympathetic stimulation to increase heart rate and contractility, and renal fluid retention to increase preload. These compensatory mechanisms may become maladaptive and can create a vicious cycle that further worsens systolic dysfunction. Vasoconstriction to maintain blood pressure increases myocardial afterload, impairing cardiac

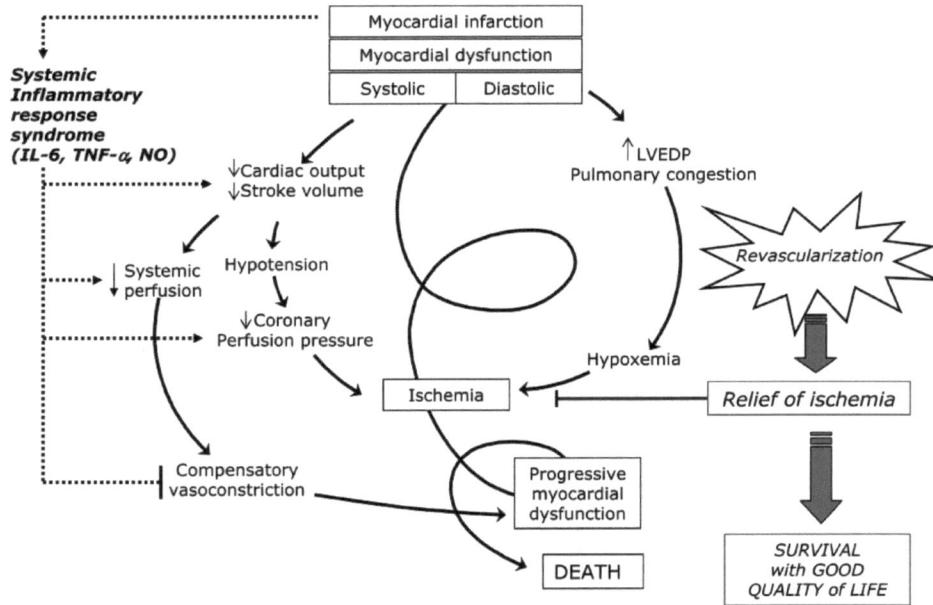

Figure 1: Current concept of CS pathophysiology-Myocardial injury causes systolic and diastolic dysfunction. A decrease in CO leads to a decrease in systemic and coronary perfusion. This exacerbates ischemia and causes cell death in the infarct border zone and the remote zone of myocardium. Inadequate systemic perfusion triggers reflex vasoconstriction, which is usually insufficient. Systemic inflammation may play a role in limiting the peripheral vascular compensatory response and may contribute to myocardial dysfunction. Whether inflammation plays a causal role or is only an epiphenomenon remains unclear. Revascularization leads to relief of ischemia. It has not been possible to demonstrate an increase in CO or LVEF as the mechanism of benefit of revascularization; however, revascularization does significantly increase the likelihood of survival with good quality of life. IL-6 indicates interleukin-6; TNF-α, tumor necrosis factor-α; and LVEDP, LV end-diastolic pressure (Reynolds & Hochman, 2008).

performance and increasing myocardial oxygen demand. Myocardial ischemia increases myocardial stiffness, increasing LV end-diastolic pressure and, thus, myocardial wall stress at a given end-diastolic volume. The increased LV stiffness limits diastolic filling and may result in pulmonary congestion, causing hypoxemia and worsening the imbalance of oxygen delivery and oxygen demand in the myocardium, resulting in further ischemia and myocardial dysfunction. The interruption of this cycle of myocardial dysfunction and ischemia forms the basis for CS therapeutic regimens. A key to understanding the pathophysiology and the treatment of CS is to realize that the areas of nonfunctional but viable myocardium can also cause or contribute to the development of CS after MI. This reversible dysfunction can be described in two main categories: stunning and hibernation. Myocardial stunning represents postischemic dysfunction that persists despite restoration of normal blood flow; myocardial performance eventually recovers completely. The direct evidence of myocardial stunning in humans has recently been obtained by demonstrating normal perfusion using positron emission tomography scanning and N-ammonia in patients with persistent wall motion abnormalities after angioplasty for acute coronary syndromes. The pathogenesis of stunning has not been conclusively established but appears to involve a combination of oxidative stress, perturbation of calcium homeostasis, and decreased myofilament responsiveness to calcium. The intensity of stunning is determined primarily by the severity of the antecedent ischemic insult. Myocardial hibernation can be seen as an adaptive response in which segments with severely reduced coronary blood flow reduce their contractile function to restore equilibrium between flow and function, minimizing the potential for ischemia or necrosis. Function in such segments can be normalized by improving blood flow. Repetitive episodes of myocardial stunning can coexist with or mimic myocardial hibernation. The consideration of myocardial stunning and hibernation is important because of their therapeutic implications. Both stunned and hibernating myocardiums retain inotropic reserve and can respond to catecholamines. The function of hibernating myocardium can improve with revascularization and function of stunned myocardium can improve in time. The notion that some myocardial tissue may recover its function has underscored the importance of expeditious initiation of supportive measures, including both medications and intraaortic balloon counterpulsation, to maintain blood pressure and cardiac output in patients with CS. The presence of reversible myocardial dysfunction also has prognostic implications, supported by data from the SHOCK trial, in which most survivors had only class I or class II heart failure (Reynolds & Hochman, 2008).

The degree of myocardial dysfunction that initiates CS is often, but not always, severe. LV dysfunction in shock reflects new irreversible injury, reversible ischemia, and damage from prior infarction. The unique position of the heart as an organ that benefits from low blood pressure via afterload reduction and also suffers from low blood pressure via compromise of coronary flow creates a situation in which changes in hemodynamic may be simultaneously beneficial and detrimental. As depicted, a decrease in coronary perfusion lowers cardiac output, which further decreases perfusion of the heart and other vital organs. Coronary flow may be additionally compromised by atherosclerosis of vessels other than the infarct artery. Metabolic derangements occur in the remote myocardium and in the infarct region. Hypoperfusion causes release of catecholamines, which increase contractility and peripheral blood flow, but catecholamines also increase myocardial oxygen demand and have proarrhythmic and myocardiotoxic effects (Reynolds & Hochman, 2008).

In light of the complex pathophysiology of CS, it is not surprising that in many cases, severe impairment of contractility does not lead to shock, and conversely, LVEF may be only moderately depressed in CS. LVEF is similar in the acute phase of CS and 2 weeks later, when functional status is quite different. Among patients in shock, however, LVEF remains a prognostic indicator. Approximately half of all CS patients have small or normal LV size, which represents the failure of the adaptive mechanism of acute dilation to maintain stroke volume in the early phase of MI. Progressive LV dilation (remodeling) in the chronic phase can be maladaptive. Serial echocardiography has demonstrated a small increase in LV end-diastolic volume in 2-week survivors of CS (15-mL change in median LV end-diastolic volume). Contractile function can be assessed with echocardiography or LV angiography. In addition, the indwelling pulmonary artery (PA) catheter allows ongoing evaluation of CO in response to changes in therapy and volume status. Diastolic function is more difficult to assess. It is likely that the abnormalities of ventricular relaxation and compliance contribute to CS in some, if not all cases (Reynolds & Hochman, 2008).

4.2 Right Ventricle

RV dysfunction may cause or contribute to CS. Predominant RV shock represents only 5% of cases of CS complicating MI. RV failure may limit LV filling via a decrease in CO, ventricular interdependence, or both. The treatment of patients with RV dysfunction and shock has traditionally focused on ensuring adequate right-sided filling pressures to maintain CO and adequate LV preload; however, patients with CS due to RV dysfunction have very high RV end-diastolic pressure, often >20 mm Hg. This elevation of RV end-diastolic pressure may result in shifting of the interventricular septum toward the LV cavity, which raises left atrial pressure but impairs LV filling due to the mechanical effect of the septum bowing into the LV. This alteration in geometry also impairs LV systolic function. Therefore, the common practice of aggressive fluid resuscitation for RV dysfunction in shock may be misguided. Inotropic therapy is indicated for RV failure when CS persists after RV end-diastolic pressure has been optimized. RV end-diastolic pressure of 10 to 15 mm Hg has been associated with higher output than lower or higher pressures, but marked variability exists in optimal values. Inhaled nitric oxide (NO) may be useful to lower pulmonary vascular resistance and promote forward flow. Both pericardiectomy and the creation of atrial septal defects have been used in extreme cases.

Shock due to isolated RV dysfunction carries nearly as high a mortality risk as LV shock. The benefit of revascularization was similar.

4.3   Cardiovascular Mechanism of Cardiogenic Shock

The main mechanical defect in cardiogenic shock is a shift to the right for the left ventricular end-systolic pressure-volume curve (Figure 2, 3) because of a marked reduction in contractility. As a result, at a similar or even lower systolic pressure, the ventricle is able to eject less blood volume per beat. Therefore, the end-systolic volume is usually greatly increased in persons with cardiogenic shock. The stroke volume is decreased, and to compensate for this, the curvilinear diastolic pressure-volume curve also shifts to the right, with a decrease in diastolic compliance. This leads to increased diastolic filling, which is associated with an increase in end-diastolic pressure. The attempt to enhance cardiac output by this mechanism comes at the cost of having a higher left ventricular diastolic filling pressure, which ultimately increases myocardial oxygen demand and causes pulmonary edema. As a result of decreased contractility, the patient develops elevated left and right ventricular filling pressures and low cardiac output. Mixed venous oxygen saturation falls because of the increased tissue oxygen extraction, which is due to the low cardiac output. This, combined with the intrapulmonary shunting that is often present, contributes to substantial arterial oxygen desaturation.

4.4   Peripheral Vasculature, Neurohormones and Inflammation in Cardiogenic Shock

Hypoperfusion of the extremities and vital organs is a hallmark of CS. The decrease in CO caused by MI and sustained by ongoing ischemia triggers release of catecholamines, which constrict peripheral arterioles to maintain perfusion of vital organs. Vasopressin and angiotensin II levels increase in the setting of MI and shock, which leads to improvement in coronary and peripheral perfusion at the cost of increased afterload, which may further impair myocardial function. Activation of the neurohormonal cascade promotes salt and water retention; this may improve perfusion but exacerbates pulmonary edema. The reflex mechanism of increased systemic vascular resistance (SVR) is not fully effective. MI can cause the systemic inflammatory response syndrome (SIRS) and suggest that inappropriate vasodilatation as part of SIRS results in impaired perfusion of the intestinal tract, which enables transmigration of bacteria and sepsis. SIRS is more common with increasing duration of shock[1] - even though levels of interleu-

---

[1] http://circ.ahajournals.org/content/117/5/686.full

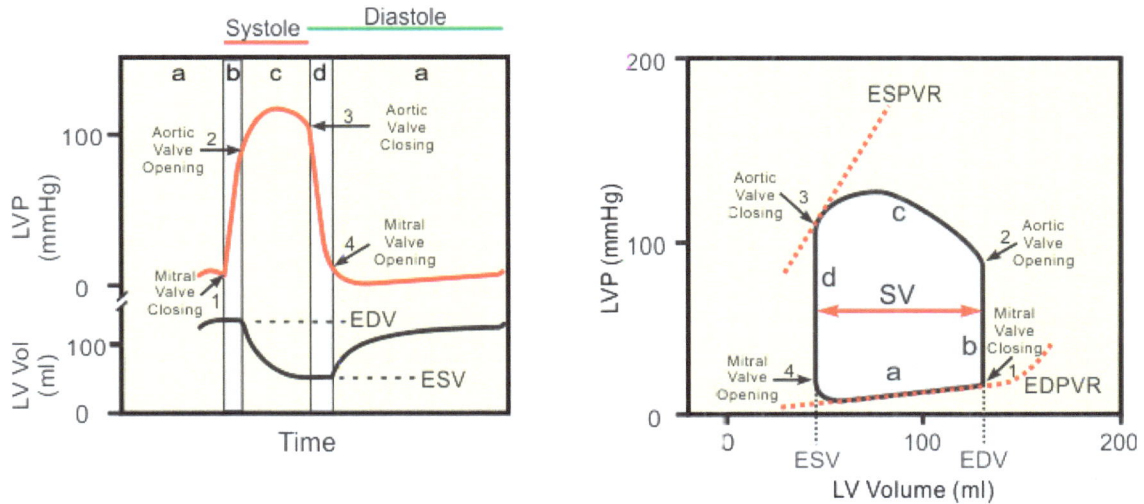

Figure 2: Left ventricular pressure-volume (PV) curves are derived from pressure and volume information found in the cardiac cycle diagram (see left panel of figure). To generate a PV curve for the left ventricle, the left ventricular pressure (LVP) is plotted against left ventricular (LV) volume at multiple time points during a complete cardiac cycle. When this is done, a PV curve is generated (right panel of figure) (Klabunde, 2011).

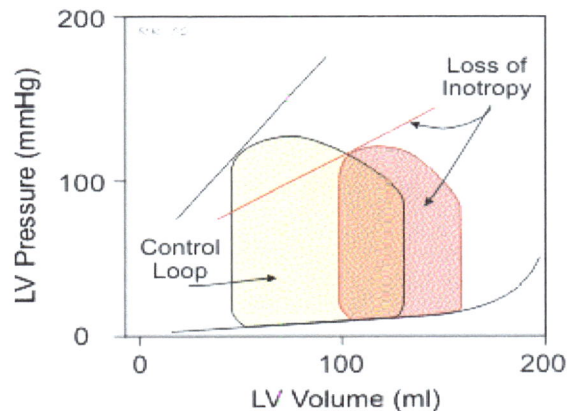

Figure 3: Effects of acute left ventricular failure (loss of inotropy) on left ventricular pressure-volume curve (Klabunde, 2011).

kin-6 and tumor necrosis factor-α have been found to be elevated on admission among MI patients who were initially in Killip class I and later developed CS (Reynolds & Hochman, 2008). Cytokine levels rise more dramatically over the 24 to 72 hours after MI. Tumor necrosis factor-α and interleukin-6 have myocardial depressant action. Tumor necrosis factor-α also induces coronary endothelial dysfunction, which may further diminish coronary flow. Other circulating factors (complement, procalcitonin, neopterin, C-reactive protein, and others) have been reported to contribute to SIRS in CS. Excess NO may also contribute to SIRS. MI is associated with increased expression of inducible NO synthase, which leads to excess NO, which causes vasodilatation, myocardial depression, and interference with catecholamine action (Reynolds & Hochman, 2008).

5   Diagnosis

CS is a state of end-organ hypoperfusion due to heart failure. Hypoperfusion may be manifest clinically by cool extremities, decreased urine output (< 20 ml/h), and/or alteration in mental status. Hemodynamic abnormalities form a spectrum that ranges from mild hypoperfusion to profound shock, and the short-term outcome is directly related to the severity of hemodynamic derangement. The definition of CS includes hemodynamic parameters: persistent hypotension (systolic blood pressure SBP < 80 to 90 mm Hg or mean arterial pressure MAP 30 mm Hg lower than baseline) with severe reduction in cardiac index (CI) (< 1.8 L $\cdot$ min^{-1} $\cdot$ m^{-2} without support or < 2.0 to 2.2 L $\cdot$ min^{-1} $\cdot$ m^{-2} with support) and adequate or elevated filling pressure (e.g. left ventricular end-diastolic pressure LVEDP > 18 mm Hg or right ventricular end-diastolic pressure RVEDP > 10 to 15 mm Hg) (Table 1). The diagnosis is usually made with the help of pulmonary artery catheterization; however, Doppler echocardiography may also be used to confirm elevation of LV filling pressures (Giannuzzi *et al.*, 1994). Echocardiography also is the technique of choice to help in diagnostic CS with estimation of LV and RV motion, kinetic disorders and valvular settings. Coronary angiography helps us to see morphology of coronary artery lesions and to perform rapid primary percutaneous coronary intervention.

Hemodynamic Parameters In Cardiogenic Shock	
SBP	< 80 to 90 mm Hg
MAP	30 mm Hg lower than baseline
CI	< 1.8 L $\cdot$ min^{-1} $\cdot$ m^{-2} without support or < 2.0 to 2.2 L $\cdot$ min^{-1} $\cdot$ m^{-2} with support
LVEDP, RVEDP	LVEDP > 18 mm Hg RVEDP > 10 to 15 mm Hg

Table 1: Diagnostic hemodynamic parameters in cardiogenic shock

6   Patient with High Risk for CS

Risk factors for development of CS in the context of MI include older age, anterior MI, hypertension, diabetes mellitus, multivessel coronary artery disease, prior MI or angina, prior diagnosis of heart failure, STEMI, and left bundle-branch block (Lindholm *et al.*, 2003).

7   Treatment

Treatment of cardiogenic shock as a complication of acute myocardial infarction includes hemodynamic stability achieved by medication therapy or circulatory and respiratory support and emergency revascularisation using PCI or surgical revascularization (CABG) (Figure 4).

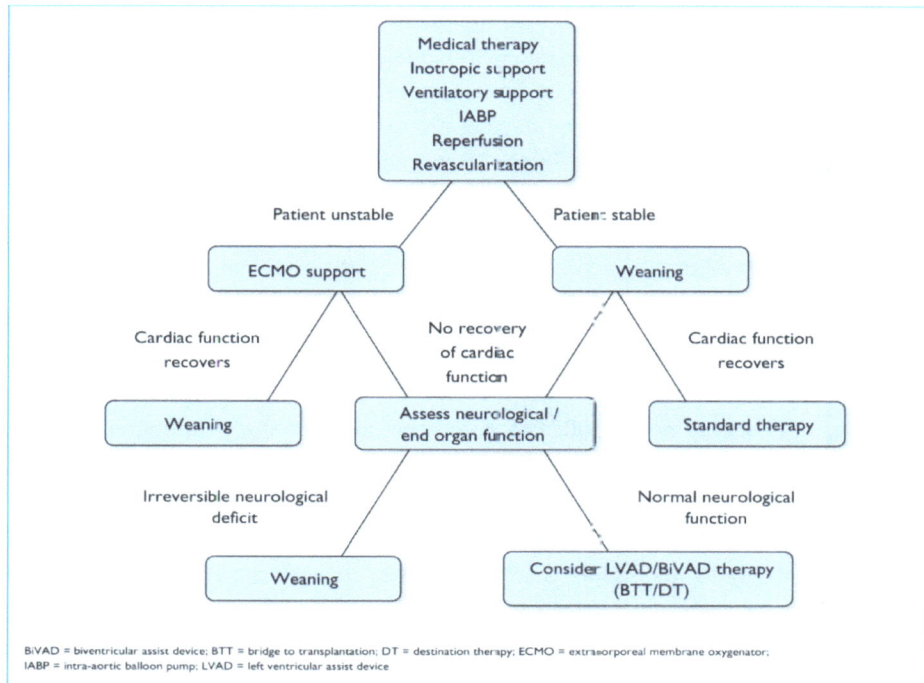

Figure 4: Treatment algorithms for acute heart failure and cardiogenic shock- After failure of initial therapy including reperfusion and revascularization to stabilize hemodynamic, temporary mechanical support using an extracorporeal membrane oxygenator should be considered. If weaning from the extracorporeal membrane oxygenator fails or heart failure persists, left ventricular assist device/biventricular assist device therapy may be considered if neurological function is not permanently impaired *Eur Heart J* 2010,31(20),2501-2555.

7.1   General Support Measures

Antithrombotic therapy with aspirin and heparin should be given as routinely recommended for MI. Clopidogrel and nowadays prasugrel or ticagrelor is indicated in all patients who undergo PCI (Steg *et al*., 2012), and on the basis of extrapolation of data from MI patients who were not in shock, it should also be useful in patients with shock as well. Negative inotropes and vasodilators (including nitroglycerin) should be avoided. Arterial oxygenation and near-normal pH should be maintained to minimize ischemia. Mechanical ventilation via mask, or endotracheal tube should be introduced. Positive end-expiratory pressure decreases preload and afterload. Mechanical ventilation also reduces work of breathing. Intensive insulin therapy improves survival in hyperglycemic critically ill patients and is recommended for use in complicated MI (Reynolds & Hochman, 2008).

7.2   Hemodynamic Management

Pulmonary artery (Swan-Ganz) catheterization is frequently performed to confirm the diagnosis of CS, to ensure that filling pressures are adequate, and to guide changes in therapy. The best use of this technique is to establish the relationship of filling pressures to cardiac output (CO) in the individual patient and supplement clinical assessment of responses with these data. Hemodynamic data, particularly cardiac output, cardiac index, have powerful short-term prognostic value (Fincke *et al.*, 2004). There has been a decline in PA catheter use. Clinical assessment with echocardiography is a reasonable alternative: Both PA systolic pressure and wedge pressure can be accurately estimated with Doppler echocardiography, and in particular, the finding of a short mitral deceleration time (≤140 ms) is highly predictive of pulmonary capillary wedge pressure ≥20 mm Hg in CS (Reynolds *et al.*, 2006). The clinical examination and chest radiograph are not reliable predictors of pulmonary capillary wedge pressure.

7.3   Pharmacological Treatment

Pharmacological support includes inotropic and vasopressor agents. Vasopressors and inotropic agents are used because of their positive hemodynamic effect, but neither of them leads to permanent symptomatic improvement, and many even reduce survival rate, which may be associated with cell dysfunction caused by these drugs (Thackray *et al.*, 2002). A recent randomised study compared norepinephrine and dopamine in cardiogenic shock. Dopamine was associated with a higher mortality rate and more adverse effects, such as arrhythmia (De Backer *et al.*, 2010). In hypotension with other signs of cardiogenic shock, norepinephrine is recommended as the first choice. It should be initially administered in low doses and gradually titrated until systolic pressure reaches values of over 80 mmHg. After that, dobutamine can be administered together with norepinephrine for better contractility (Steg *et al.*, 2012).

7.4   Reperfusion

The survival benefit of early revascularization in CS, reported in several observational studies, was shown convincingly in the randomized SHOCK trial, which found a 13% absolute increase in 1-year survival in patients assigned to early revascularization (Reynolds & Hochman, 2008). Revascularization could be percutaneous or surgical. Percutaneous coronary intervention is superior to fibrinolytic therapy. Fibrinolysis is recommended if PCI is not feasible or if delayed.

Stenting and glycoprotein IIb/IIIa inhibitors were independently associated with improved outcomes in patients undergoing PCI for CS in multiple registries, including the large ACC-National Cardiovascular Data Registry (Klein *et al.*, 2005).

The optimal revascularization strategy (i.e., percutaneous or surgical, single or multivessel PCI) for patients with multivessel coronary artery disease and CS is not clear. This is of particular importance because multivessel disease is common. According to the ACC/AHA guidelines for revascularization in shock, in patients with multivessel disease, revascularization of the noninfarct related artery may be necessary to maximize myocardial perfusion. Alternatively, in patients with multivessel disease and particularly left main disease, emergency CABG as a primary reperfusion strategy may be preferred (Levine *et al.*,   2011).   The ability to achieve complete revascularization may   be   strongly   associated with improved in-hospital survival in patients with cardiogenic shock (Hussain *et al.*, 2011).

7.5   Mechanical Circulatory Support: Intraaortic Balloon Pump

Intraaortic balloon pump (IABP) remains the most widely used circulatory assist device in crtically ill patients with heart diseases. Counterpulsation is the term that describes balloon inflation in diastole and deflation in early systole (Figures 5, 6). That improves coronary and peripheral perfusion via diastolic balloon inflation and augments LV performance via systolic balloon deflation with an acute decrease in afterload. Accurate timing of inflation and deflation provides optimal support (Ramanathan *et al.*, 2011).

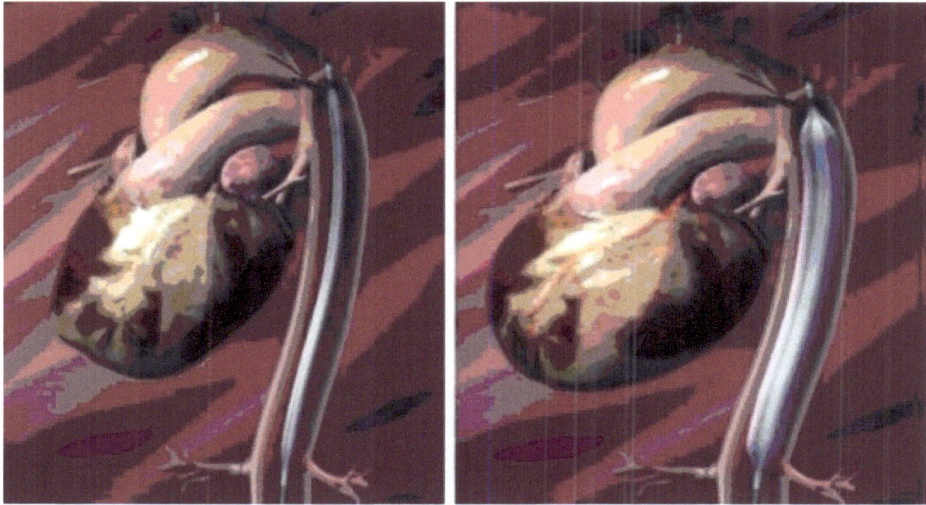

Figure 5: Intra-aortic balloon pump, which is inserted into the descending aorta between the arch vessels and renal arteries. Intraaortic balloon deflation and inflation

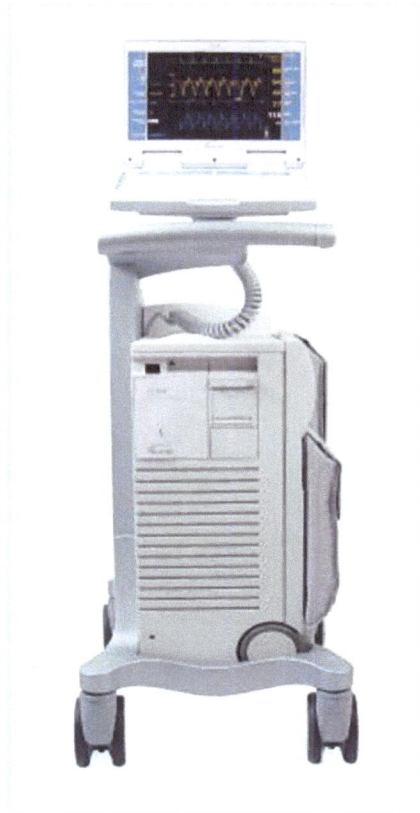

Figure 6: Intraaortic balloon pump console (Maquet Cardiopulmonary AG, Hirrlingen, Germany).

The primary goal of IABP treatment is to improve ventricular performance of failing heart by facilitating an increasing myocardial oxygen supply and decrease myocardial oxygen demand. Although these effects are predominantly associated with enhancement of LV performance, IABP may also have favorable effects on RV function by complex mechanisms including accentuation RV myocardial blood flow, unloading of LV causing reduction in left atrial and pulmonary vascular pressure and RV afterload (Miller, 2011). Not every patient has a hemodynamic response to IABP; response predicts better outcome (Ramanathan *et al.*, 2011). TACTICS study showed that IABP does not contribute to reduction of intra-hospital mortality, but it brings about improvement in six-month mortality rate (Ohman *et al.*, 2005). Recent meta-analyses evidenced in relation to survival rate when using IABP in cardiogenic shock (Bahekar *et al.*, 2012). IABP-SHOCK II study showed that use of intraaortic balloon counterpulsation did not significantly reduce 30-day mortality in patients with cardiogenic shock complicating acute myocardial infarction for whom an early revascularization strategy was planned (Thiele *et al.*, 2012). IABP support should be instituted as quickly as possible, even before any transfer for revascularization if a skilled operator is available and insertion can be performed quickly. Complications associated with IABP are less common in the modern era; in the largest series, the overall and major complication rates were 7.2% and 2.8%, respectively. Risk factors for complications include female sex, small body size, and peripheral vascular disease (Urban *et al.*, 2004). IABP therapy is considered to be a class IIb indication (European Society of Cardiology guidelines) for the management of cardiogenic shock (Steg *et al.*, 2012).

7.6   Mechanical Circulatory Support: Ventricular Assist Devices

In profound cardiogenic shock, blood flow and perfusion pressure must be restored urgently to prevent permanent damage to the brain, liver, kidneys, and gut. Adequate right ventricular function is necessary to avoid central venous hypertension and end-organ venous congestion. In mechanical engineering, a failing pump is repaired or replaced provided that the rest of the system remains in working order. The same strategy can be applied in patients with heart failure using modern circulatory support technology. The landmark REMATCH study (Rose *et al.*, 2001; Westaby *et al.*, 2012) established a long-term role for left ventricular assist devices (LVADs) to relieve symptoms and improve longevity in terminally ill patients with cardiomyopathy who were not eligible for a cardiac transplant. Temporary mechanical circulatory support with LV assist devices (LVADs) is theoretically appealing to interrupt the vicious spiral of ischemia, hypotension, and myocardial dysfunction, allowing for recovery of stunned and hibernating myocardium and reversal of neurohormonal derangements. Device-related complications and irreversible organ failure remain major limitations. LVAD support involves circulation of oxygenated blood through a device that drains blood from the left side of the heart and returns blood to the systemic arteries with pulsatile or continuous flow. A variety of surgically implanted continuous-flow and pulsatile blood pumps have proven to be very effective postinfarction (Westaby *et al.*, 2012). The advantage of these devices is that central cannulation of atria, ventricles, and great arteries can bypass and unload the failing ventricle and provide blood flow of up to 10 l/min. For left ventricular support, the ventricular assist device (VAD) drains the left atrium or ventricle and pumps blood into the aorta. For right ventricular bypass, the right atrium is normally used for VAD inflow with blood pumped into the main pulmonary artery, thereby avoiding peripheral vascular complications. Outcome depends on myocardial viability following revascularization, pre-existing left ventricular dysfunction, and potential for recovery in stunned or hibernating myocardium. In contrast to percutaneously inserted systems, all centrally implanted pumps can be kept *in situ* for periods ranging from weeks to several years. Temporary pumps can be replaced by long-term implanted LVADs if the native heart does not recover (Westaby *et al.*, 2012).

Data from the US INTERMACS provides important insights into the overall success of blood pumps in cardiogenic shock (Holman *et al.*, 2009). Shock accounted for 42% of 483 VAD implants and, not surprisingly, these patients had a worse survival profile than those who underwent elective destination therapy. Patients who only required left ventricular support had the best outlook (50% survival at 12 months). When biventricular support was needed, survival fell to 35%. Prognosis was poor for those receiving isolated right ventricular support or a total artificial heart (Holman *et al.*, 2009).

Percutaneous LVADs are also available. Shock may already be apparent at the time of pPCI, or can be predicted from angiographic or echocardiographic findings. In both circumstances, two percutaneously implanted blood pumps are available to the cardiologist without the need for immediate intervention by surgeons. The Tandem Heart (Cardiac Assist, Inc, Pittsburgh, PA) (Figure 7) removes blood from the left atrium using a cannula placed through the femoral vein and into the left atrium via transseptal puncture. Blood is then returned to a systemic artery, usually the femoral, with retrograde perfusion of the abdominal and thoracic aorta (Reynolds & Hochman, 2008). Another percutaneous device, the Impella 2.5 (Abiomed, Inc, Danvers, Mass) (Figure 8) pulls blood from the left ventricle through an inlet area near the tip and expels blood from the catheter into the ascending aorta. The pump can be inserted via a standard catheterization procedure through the femoral artery, into the ascending aorta, across the valve and into the left ventricle (Henriques *et al.*, 2006). Extracorporal membrane oxygenation (ECMO) (Figure 9) is used to sustain physiological levels of blood flow in cardiogenic shock, as a rescue system during cardiopulmonary resuscitation and to provide both cardiac and pulmonary support for patients with hypoxia (Smedira *et al.*, 2001). An ECMO circuit consists of a centrifugal blood pump, membrane oxygenator, and a heparin-coated circuit. ECMO is the simplest and most-rapid method of restoring systemic blood flow and, with contemporary peripheral arteriovenous cannulation techniques, can now be used in the catheterization laboratory or emergency room (Westaby *et al.*, 2012). Cannulation of the femoral artery and vein are achieved rapidly by the Seldinger technique, using specifically designed perfusion cannulas over a guidewire, even during cardiac massage or PPCI. The tip of the femoral arterial cannula is advanced to the aortoiliac junction and the venous drainage pipe advanced into the lower right atrium. Systemic heparinization is used to achieve an activated clotting time of 150–180 s. Flow rates are initiated at 2–3 l/min using dopamine to raise mean blood pressure to > 55 mmHg. Once the circuit is established, the flow rate can be progressively increased to 3.5–4.0 l/min, thus restoring a normal cardiac index and mean blood pressure to >70 mmHg (Westaby *et al.*, 2012). Because venoarterial ECMO increases left ventricular afterload and wall stress, cardiac contractility must be maintained to avoid left ventricular distension, clot on the akinetic myocardium, or pulmonary hypertension using an IABP and inotropes (Westaby *et al.*, 2012). ECMO can provide an effective bridge to urgent cardiac transplantation or to prolonged LVAD support.

Mechanical circulatory support can sustain life during profound postinfarction cardiogenic shock and is an important adjunct to coronary angioplasty in rapidly deteriorating patients. Neither the IABP nor percutaneously inserted LVADs have been shown to improve survival in established cardiogenic shock. By contrast, both ECMO and centrally implanted blood pumps show the capacity to salvage more than half of those patients who would otherwise die (Westaby *et al.*, 2012).

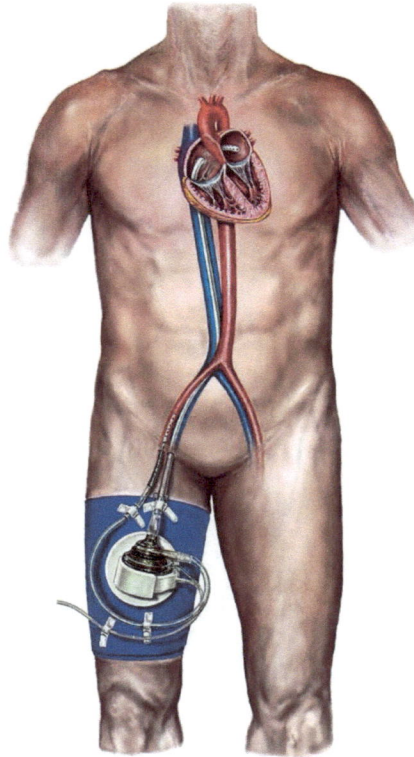

Figure 7: The Tandem Heart LV Device- TandemHeart® (Cardiac Assist, Inc., Pittsburgh, PA, USA). A cannula is inserted percutaneously through the right femoral vein and advanced towards the right atrium, where it is introduced by transatrial septal perforation. A cannula in either femoral artery then provides left heart bypass.

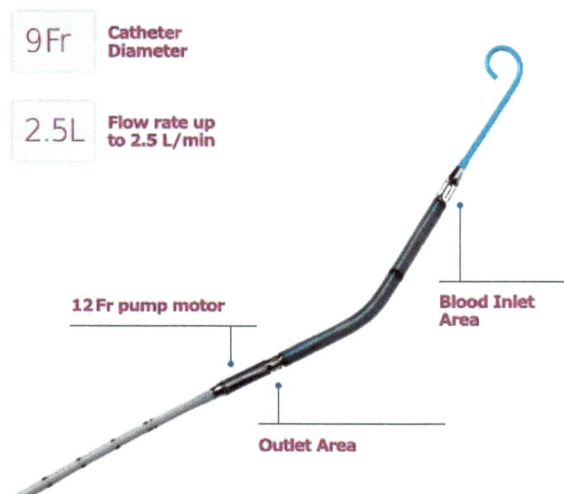

Figure 8: Impella 2,5 (Abiomed, Inc, Danvers, Mass). This device is percutaneously inserted via the femoral artery and positioned across the aortic valve.

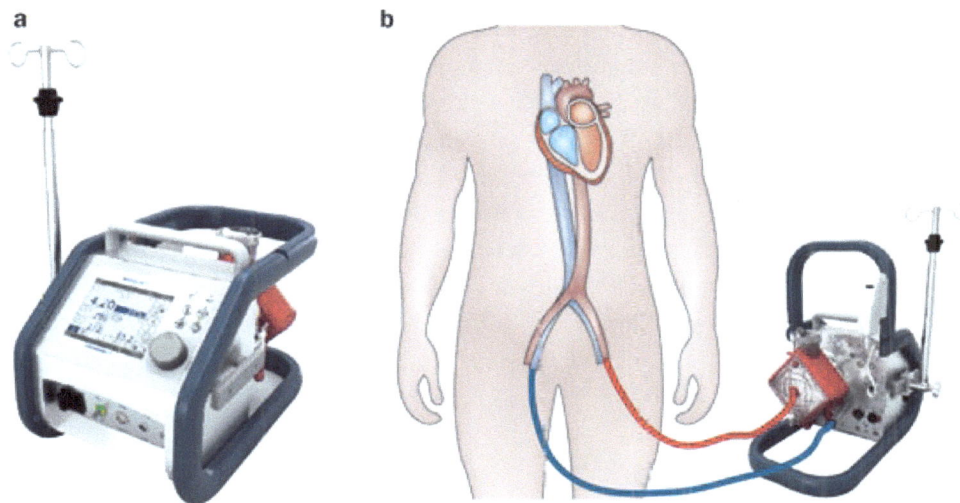

Figure 9: The Maquet Cardiohelp® (Maquet Cardiopulmonary AG, Hirrlingen, Germany) hybrid pump oxygenator. **(a)** The device is compact and easily portable, with a total weight of only 9 kg. **(b)** Veno-arterial extracorporeal membrane oxygenation (ECMO) is established by cannulation of a femoral vein and artery using the Seldinger technique. To expedite interhospital transfer these vessels can be located with guidewires before arrival of the outreach team. The cannulas can then be inserted rapidly to begin ECMO before transport by air or ground ambulance. Images of the Cardiohelp®device courtesy of © Maquet Cardiopulmonary AG. Westaby. S., Anastasiadis, K., Wieselthaler, G.M. (2012) Cardiogenic shock in ACS. Part 2: Role of mechanical circulatory support. *Nat Rev Cardiol.* 10; 9(4):195-208.

7.7   Treatment of CS due to Mechanical Complications after MI

Mechanical complications of MI, including rupture of the ventricular septum, free wall, or papillary muscles, cause 12% of CS cases; of these, ventricular septal rupture (VSR) has the highest mortality, 87% Hoefer *et al.*, 2006). Timely repair of mechanical complications associated with CS is critical for survival. Repair of VSR and free wall rupture present technical difficulties to the surgeon because of the need to suture in an area of necrotic myocardium. Repair of papillary muscle rupture does not involve necrotic myocardium in suture lines, and mortality associated with this repair is lower. The unpredictability of rapid deterioration and death with VSR and papillary muscle rupture makes early surgery necessary even though there may be apparent hemodynamic stabilization with IABP. Percutaneous VSR repair has been reported for simple and complex defects (Menon *et al.*, 2000) and after failure of surgical repair (Schiele *et al.*, 2003). One limitation of this approach is that ventricular septal defect sizing may be technically difficult, and healing of the infarcted myocardium may increase the size of the ventricular septal defect, leading to device malapposition or even embolization. The use of devices with diameter larger than the ventricular septal defect has been associated with relatively good outcome (Cutfield *et al.*, 2005).

7.8   Management of Special Conditions

The treatment of certain conditions that lead to CS is marked by important differences from management of CS due to LV failure. The recognition of LV outflow obstruction is critical in patients with hypotension, because diuretics and inotropic agents exacerbate obstruction. Treatment of CS with hypertrophic obstructive cardiomyopathy includes volume resuscitation. Outflow obstruction may also be seen in some cases of tako-tsubo cardiomyopathy when extensive akinesis/dyskinesis of apical zones occurs with hyperkinesis of remaining myocardium. Therapy is guided by echocardiography and clinical response. IABP may provide circulatory support. β-Blockade is often not indicated in this circumstance because it exacerbates LV dysfunction. Vasopressors and inotropes improve function in the stunned myocardium and may therefore be useful when outflow obstruction is not visualized. Low doses should be initiated, with careful monitoring of the response (Reynolds & Hochman, 2008).

8   CS as an Iatrogenic Illness

Approximately three fourths of patients with CS complicating MI develop shock after hospital presentation (Holzer *et al.*, 2004). In some, medication use contributes to the development of shock. Several different classes of medications used to treat MI have been associated with shock, including β-blockers, angiotensin-converting enzyme inhibitors, nitrates and morphine. Although early use of each of these medications is associated with only a small excess risk of CS, the large number of patients treated with these therapies translates into a substantial potential number of events (Jeger *et al.*, 2006; Meine *et al.*, 2005). The timing of CS (early after medication initiation) in the placebo-controlled, randomized trials of β-blockade and angiotensin-converting enzyme inhibition combined with their mechanisms of action indicate that they may contribute to CS development in those at high risk. Diuretics may also cause or contribute to shock in patients with MI (Chen *et al.*, 2005; Hochman, 2003). Acute pulmonary edema is a state of redistribution of intravascular volume into extracellular space in the lungs. When hemodynamic stability is tenuous, the additional decrease in plasma volume caused by diuretics in patients without prior heart failure may induce shock. Tachycardia is often compensatory for lower stroke volume but is not appreciated as such. Treatment with β-blockade lowers heart rate and stroke volume, leading to frank shock. Decompensation may also occur when patients who are reliant on compensatory vasoconstriction are treated with angiotensin-converting enzyme inhibitors, particularly intravenously and early. Nitrates would be expected to have a similar effect but did not in the only systematic study, which used oral, low-dose treatment. Volume expansion may be deleterious when used to excess or when RV filling pressure is already elevated, because the RV may become volume overloaded with shift of the septum causing impairment in LV filling and contraction. A trial of a low diuretic dose coupled with low-dose nitrates and positional measures to decrease preload (e.g., seated position with legs down) should be attempted in patients with MI and pulmonary edema to avoid precipitating shock (Reynolds & Hochman, 2008).

8   Conclusion

CS following acute myocardial infarction is a potentially treatable illness with a reasonable chance for fully recovery. An early invasive approach can increase short- and long-term survival and can result in excellent quality of life. Revascularization is associated with some benefit at every level of risk.

References

Babaev, A., Frederick, P.D., Pasta, D.J., et al. (2005). Trends in management and outcomes of patients with acute myocardial infarction complicated by cardiogenic shock. JAMA, 294(4), 448–454.

Bahekar, A., Singh, M., Singh, S., et al. (2012). Cardiovascular outcomes using intra-aortic balloon pump in high-risk acute myocardial infarction with or without cardiogenic shock: a meta-analysis. J Cardiovasc Pharmacol Ther, 17(1), 44–56.

Chen, Z.M., Pan, H.C., Chen, Y.P., et al. (2005). Early intravenous then oral metoprolol in 45,852 patients with acute myocardial infarction: randomized placebo-controlled trial. Lancet. 366(9497), 1622–1632.

Cutfield, N.J., Ruygrok, P.N., Wilson, N.J., et al. (2005). Transcatheter closure of a complex postmyocardial infarction ventricular septal defect after surgical patch dehiscence. Intern Med J, 35(2), 128–130.

De Backer, D., Biston, P., Devriendt, J., et al. (2010). Comparison of dopamine and norepinephrine in the treatment of shock. N Engl J Med, 362, 779–89.

Fincke, R., Hochman, J.S., Lowe, A.M., et al. (2004). Cardiac power is the strongest hemodynamic correlate of mortality in cardiogenic shock: a report from the SHOCK trial registry. J Am Coll Cardiol, 44(2), 340–348.

Fox, K.A., Anderson, F.A. Jr, Dabbous, O.H., et al. (2007). Intervention in acute coronary syndromes: do patients undergo intervention on the basis of their risk characteristics? The Global Registry of Acute Coronary Events (GRACE). Heart, 93(2), 177–182.

Gianni, M., Dentali, F., Grandi, A.M., et al. (2006). Apical ballooning syndrome or takotsubo cardiomyopathy: a systematic review. Eur Heart J, 27(13), 1523–1529.

Giannuzzi, P., Imparato, A., Temporelli, P.L. et al. (1994). Doppler-derived mitral deceleration time of early filling as a strong predictor of pulmonary capillary wedge pressure in postinfarction patients with left ventricular systolic dysfunction. J Am Coll Cardiol, 23(7), 1630–1637.

Hasdai, D., Harrington, R.A., Hochman, J.S., et al. (2000). Platelet glycoprotein IIb/IIIa blockade and outcome of cardiogenic shock complicating acute coronary syndromes without persistent ST-segment elevation. J Am Coll Cardiol, 36(3), 685–692.

Henriques, J.P., Remmelink, M., Baan, J. Jr, et al. (2006). Safety and feasibility of elective high-risk percutaneous coronary intervention procedures with left ventricular support of the Impella Recover LP 2.5. Am J Cardiol, 97(7), 990–992.

Hochman, J.S. (2003). Cardiogenic shock complicating acute myocardial infarction: expanding the paradigm. Circulation, 107(24), 2998–3002.

Hoefer, D., Ruttmann, E., Poelzl, G., et al. (2006). Outcome evaluation of the bridge-to-bridge concept in patients with cardiogenic shock. Ann Thorac Surg, 82(1), 28–33.

Holman, W. L. et al. (2009) INTERMACS: interval analysis of registry data. J Am Coll Surg, 208(5), 755–761.

Holzer, R., Balzer, D., Amin, Z., et al. (2004). Transcatheter closure of postinfarction ventricular septal defects using the new Amplatzer muscular VSD occluder: results of a U.S. registry. Catheter Cardiovasc Interv, 61(2), 196–201.

Hussain, F., Philip, R.K., Ducas, A.R. et al. (2011). The ability to achieve complex revascularization is associated with improve in-hospital survival in cardiogenic shock due to myocardial infarction: Manitoba cardiogenic shock registry investigators, Catheter cardiovasc Interv, 78(4), 540–548

Jeger, R.V., Harkness, S.M., Ramanathan, K., et al. (2006). Emergency revascularization in patients with cardiogenic shock on admission: a report from the SHOCK trial and registry. Eur Heart J, 27(6), 664–670.

Klabunde, R.E. (2011) Cardiovascular Physiology Concepts; 2nd edition; Lippincott Williams & Wilkins ISBN 9781451113846

Klein LW, Shaw RE, Krone RJ, et al. (2005). *Mortality after emergent percutaneous coronary intervention in cardiogenic shock secondary to acute myocardial infarction and usefulness of a mortality prediction model. Am J Cardiol, 96(1), 35–41.*

Levine, G.N., Bates, E.R., Blankenship, J.C., et al. (2011). *ACCF/AHA/SCAI Practice Guideline for Percutaneous Coronary Intervention, Circulation, 124(23), e574-e651*

Lindholm, M.G., Kober, L., Boesgaard, S., et al. (2003). *Cardiogenic shock complicating acute myocardial infarction: prognostic impact of early and late shock development. Eur Heart J, 24(3), 258–265.*

Meine, T.J., Roe, M.T., Chen, A.Y., et al. (2005). *Association of intravenous morphine use and outcomes in acute coronary syndromes: results from the CRUSADE Quality Improvement Initiative. Am Heart J, 149(6), 1043–1049.*

Menon, V., Webb, J.G., Hillis, L.D., et al. (2000). *Outcome and profile of ventricular septal rupture with cardiogenic shock after myocardial infarction: a report from the SHOCK Trial Registry: Should we emergently revascularize Occluded Coronaries in cardiogenic shock? J Am Coll Cardiol, 36(3s1), 1110–1116.*

Miller, R.D. *Miller's anesthesia. In: Nyhan D Johns RA eds. (1991/2007). Anesthesia for Cardiac Surgery. Elsevier*

Ohman, E.M., Nanas, J., Stomel, R.J., et al., for the TACTICS Trial (2005). *Thrombolysis and counterpulsation to improve survival in myocardial infarction complicated by hypotension and suspected cardiogenic shock or heart failure: results of the TACTICS Trial. J Thromb Thrombolysis, 19(1), 33-39.*

Ramanathan, K., Farkouh, M.E., Cosmi, J. et al. (2011). *Rapid complete reversal of systemic hypoperfusion after intra-aortic balloon pump counterpulsation and survival in cardiogenic shock complicating an acute myocardial infarction. Am Heart J, 162(2):268-75.*

Reynolds, H.R., Anand, S.K., Fox, J.M., et al. (2006). *Restrictive physiology in cardiogenic shock: observations from echocardiography. Am Heart J, 151(4), 890 e9–e15.*

Reynolds, H.R., Hochman, J.S. (2008). *Cardiogenic Shock Current Concepts and Improving Outcomes. Circulation, 117(6), 686-697*

Rose, E.A. et al. (2001). *Long-term use of a left ventricular assist device for end-stage heart failure. N Engl J Med 345, 1435–1443.*

Schiele, T.M., Kozlik-Feldmann, R., Sohn, H.Y., et al. (2003). *Transcatheter closure of a ruptured ventricular septum following inferior myocardial infarction and cardiogenic shock. Catheter Cardiovasc Interv, 60(2), 224–228.*

Sharma, S., Zevitz, M. (2005). *Cardiogenic shock. eMedicine. Available at: http://www.emedicine.com/med/topic285.htm*

Smedira, N.G. et al. (2001). *Clinical experience with 202 adults receiving extracorporeal membrane oxygenation for cardiac failure: survival at five years. J Thorac Cardiovasc Sug 122(1), 92–102.*

Steg., G., James, S. K., Atar, D., et al. (2012). *ESC Guidelines for the management of acute myocardial infarction in patients presenting with ST-segment elevation. European Heart Journal, 33(20), 2569–2619.*

Thackray, S., Easthaugh, J., Freemantle, N., et al. (2002). *The effectiveness and relative effectiveness of intravenous inotropic drugs acting through the adrenergic pathway in patients with heart failure-a meta-regression analysis. Eur J Heart Fail,4(4),515–529.*

Thiele, H., Zeymer, U., Neumann, F.J., et al. for the IABP-SHOCK II trial investigators (2012). *Intraaortic balloon support for myocardial infarction with cardiogenic shock. N Engl J Med, 367,1287-96*

Thom, T., Haase, N., Rosamond, W., et al. (2006). *Heart disease and stroke statistics—2006 update: a report from the American Heart Association Statistics Committee and Stroke Statistics Subcommittee. Circulation, 113(6), e85–e151.*

Urban, P.M., Freedman, R.J., Ohman, E.M., et al. (2004). *In-hospital mortality associated with the use of intra-aortic balloon counterpulsation. Am J Cardiol, 94(2), 181–185.*

Westaby, S., Anastasiadis, K., Wieselthaler, G.M. (2012) *Cardiogenic shock in ACS. Part 2: Role of mechanical circulatory support. Nat Rev Cardiol, 10,9(4), 195-208.*